Nutrition and Metabolism of the Surgical Patient, Part II

Guest Editors

STANLEY J. DUDRICK, MD, FACS
JUAN A. SANCHEZ, MD, MPA, FACS

SURGICAL CLINICS
OF NORTH AMERICA

www.surgical.theclinics.com

Consulting Editor
RONALD F. MARTIN, MD

August 2011 • Volume 91 • Number 4

SAUNDERS an imprint of ELSEVIER, Inc.

W.B. SAUNDERS COMPANY

A Division of Elsevier Inc.

1600 John F. Kennedy Blvd., Suite 1800, Philadelphia, PA 19103-2899

http://www.surgical.theclinics.com

SURGICAL CLINICS OF NORTH AMERICA Volume 91, Number 4
August 2011 ISSN 0039–6109, ISBN-13: 978-1-4557-7994-9

Editor: John Vassallo, j.vassallo@elsevier.com

Developmental Editor: Donald Mumford

Surgical Clinics of North America (ISSN 0039–6109) is published bimonthly by Elsevier Inc., 360 Park Avenue South, New York, NY 10010-1710. Months of publication are February, April, June, August, October, and December. Business and Editorial Offices: 1600 John F. Kennedy Blvd., Suite 1800, Philadelphia, PA 19103-2899. Periodicals postage paid at New York, NY and additional mailing offices. Subscription prices are $311.00 per year for US individuals, $532.00 per year for US institutions, $152.00 per year for US students and residents, $381.00 per year for Canadian individuals, $661.00 per year for Canadian institutions, $429.00 for international individuals, $661.00 per year for international institutions and $210.00 per year for Canadian and foreign students/residents. To receive student/resident rate, orders must be accompanied by name of affiliated institution, date of term, and the *signature* of program/residency coordinator on institution letterhead. Orders will be billed at individual rate until proof of status is received. Foreign air speed delivery is included in all *Clinics* subscription prices. All prices are subject to change without notice. POSTMASTER: Send address changes to *Surgical Clinics*, Elsevier Health Sciences Division, Subscription Customer Service, 3251 Riverport Lane, Maryland Heights, MO 63043. **Customer Service (orders, claims, online, change of address): Telephone: 1-800-654-2452 (U.S. and Canada); 314-447-8871 (outside U.S. and Canada). Fax: 314-447-8029. E-mail: journalscustomerservice-usa@elsevier.com (for print support); journalsonline support-usa@elsevier.com (for online support).**

Reprints. For copies of 100 or more, of articles in this publication, please contact the Commercial Reprints Department, Elsevier Inc., 360 Park Avenue South, New York, New York 10010-1710. Tel. (212) 633-3812, Fax: (212) 462-1935, e-mail: reprints@elsevier.com.

The Surgical Clinics of North America is also published in Spanish by McGraw-Hill Interamericana Editores S.A., P.O. Box 5-237 06500 Mexico D.F. Mexico; and in Portuguese by Interlivros Edicoes Ltda., Rua Comandante Coelho 1085, CEP 21250, Rio de Janeiro, Brazil; and in Greek by Paschalidis Medical Publications, Athens Greece.

The Surgical Clinics of North America is covered in *MEDLINE/PubMed (Index Medicus)*, *EMBASE/Excerpta Medica*, *Current Contents/Clinical Medicine*, *Current Contents/Life Sciences*, *Science Citation Index*, and *ISI/BIOMED*.

Printed and bound by CPI Group (UK) Ltd, Croydon, CR0 4YY

Transferred to Digital Print 2011

Contributors

CONSULTING EDITOR

RONALD F. MARTIN, MD
Staff Surgeon, Department of Surgery, Marshfield Clinic, Marshfield, Wisconsin; Clinical Associate Professor, University of Wisconsin School of Medicine and Public Health, Madison, Wisconsin; Colonel, Medical Corps, United States Army Reserve

GUEST EDITORS

STANLEY J. DUDRICK, MD, FACS
Chairman Emeritus and Program Director Emeritus, Department of Surgery, Saint Mary's Hospital, Waterbury; Professor of Surgery, Department of Surgery, Yale University School of Medicine, New Haven, Connecticut

JUAN A. SANCHEZ, MD, MPA, FACS
Chairman and Program Director, Department of Surgery, Saint Mary's Hospital, Waterbury; Assistant Professor of Surgery, Department of Surgery, University of Connecticut School of Medicine, Farmington, Connecticut

AUTHORS

JOHN C. ALVERDY, MD
Sarah and Harold Lincoln Thompson Professor, Executive Vice Chair, Professor of Surgery, Department of Surgery, University of Chicago Pritzker School of Medicine, University of Chicago Medical Center, Chicago, Illinois

ERICA M. CARLISLE, MD
Surgical Research Fellow, Resident in General Surgery, University of Chicago Pritzker School of Medicine, University of Chicago Medical Center, Chicago, Illinois

EDWARD M. COPELAND III, MD
Chairman Emeritus and Distinguished Professor of Surgery, Department of Surgery, University of Florida College of Medicine, Gainesville, Florida

JOHN M. DALY, MD
Emeritus Dean, Department of Surgery, Temple University School of Medicine and Temple University Hospital; Harry C. Donahoo Professor of Surgery, Philadelphia, Pennsylvania

STANLEY J. DUDRICK, MD, FACS
Chairman Emeritus and Program Director Emeritus, Department of Surgery, Saint Mary's Hospital, Waterbury; Professor of Surgery, Department of Surgery, Yale University School of Medicine, New Haven, Connecticut

KAZUHIKO FUKATSU, MD, PhD
Associate Professor, Surgical Center, Department of Surgery, The University of Tokyo Hospital, Tokyo, Japan

JOHN P. GRANT, MD
Professor of Surgery, Duke University Medical Center, Durham, North Carolina

SENTHIL JAYARAJAN, MD
Resident in General Surgery, Department of Surgery, Temple University School of Medicine, Philadelphia, Pennsylvania

HAYTHAM M.A. KAAFARANI, MD, MPH
Chief Resident, Department of Surgery, Tufts Medical Center and Tufts University School of Medicine, Boston, Massachusetts

KENNETH A. KUDSK, MD
Professor of Surgery, Veterans Administration Surgical Services, William S. Middleton Memorial Veterans Hospital; Department of Surgery, University of Wisconsin School of Medicine and Public Health, Madison, Wisconsin

JAMES H. MEHAFFEY, BS
MS3, The Brody School of Medicine at East Carolina University, Greenville, North Carolina

MICHAEL J. MOROWITZ, MD
Assistant Professor of Surgery, Division of Pediatric General and Thoracic Surgery, University of Pittsburgh School of Medicine, Children's Hospital of Pittsburgh of UPMC, Pittsburgh, Pennsylvania

J. ALEXANDER PALESTY, MD, FACS
Assistant Clinical Professor of Surgery, Department of Surgery, University of Connecticut School of Medicine, Farmington, Connecticut; Director of Surgical Oncology, Department of Surgery, Saint Mary's Hospital/Yale Affiliate, Waterbury, Connecticut

MELISSA S. PHILLIPS, MD
Laparoendoscopic Fellow, Department of Surgery, University Hospitals Case Medical Center, Case Western Reserve University, Cleveland, Ohio

JOSE MARIO PIMIENTO, MD
Fellow, Surgical Oncology, Moffitt Cancer Center and Research Institute, Department of Surgery, Tampa, Florida

JEFFREY L. PONSKY, MD
Oliver H. Payne Professor and Chairman, Department of Surgery, University Hospitals Case Medical Center, Case Western Reserve University, Cleveland, Ohio

WALTER J. PORIES, MD, FACS
Professor of Biochemistry, Adjunct Professor of Exercise and Sport Science, Director of Metabolic Institute, Professor of Surgery, Division of Bariatric Surgery, Department of Surgery, The Brody School of Medicine at East Carolina University, East Carolina University, Greenville, North Carolina; Adjunct Professor of Surgery, Uniformed Services, University of the Health Sciences, Bethesda, Maryland

KRISTEN M. RHODA, RD
Registered Dietitian, Intestinal Rehabilitation and Transplant, Digestive Disease Institute, Cleveland Clinic, Cleveland, Ohio

JOHN L. ROMBEAU, MD
Professor, Department of Surgery, Temple University School of Medicine, Temple University Hospital, Philadelphia, Pennsylvania

JUAN A. SANCHEZ, MD, MPA, FACS
Chairman and Program Director, Department of Surgery, Saint Mary's Hospital, Waterbury; Assistant Professor of Surgery, Department of Surgery, University of Connecticut School of Medicine, Farmington, Connecticut

LISE L. SANCHEZ, RD
Clinical Dietitian, Department of Food and Nutrition, Bridgeport Hospital, Bridgeport, Connecticut

SCOTT A. SHIKORA, MD
Professor of Surgery, Tufts Medical Center and Tufts University School of Medicine; Chief, General and Bariatric Surgery, Tufts Medical Center, Boston, Massachusetts

KYLE M. STATON, BS
MS3, The Brody School of Medicine at East Carolina University, Greenville, North Carolina

EZRA STEIGER, MD
Professor of Surgery, Cleveland Clinic Lerner College of Medicine of Case Western Reserve University; Consultant in General Surgery and Gastroenterology, Intestinal Rehabilitation and Transplant, Digestive Disease Institute, Cleveland Clinic, Cleveland, Ohio

SIDNEY J. STOHS, PhD
Dean Emeritus, Creighton University Medical Center, Omaha, Nebraska; Frisco, Texas

SREE SURYADEVARA, MD
Nutrition Fellow, Nutrition Support Team, Digestive Disease Institute, Cleveland Clinic, Cleveland, Ohio

I. JANELLE WAGNER, MD
Clinical Instructor in Surgery, Department of Surgery, Temple University School of Medicine, Temple University Hospital, Philadelphia, Pennsylvania

Contents

> The early development of total parenteral nutrition and its evolution as an adjunct to the nutritional, metabolic, and antineoplastic therapy of cancer patients is described. Examples related to the sine wave of responses to new data and discovery are placed in context to understand better past, present, and how and where to proceed in the future to achieve optimal results from multimodal comprehensive management of patients with malignancies. Practical and philosophic thoughts are proffered to justify continued, intensified, logical, controlled clinical studies directed toward establishing the most rational, safe, and effective use of total parenteral nutrition in treating patients with cancer.

> Malnutrition has marked consequences on surgical outcomes. Adequate nutrition is important for the proper functioning of all organ systems, particularly the immune system. Determination of the type and amount of nutrient supplementation and the appropriate route of nutrient delivery is essential to bolster the immune system and enhance the host's response to stress. Correct administration of immunonutrients could lead to reductions in patient morbidity following major surgery, trauma, and critical illness.

> The human intestine contains huge amounts of nonpathologic bacteria surviving in an environment that is beneficial to both the host and the bacterial populations. When short pauses in oral intake occur with minimal alterations in the mucosa-microbial interface, critical illness, with its attendant acidosis, prolonged gastrointestinal tract starvation, exogenous antibiotics, and breakdown in mucosal defenses, renders the host vulnerable to bacterial challenge and also threatens the survival of the bacteria. This review examines the altered innate and adaptive immunologic host defenses that occur as a result of altered oral or enteral intake and/or injury.

bariatric and obese nonbariatric patients in increasing numbers. This patient population presents several difficulties from the medical and surgical management perspectives. In particular, nutrition of the bariatric patient and critically ill obese patient is challenging. A clear understanding of the nutritional assessment and unique management strategies available for the bariatric and the critically ill obese patient is essential to provide them with the safest and most effective care.

The importance of the preoperative nutritional status of cardiothoracic surgical patients in determining outcomes is demonstrated and discussed. Demographic, anthropometric, and biochemical changes in patients undergoing cardiothoracic surgery increase the importance of identifying those at risk for postoperative complications resulting from malnutrition. The interrelationships of chronic heart failure, cardiac cachexia, nutritional status, and nutritional support are identified and emphasized. The complexities of myocardial energetics and metabolism are outlined together with the nutrient needs for patients undergoing cardiac, pulmonary, or other intrathoracic operative procedures.

Surgery in geriatric patients is accompanied by increases in morbidity and mortality, increases in functional abnormalities and poor outcomes, and increases in severe malnutrition, compared with surgery of similar magnitude in nongeriatric patients. Hospitalized elderly patients are at significant risk of presenting with, or developing, protein-energy and other nutrient deficiencies. However, nutritional assessment of older geriatric patients, 65 to 100 years of age, is a challenging task because of lack of adequate age-specific reference data in this diverse and heterogeneous population. Dietary counseling and conscientious, aggressive nutritional support are required for optimal metabolic and surgical care of this age group.

The importance of adequate nutrition has long been established in the surgical patient population. Enteral nutrition provides the safest, most cost-effective approach with endoscopic and surgical options for permanent access. Parenteral nutrition should be reserved for patients in whom enteral nutrition is contradicted. This article summarizes the routes of access for both enteral and parenteral nutrition as well as the indications, procedural pearls, and complications associated with each approach.

Home parenteral nutrition is a life-saving treatment for many patients with intestinal failure. Expert placement and care of the vascular access device reduces the incidence of access-related complications. Careful monitoring of fluid, electrolyte, and macronutrient and micronutrient status can minimize major organ dysfunction and metabolic complications. A multi-disciplined, integrated nutrition support team can allow patients with intestinal failure who need home parenteral nutrition maintain a near-normal life.

This article presents an overview of the current knowledge, status, and use of supplements by patients before surgical operations, together with the benefits expected of the supplements by the patients. The indications, potential advantages and disadvantages, and the relationships with various aspects of the preoperative preparation and postoperative management of surgical patients are discussed, with emphasis on the significant percentage of this population that is deficient in fundamental nutrients. Recent revisions and recommendations for some of the macronutrients are presented, together with a summary of federal regulations and an oversight of supplements.

The most significant events and discoveries regarding the development of enteral nutrition (EN) dating back to 1500BC are chronicled. A more detailed description and discussion of subsequent more recent progress during the past two decades is focused primarily on 3 of the most dynamic areas of endeavor: tight glycemic control; timing and combining of EN and total parenteral nutrition to meet early target nutrition goals in intensive care unit patients; and the role, advances, and future of immunonutrition. An abridged classification of solutions for enteral feeding, and a brief outline of key prudent oral dietary guidelines are also presented.

THE CLINICS ARE NOW AVAILABLE ONLINE!

Access your subscription at:
www.theclinics.com

Foreword

Nutrition and Metabolism of the Surgical Patient, Part II

This issue of *Surgical Clinics of North America* will complete this two part series led by Drs Dudrick and Sanchez. The issues comprise expert, concise reviews by some of the thought leaders in our discipline. It is somewhat difficult to introduce a topic to the readership at the "intermission," so perhaps it would be better to reflect on what the efforts that led us to these issues may have taught us beyond what we can read from the pages.

Science has a long history of allowing one to see further than others before by "standing on the shoulders of giants." Ironically, that great line attributed to Newton, and quoted by so many, may have been intended as an insult to the short, physical stature of the Royal Astronomer during Newton's time. Ironic backhanded compliments aside, it is generally accepted that many of the great developments are based on the foundations of discovery that precede our efforts. In the case of the development of our understanding of nutrition, this is clearly the case. In the particular case of total parenteral nutrition, not only did we need to develop an understanding of the fundamental building blocks of nutrition, but we also needed to develop a method of creating solutions that could be infused into a human safely and the technology to deliver them to the central circulation. For many of the people who worked in this field, not only did they expand the work of their predecessors but doggedly advanced contributions built on their previous advances. Nearly any of the independent developments that are covered in these two issues of the *Clinics* would be worthy of significant recognition.

Recognition for effort in surgery has been perhaps spotty. There are certainly examples of procedures that are credited to individuals that were well described years prior: the "Graham" patch leaps to mind as it first appeared in the United States literature 10 years after Cellen-Jones published his account in the *British Journal of Surgery*. There are probably many discoveries that were made by fellows, residents, junior staff people, and others that are credited to senior professors as well (not naming any names here). In the case of the development of surgical nutrition it is clear to me that Dr Stan Dudrick's accomplishments are real and truly attributed to him. There is no doubt that he did not work alone in a vacuum but his lifetime of singular dedicated progress has fundamentally changed all of our understanding of nutrition. In my opinion, he is deserving of the highest recognition that can be awarded for his efforts.

I am reasonably confident that I shall not have any influence over the awarding of Nobel prizes, the Presidential Medal of Freedom, or knighthoods, but if I were to ever have such influence, I would suggest that Dr Dudrick be considered for any of these. For our part at the *Clinics* what we can offer Dr Dudrick is the opportunity and a platform to collect a group of experts to tell their story as they feel they should. It has been our very great honor to work with him and his colleagues. And as should be a lesson for all of us, by doing what we can for Drs Dudrick, Sanchez, and their

Surg Clin N Am 91 (2011) xiii–xiv
doi:10.1016/j.suc.2011.06.003
0039-6109/11/$ – see front matter © 2011 Elsevier Inc. All rights reserved.

colleagues, we find ourselves all the more enriched. These two issues of the *Surgical Clinics* should serve as a compendium that one can turn to for a very long time on matters of nutrition.

Ronald F. Martin, MD
Department of Surgery
Marshfield Clinic
1000 North Oak Avenue
Marshfield, WI 54449, USA

E-mail address:
martin.ronald@marshfieldclinic.org

Preface

Nutrition and Metabolism of the Surgical Patient, Part II

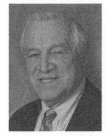 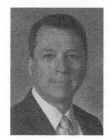

Stanley J. Dudrick, MD   Juan A. Sanchez, MD
Guest Editors

This issue of *Surgical Clinics of North America* is the second volume of a two-part set devoted to nutrition and metabolism of surgical patients, and represents a compilation of topics covering a broad range of important clinical information gleaned from basic and clinical investigators throughout the world by an expert group of authors who have contributed throughout their professional careers to this vital field of endeavor. We are most grateful for the knowledge, experience, expertise, judgment, and wisdom, which they have been willing to share with us unselfishly and collegially in our mutual efforts to advance and optimize the art and science of nutritional support in the comprehensive management of surgical patients. What a privilege it has been to be able to cooperate, collaborate, and communicate with so many colleagues in the greater medical and surgical community throughout the past several decades, but especially with our author-partners in this venture, who have all made unique scientific contributions during this special period of extraordinary and unprecedented discovery and advancement in virtually every aspect of basic and clinical surgical research. Our mutual rewards have been to experience the joy and satisfaction of the effective practical translation of the newly acquired knowledge and technology to the solution or amelioration of difficult and complex patient problems.

The current strategies of comprehensive nutritional and metabolic support of the entire patient generally, and of the primary organ systems specifically, including the cardiovascular, pulmonary/respiratory, gastrointestinal, hepato-pancreatic, renal, endocrine, and central nervous system, must continue to progress and advance further to the cellular and subcellular levels if the ultimate goal of providing optimal nutritional, metabolic, immunologic, neuroendocrine, pharmacologic, and interventional support

Surg Clin N Am 91 (2011) xv–xvii
doi:10.1016/j.suc.2011.06.002
0039-6109/11/$ – see front matter © 2011 Elsevier Inc. All rights reserved.

surgical.theclinics.com

for all patients under all conditions at all times is to be fully realized. The countless intricate relationships among the multiple nutrient substrates, body composition and performance, cellular and molecular biology, immunology (immunoaugmentation and immunosuppression), and human genomics and epigenomics; and their identification, classification, understanding, and potential beneficial applications to the management of complex and/or critically ill patients have undoubtedly presented new and greatly expanded frontiers for basic and clinical investigation throughout this 21st century and beyond. In part, this volume reports upon the progress of these promising possibilities and demonstrates clearly that knowledge of, and the judicious practice of, clinical nutrition and metabolism require the most sophisticated integration of clinical skills and acumen with the basic science disciplines of biology, chemistry, physics, immunology, genomics, pharmacology, interventional therapeutics, and hybrids of these fundamental disciplines. Measures for reducing the morbidity and mortality associated with all major pathophysiologic conditions, and their management by improving the nutritional and metabolic status of patients, have expanded vastly from the simple peripheral intravenous infusion of isotonic carbohydrate, electrolyte, and water-soluble vitamin solutions to the complex and sophisticated parenteral and enteral provision of most or all of the nutrient requirements in virtually all clinical situations. Today, clinical nutrition is progressing rapidly toward the provision of optimal nutrient substrates to individual cells and/or groups of cells, whether normal or compromised by disease, disorders, or age, and in reality represents the practice of clinical biochemistry. The continuing identification and classification of genetic control of all metabolic events in human beings is well on its way, and upon the realization of its full potential, nutritional support will require an unprecedented degree of precision; this molecular biological revolution will transform the practice of medicine and surgery forever.

It has been gratifying to witness the growth and development of cherished and productive personal and professional relationships that have been spawned by the mutual interests, cooperation, and collaboration among basic and clinical scientists throughout the world. This issue is exemplary, tangible evidence of some of the most objective successes of the multiple endeavors of our contributing colleagues. Together with Part I, it is intended to serve as a state-of-the-art resource that might prove useful to all who are interested in multiple and complex areas of nutrition and metabolism in order to help provide the best and most comprehensive care for their patients.

Finally, we are most grateful to the multiple authors who have shared their special knowledge, experience, skills, and philosophy, together with their invaluable contributions of time, talent, and effort, in order to produce this relevant and up-to-date educational tome. We greatly appreciate the outstanding opportunity, advice, and wisdom received from our respected colleague, Ronald F. Martin, MD, Consulting Editor of *Surgical Clinics of North America*, who invited us to serve as guest editors of this issue. Subsequently, his assistance, guidance, counsel, confidence, and patience have been most encouraging, supportive, and exceptional. Additionally, we are deeply indebted to John Vassallo, Associate Publisher, Elsevier, who has been an exacting, indefatigable, and ever-present professional while providing expert assistance in every important decision throughout the production of this volume. We are especially grateful to the otherwise unacknowledged heroic efforts and contributions of our Executive Assistant, Joan Reeser, who guaranteed excellence, timeliness, consummate technical, editorial, and cognitive expertise, and eternal optimism and cheerfulness as we toiled together systematically and unrelentingly to complete the countless tasks essential to the success of this venture. Finally, our sincere thanks and love to Terry and Lise for their unselfish and unfailing contributions, support, and sacrifices, willingly made so that we could undertake this challenging, but gratifying, editorial challenge.

Stanley J. Dudrick, MD
Chairman Emeritus and Program Director Emeritus
Department of Surgery
Saint Mary's Hospital
56 Franklin Street
Waterbury, CT 06706, USA

Juan A. Sanchez, MD
Chairman and Program Director
Department of Surgery
Saint Mary's Hospital
56 Franklin Street
Waterbury, CT 06706, USA

E-mail addresses:
sdudrick@stmh.org (S.J. Dudrick)
juan.sanchez@stmh.org (J.A. Sanchez)

Total Parenteral Nutrition and Cancer: From the Beginning

Edward M. Copeland III, MD[a],*, Jose Mario Pimiento, MD[b],
Stanley J. Dudrick, MD[c,d]

KEYWORDS

• TPN • Cancer • History

Before 1972, total parenteral nutrition (TPN) was used sparingly in patients with cancer for fear of stimulating tumor growth or inducing septicemia via the indwelling subclavian catheters. The immune incompetence and the infectious consequences of malnutrition have been well characterized since that time. As a fellow in surgical oncology at the University of Texas MD Anderson Hospital (MDAH) in 1971, the first author of this article (Dr Copeland) observed that there often were patients who were candidates for antineoplastic therapy but were denied treatment because of the advanced degree of their malnutrition. With the arrival of Stanley J. Dudrick, MD, as the first Chairman of the Department of Surgery at the then new University of Texas Medical School at Houston in 1972, the motivation and expertise to attempt to replenish these patients nutritionally was available. Dr Copeland was invited to join the faculty and assigned as head of medical school surgical service at the MDAH and was fortunate to have Bruce MacFadyen, MD, later Chairman of the Department of Surgery at the Medical College of Georgia, as his assigned resident. With this team in place, it was felt justified to offer TPN to malnourished cancer patients who did not have an adequately functioning gastrointestinal tract available for enteral nutrition and who were candidates for antineoplastic therapy, consisting of surgery, chemotherapy, and/or radiation therapy. Stimulation of tumor growth and infectious complications, although not insignificant, were of lesser consequence, because without TPN support, cancer treatment would have been denied. Together with the leaders of the institution, we undertook the

The authors have nothing to disclose.
[a] Department of Surgery, University of Florida College of Medicine, 1600 Southwest Archer Road, Gainesville, FL 32607, USA
[b] Moffitt Cancer Center and Research Institute, Department of Surgery, 12902 Magnolia Drive, Tampa, FL 33612, USA
[c] Department of Surgery, Saint Mary's Hospital, 56 Franklin Street, Waterbury, CT 06706, USA
[d] Department of Surgery, Yale University School of Medicine, 333 Cedar Street, New Haven, CT 06510, USA
* Corresponding author.
E-mail address: copelem@surgery.ufl.edu

doi:10.1016/j.suc.2011.04.003
0039-6109/11/$ – see front matter
surgical.theclinics.com

challenge of providing treatment with TPN as a novel opportunity to rehabilitate these patients nutritionally, and, therefore, to allow them to receive the cancer treatment for which they would have been candidates had they not been severely malnourished.

In 1974, at the American College of Surgeons annual clinical congress, we reported a 2.2% incidence of catheter-related sepsis in this cadre of cancer patients.[1] Duration of TPN was 10 days or longer, and 48% of patients had white blood cell counts below 2500 cells per mm^3 for an average time of 7.2 days. During this trial, no stimulation of tumor growth was observed clinically. The conclusion reached from this study was, "The low rate of microbial complications is the result of strict adherence to aseptic techniques in preparation of the solutions, insertion of the catheter, and long term maintenance of the delivery system." It would behoove physicians in 2011 to pay close attention to these results and the reasons for their achievement. In contrast, a recent article by Brown and associates[2] questions the need for chest roentgenograms after fluoroscopically guided insertion of a subclavian central venous port as an example of a deviation from standard of care. In their study the chest roentgenogram was deemed unnecessary. Nevertheless, delayed and potentially disastrous pneumothoraces after discharge from the surgical suite have been avoided by information gained from a good-quality chest roentgenogram before discharge during the previous 35 years.

Also in 1974, our clinical results with the use of TPN, in a series of 120 patients with a cross-section of oncologic diseases, were presented at the Association for Academic Surgery.[3] Our simple definition of malnutrition was a serum albumin below 3 g/dL% and a recent weight loss of at least 10 lb below ideal or usual body weight. A more comprehensive definition of malnutrition has been refined since that time; nevertheless, in most studies of TPN in cancer patients, malnutrition is poorly defined, and well-nourished patients are often found among both the randomized and control subjects in published studies. The results of TPN in well-nourished patients include weight gain as fat and water and an iatrogenic increase of catheter and metabolic complications. An observation in patients with large tumor burdens in the study was the continuation of weight loss while receiving an enteral diet containing a normal caloric content based on current body weight. The addition of TPN allowed for a gain in strength and lean body mass without stimulation of additional tumor growth. We postulated that the tumor had likely been growing at the expense of the body cell mass, a concept later proved in the laboratory. Tumors, at least in animal models, grow at a maximal rate and preferentially extract nutrients that normally are available for host nutritional maintenance and repletion. With TPN, additional nutrients become available for host cell use because extraction of host nutrients by the tumor cells is at, or close to, maximum. This observation is best demonstrated by the studies on differential glutamine use between host and tumor cells reported by Souba and colleagues.[4]

Our attention subsequently turned to the etiology of depressed cell-mediated immunity in cancer patients. Dudrick's group had already demonstrated, in patients without cancer, that malnutrition resulted in a depression of cell-mediated immunity, which could be reversed by adequate nutritional repletion.[5] We used a battery of 5 recall skin test antigens to test cellular immunity both before and after nutritional repletion with TPN (again in patients who met the criteria for administering TPN). Cellular immunity could be restored even in patients whose tumors persisted and did not respond to oncologic therapy. This observation demonstrated that, in these patients, the tumor was not the cause of the depressed immunity; rather, malnutrition was the cause.[6]

Surgeons specializing in the treatment of patients with head and neck cancer had noted that cell-mediated immunity often returned toward normal after the surgical removal of the cancer. What these investigators failed to consider was the enteral nutritional replenishment, often via feeding tubes, that had been provided preoperatively.

Immunologic evaluation had been done before preoperative nutritional repletion and after surgical removal of the cancer. The flaw in this study design was that immune evaluation occurred after nutritional repletion but before the surgery. We turned our attention to this issue and showed that nutritional repletion preoperatively, not the removal of the cancer, was the reason for restoration of cell-mediated immunity.[7]

Patients with head and neck cancers are often heavy smokers and alcohol drinkers and often have chronic malnutrition because of inadequate and unbalanced nutritional intake. In the course of studying a subset of patients with head and neck cancers, we noted a form of malabsorption that prevented assimilation of nutrients across the gastrointestinal mucosa, because any attempt to use the enteral route resulted in diarrhea. Nevertheless, use of the gastrointestinal tract was continued during treatment with TPN under the assumption that its use and stimulation was likely beneficial.[8] Diarrhea abated when patients became anabolic. Now it is known that malnutrition results in malabsorption. Characteristically, the columnar cells of the mucosa become cuboidal; the brush border enzymes responsible for nutrient assimilation are depressed; and various transport mechanisms across the luminal barrier of the gastrointestinal mucosa function minimally. Many of these morphologic and physiologic changes can be reversed and/or prevented by specialized TPN solutions, even, somewhat, the injury to the small bowel caused by abdominal radiation. The importance of maintaining some enteral nutrition cannot be overemphasized. The functional gut does not atrophy and maintains its immune competence. These fundamental experimental observations were made in collaboration with several investigators, including Daly and colleagues,[9] Souba and colleagues,[10] Klimberg and colleagues,[11] Ota and colleagues,[12] Johnson and colleagues,[13] and Castro and colleagues.[14]

Our next task was to convince the nursing supervisor at MDAH, Renalda Hilkemyer, RN, to provide a nurse totally responsible for TPN. There were no TPN teams in 1974 in any categorical cancer institute. Under her supervision, 2 surgical floors were identified for studies, and on 1 of the floors, staff nurses, among their other administrative and patient duties, changed the central venous catheter dressings and the intravenous tubing and were responsible for other required aseptic and antiseptic maneuvers. On the other floor, one of the laboratory assistants was responsible for these duties. The catheter sepsis and metabolic complication rates were significantly lower on the floor on which the laboratory assistant was responsible for TPN.[15] Subsequent to that unequivocal clinical demonstration, MDAH has had a dedicated team to provide care for patients receiving TPN. A great deal of the credit for the success of Dr Copeland as an academic surgeon must be attributed to 3 of these nurses. Mary Ann Rapp, RN,[16] maintained comprehensive data on all of these patients, allowing evaluation of the effects of TPN. Louise Cox, RN, MSN,[17] initiated the first home TPN program at a categorical cancer institute. She developed the criteria and the teaching principles and methods still used today. Sandra Norman, RN, was the consummate nurse clinician, even though there was no such designated title at the time. She established the catheter insertion clinic at the MDAH that is in existence and use to this day.

Cachectic patients with cancer exhibit a much narrower safe therapeutic margin for tolerating chemotherapy than well-nourished hosts in the early stages of metastatic disease, and malnutrition often eliminates such patients as candidates for adequate oncologic treatment. This was documented by Copeland and colleagues[18,19] more than 30 years ago in a group of 58 nutritionally depleted patients with cancer who had been denied adequate antitumor therapy because of the fear of complications related to malnutrition or inanition. After an average of 3 to 4 weeks of nutritional rehabilitation, primarily in the form of TPN, 52 patients gained an average of 6.8 lb, whereas 6 patients lost an average of 7 lb. The patients then received chemotherapeutic regimens in accordance with established protocols at that time for their tumor types and stages, and a 36% response rate was obtained in these 58 nutritionally depleted patients who otherwise would have been denied an adequate course of antineoplastic therapy. A 50% reduction in measurable tumor metastases occurred in 21 of the patients, and a 25% reduction occurred in another 3 patients. The conclusion of this study was that intravenous hyperalimentation, as TPN was known at that time, can be a valuable adjunct to cancer chemotherapy by improving the nutritional status, increasing the total deliverable dose of anticancer agent per unit of time, and reducing the incidence and severity of the toxic gastrointestinal side effects without adversely stimulating malignant cell growth or producing septic complications.[18,19]

It was never our intent to suggest that TPN was a potentiator of any cancer treatment. TPN was given primarily as a nutritional supplement to allow indicated cancer therapy to be provided. Several randomized controlled trials, many of which include well-nourished patients in their cohorts, have attempted to show a response advantage for patients receiving TPN. If the patients could tolerate a full course of therapy without requiring TPN support, there was no survival advantage in the TPN groups. In some of the studies, an increase in infectious complications occurred in the TPN groups. This latter result is no surprise because most of the patients were not TPN candidates by the established criteria. Why risk exposing patients with cancer to the recognized complications of TPN if no therapeutic advantages are expected?

From 1972 to 1982 was somewhat of a golden age of health care during which patients could be hospitalized for long enough periods of time to treat their conditions optimally and to evaluate the pros and cons of TPN. Few clinical studies of TPN emanate from this country today. Hasenberg and colleagues[20] from Germany recently published a prospective, randomized controlled trial of malnourished patients with advanced colorectal cancers undergoing appropriate chemotherapy. Both groups were fed an appropriate enteral diet, but nutritional intake of 1 group was supplemented by outpatient TPN. In the 60-week trial, the control group, body mass fell by week 6; serum albumin dropped significantly; quality-of-life measures were deteriorated by week 16; chemotherapy-associated side effects were higher, and survival was worse. The original follow-up was too short to evaluate survival, but the other salutary effects of parenteral nutrition noted by the Hasenberg group were observed and reported by us in the 1970s.

In 2010, Burnette and Jatoi[21] from the Mayo Clinic published guidelines for parenteral nutrition in cancer patients. They stated that the role for TPN in patients with metastatic malignancies "has changed over the years." They go on to state, "Once considered the panacea, this invasive intervention is now approached with great caution when prescribed to patients with incurable malignancies." The term, *routine administration*, for such patients is used. They go on to describe the indication for the use of TPN in such patients as, "malnourished individuals with a predictable positive outcome from chemotherapy when enteral nutrition is not a viable option." Does this indication seem familiar? It is a de facto restatement of our indications from the 1970s; however, the earliest reference in their manuscript is 2005, and our seminal efforts in this area were completely ignored in their guidelines.

Where did things go wrong? Who decided that TPN was a panacea for patients with metastatic malignancies? Certainly not us! We published simple observations that TPN could be of nutritional value when all other methods of nutritional maintenance and/or repletion were ineffective or exhausted in cancer patients who had a viable treatment regimen available to them.

Treatment with TPN for cancer patients began to be misconstrued at the MDAH in the late 1970s and early 1980s. TPN was developed by Stanley J. Dudrick, MD, and

Jonathan E. Rhoads, MD, both surgeons. Consequently, the candidates for TPN and its administration historically were controlled by surgeons when TPN was initiated at an institution. Dr Copeland decided who were to be the candidates for TPN and supervised the program at MDAH. Once the value of TPN was observed by members of the medical oncology service, they began their own TPN program when several of their patients were turned down by us because of lack of proper indications. A good example of this indiscretion is a study done by Samuels and colleagues.[22] Vinblastine and bleomycin was a new drug combination for the treatment of testicular carcinoma. This is a disease of young, healthy men, and they often become malnourished during treatment. The protocol was designed to use TPN to allow more cycles of chemotherapy to be administered closer together. Not a bad idea, but one that predictably would not work. Patients could easily recover after one treatment cycle for the next course of chemotherapy with oral intake. Patients in this series treated with TPN did not have better response rates, and, moreover, infectious complications were increased. Both of these outcomes were predictable. In evaluating the data from this study, we made the observation that any survival advantage for TPN was in the patients who did not respond to chemotherapy.

In fairness to our medical oncology colleagues of that day, observations were made in patients with lung cancer that suggested that well-nourished patients at the outset of chemotherapy, and those malnourished patients who were nutritionally replenished with TPN, had better responses to chemotherapy than their malnourished counterparts.[23,24] The Hasenberg trial (discussed previously) lends some credibility to this hypothesis, but a study required yet to prove it must be done as carefully as Hasenberg and colleagues' study.[20]

In the surgical patients with cancer, none of our observations on the value of nutritional replenishment with TPN either preoperatively or postoperatively were randomized.Indicators of anabolism were maintained, however, and patients who gained lean body mass had better surgical outcomes than those who did not. Two proper randomized trials, 19 years apart, must be disucssed. In 1981, Muller and colleagues[25] from Germany evaluated the efficacy of TPN in patients undergoing major operations for abdominal malignancies. Malnutrition was appropriately defined, nutritional values were appropriately selected and determined longitudinally, and outcomes were stratified. TPN was maintained for 10 days preoperatively and at least 3 days postoperatively. Skin test reactivity, retinol binding protein, prealbumin, transferrin, and IgG improved in the TPN group but declined in the control group. The control group had significantly more deaths and major complications, primarily pneumonia and anastomotic breakdown, than the TPN group. Similar results were obtained in 2000 by Bozzetti and colleagues[26] from Italy, who randomized malnourished patients with stomach or colorectal cancer to TPN versus control groups. Infectious complications in the two groups were 37% versus 57%, and noninfectious complications were 12% versus 34%, respectively. Four patients in the control group died. Hospitalization was significantly longer for the TPN group by 6 days. Who is to decide whether or not this 6-day prolongation of hospital stay justified the resultant better outcomes?

Neumeyer and associates[27] have shown convincingly that early and sufficient feeding, when indicated, reduces length of stay and hospital charges in surgical patients. Brennan and coworkers have established in a randomized controlled trial of patients undergoing major pancreatic procedures for malignancy that the administration of TPN, beginning on day 1 postoperatively, provided no benefit over control patients who were treated in a standard fashion.[28] In this patient population, TPN should be reserved for patients malnourished preoperatively or those who develop abdominal complications postoperatively that lead to malnutrition. Our group agrees with Brennan's group that TPN should not be used routinely in patients undergoing major pancreatic resections for malignancy.

Multiple studies have now shown that morbidity and mortality secondary to multiple surgical procedures are reduced in high volume centers, such as Memorial Sloan-Kettering Cancer Center, in which Brennan and his colleagues work. It is often hard to separate the technical and judgmental abilities of the surgeons who perform the surgical procedures in randomized trials. If surgical complication rates are low among the patients of a particular surgical group, the numbers of patients within randomized trials must necessarily be large to define differences between randomized and control groups. An institution having a low complication rate, virtually regardless of nutritional status, is unlikely to identify differences in incidence of complications, whether or not TPN is used. Other measures, such as gastric emptying, length of stay, quality of life after return from the hospital, and hospital costs, should be investigated, some of which have been reported in the study by Neumeyer and her colleagues.[27] Their study was comprised of patients from 8 hospitals in which 1007 patients underwent abdominal procedures. Nutritional support (>60% of protein and calorie requirements) was administered to 183 of these patients. From a study of this size, when analyzed for more than 800 components of detailed patient care, outcome measures, and processes within a system, meaningful data on clinical practice environment can be reliable, even though the patients were not randomized.

Wong, from Hong Kong, is regarded internationally as one of the premier hepatobiliary surgeons and recognized as having the best outcomes. His group randomized patients undergoing resection for hepatocellular carcinoma to TPN for 8 days both preoperatively and postoperatively along with their oral intake. The control group did not have additional nutritional supplementation with TPN. This study lessens the variable of surgical techniques and judgment from the study because all of the patients were operated upon by Wong and his group. In every measured parameter, the TPN group was significantly better than the enteral group. TPN was most beneficial for patients who had cirrhosis. No patients were malnourished preoperatively. These patients may be a special group who undergo hepatic resection and require additional nutrients to maintain weight, liver regeneration, and hepatic function to generate appropriate plasma levels of acute phase proteins, such as transferrin, prealbumin, and retinol-binding protein.[29]

A meta-analysis of randomized controlled trials of patients with critical illness and cancer was supported by Heys and colleagues[30] from Scotland. All patients had functional gastrointestinal tracts. The control group received standard enteral diets, and the experimental group received supplemental enteral nutrition fortified with key nutrients, such as glutamine, arginine, and branched-chain amino acids. Significant reductions in mortality and in morbidity were identified in the supplemented group together with a reduction of hospitalization by 2.5 days.

A trend is apparent. Interest in the nutritional repletion of malnourished cancer patients continues overseas, and the gastrointestinal tract is the preferred method of nutritional repletion and maintaince if available. For anyone using TPN, it is advisable to visit or revisit the experiences of our group that were published in the 1970s and 1980s. The most striking study to underline this recommendation is the outcome of the Veterans Affairs randomized trial of malnourished patients who required laparotomy or noncardiac thoracotomy.[31] The patients were randomized to TPN versus standard nutritional and fluid maintenance and were stratified by measured nutritional status into borderline, moderate, and severe malnutrition. Only the severely malnourished group had a significant reduction in morbidity with the use of TPN. Noninfectious complications (primarily wound healing) occurred in 5.3% of the TPN group and in 42.9% of the control group. Infectious complications in these 2 groups of severely malnourished patients were the same. Infectious complications in the mildly malnourished patients were significantly increased in the TPN group, once again demonstrating that patients who are not candidates for TPN should not receive it and be exposed to the complications of the technique.

A major difficulty during the early development and application of TPN in the management of cancer patients seems to have been, and continues to be, an inherent resistance among medical oncologists to add or include this important modality in their various protocols. Their usual rationalization is that adding nutritional support to patient management would introduce a confounding factor to their original protocols. The time is long overdue to overcome this negative attitude and to carry out prospective, controlled studies in comparable cancer patients to measure the effects of malnutrition and its correction or amelioration in cancer patients when the nutritional support regimen is tailored, formulated, conducted, and/or supervised by a competent nutritional support team. Virtually none of the studies reported in the literature during the past decade or more satisfies these criteria and is, therefore, fundamentally flawed. Until this unacceptable situation is corrected, the optimal nutritional support of cancer patients will be compromised and will not reach its full adjunctive therapeutic potential.

One of the studies most frequently cited in this area provided 35 kcal/kg per day to all the cancer patients. Perhaps the results would have been better if the caloric ration had been increased up to 45 kcal/kg per day in patients who required and tolerated this caloric level, together with a concomitant increase in amino acid nitrogen.[32] It has seemed to be prudent, in our experience, to maximize parenteral nutritional support rather than simply following boilerplate recommendations, as if every patient were exactly the same. Malnourished or cachectic cancer patients are the same persons they were when in optimal nutritional condition and health, but the body cell mass does not act, react, or respond in the same manner under both sets of circumstances. More simply stated, patients with cancer are not the same nutritionally or metabolically as they had been when they were cancer-free, and this must be taken into consideration in performing their treatment. Optimal results cannot be obtained uniformly with any therapeutic endeavor in malnourished or cachectic patients. Their systems require adequate nutrient substrates at all times to function at their maximum potential. Because infection associated with parenteral nutrition has been the single most important impediment to its optimal application in critically ill patients and in cancer patients, and has been related primarily to catheter and other related administrative aspects of the technique, it is of paramount importance that dedicated and competent nutritional support teams are actively and conscientiously engaged in the comprehensive management of cancer patients daily.

The techniques used for providing optimal specialized nutritional support must be applied just as conscientiously and competently as, for example, the management of blood sugar levels in critically ill patients, especially postoperatively, in intensive care situations. A fundamental problem with providing nutritional support is that caregivers, especially physicians and surgeons, have become virtually too familiar and comfortable with the existence of the technology without mastering the essential principles and practices mandatorily associated with the desired optimal outcomes. In some quarters, TPN is still considered for use primarily as a last ditch effort rather than having been applied earlier and more rationally in the clinical course. Inevitably, the conclusion drawn from this predictably suboptimal experience is, "the TPN doesn't work." TPN is not holy water and should be used prudently and judiciously when indicated for patients who are significantly malnourished and who cannot otherwise obtain adequate nutrition in a timely manner.

Finally, the composition of TPN is so variable in different institutions that it is difficult or impossible to derive meaningful data from meta-analysis, which has been used so frequently to discredit its use. The meta-analysis of nutritional support using parenteral and enteral techniques has been flawed and has propagated more misinformation than useful information. Moreover, meta-analysis is to science what alchemy is to chemistry; it is pseudoscience rather than real science. In the frequently quoted study by Brennan and colleagues,[28] the data are flawed by the facts that patients were included in the study and randomized without regard to their nutritional status; all of the patients received the same parenteral nutrition regimen providing 2000 calories, an inordinately high fat content approaching 60% of total calories, and inadequate protein; the TPN was administered autonomously by the medical TPN team, and the composition and ratios of the components of the parenteral diet would not be considered a healthy diet if given by mouth or enterally. This study has resulted in a widespread attitude among oncologic surgeons that parenteral nutritional support not only is unnecessary as an adjunct to the management of all patients with pancreatic malignancies but also may be contraindicated. This is not only an invalid but also a dangerous attitude because there are patients at various stages of pancreatic cancer and its treatment who can benefit from parenteral nutritional support when enteral or oral nutritional support cannot be provided adequately or at all.

The consensus statement published in 1997 by the American Society for Parenteral and Enteral Nutrition represents the best published principles in this area to date.[33] Our primary modification of the statement is that we feel that parenteral nutrition should be either strongly considered or mandated 5 to10 days after operation for patients still unable to eat or tolerate enteral feedings rather than merely considered, which to us is a bit too soft, weak, or polite. Too often, clinicians tend to put off or delay the initiation of specialized nutritional support postoperatively "to see how the patient feels tomorrow" in the hope that patients will then begin to ingest adequate nutrients. The tomorrows often become successive, however, so that by the time the specialized nutritional support technologies are initiated or fully undertaken, the nutritional status of the patient has deteriorated to a severe state, which can be difficult or impossible to overcome nutritionally. To emphasize this common error in clinical judgment, we reinforce the teaching of prudent application of specialized nutritional support postoperatively to students and residents by relating to them the anecdote of a local pub, which has a sign behind the bar that states, "free beer tomorrow." The catch is that if one returns tomorrow for the free beer advertised by the sign, the bartender points out that the sign still says, "free beer tomorrow." The tomorrow never becomes today, and the beer never becomes free. Unfortunately, in a clinical situation, patients pay the price for this conundrum.

As a professor and mentor of ours once said, "the closer you get to being history, the more you will learn to appreciate it." Having lived through the development of TPN by Dudrick and colleagues and the application of the technique to cancer patients, we can attest to the wisdom of this advice. We hope that the readers of this understand and appreciate the meaning of this insight as well.

REFERENCES

1. Copeland EM, MacFadyen BV Jr, McGown C, et al. The use of hyperalimentation in patients with potential sepsis. Surg Gynecol Obstet 1974;138:377–80.

2. Brown JR, Slomski C, Saxe AW. Is routine postoperative chest X-ray necessary after fluoroscopic-guided subclavian central venous port placement? J Am Coll Surg 2009;208:517–9.
3. Copeland EM, MacFadyen BV Jr, Dudrick SJ. Intravenous hyperalimentation in cancer patients. J Surg Res 1974;16:241–7.
4. Austgen TR, Dudrick PS, Sitren H, et al. The effect of glutamine-enriched total parenteral nutrition on tumor growth and host tissues. Ann Surg 1992;215:107–13.
5. Law DK, Dudrick SJ, Abdou NI. Immunocompetence of patients with protein-calorie malnutrition. Ann Intern Med 1973;79:545–50.
6. Copeland EM, MacFadyen BV Jr, Dudrick SJ. Effect of intravenous hyperalimentation on established delayed hypersensitivity in the cancer patient. Ann Surg 1976;184:60–4.
7. Daly JM, Dudrick SJ, Copeland EM. Intravenous hyperalimentation: effect on delayed cutaneous hypersensitivity in cancer patients. Ann Surg 1980;192:587–92.
8. Copeland EM, Daly JM, Dudrick SJ. Nutritional concepts in the treatment of head and neck malignancies. Head Neck Surg 1979;1:350–63.
9. Daly JM, Reynolds HM, Rowlands BJ, et al. Tumor growth in experimental animals: nutritional manipulation and chemotherapeutic response. Ann Surg 1980;191:316–22.
10. Souba WW, Strebel FR, Bull JM, et al. Interorgan glutamine metabolism in tumor-bearing rats. J Surg Res 1988;44:720–6.
11. Klimberg VS, Souba WW, Salloum RM, et al. Glutamine-enriched diets support muscle glutamine metabolism without stimulating tumor growth. J Surg Res 1990;48:319–23.
12. Ota DM, Copeland EM, Strobel HW, et al. The effect of protein nutrition on host and tumor metabolism. J Surg Res 1977;22:181–8.
13. Johnson LR, Copeland EM, Dudrick SJ, et al. Structural and hormonal alterations in the gastrointestinal tract of parenterally fed rats. Gastroenterology 1975;68:1177–83.
14. Castro GA, Copeland EM, Dudrick SJ, et al. Intestinal disaccharidase and peroxidase activity in parenterally nourished rats. J Nutr 1975;105:776–81.
15. Copeland EM, MacFadyen BV Jr, Dudrick SJ. Prevention of microbial catheter contamination in patients receiving hyperalimentation. South Med J 1974;67:303–7.
16. Rapp MA, Hilkemeyer R, Copeland EM, et al. Hyperalimentation: special nutrition therapy for the cancer patient. Magazine. RN 1976;39:55–61.
17. Ota DM, Cox LC, Martin S, et al. Ambulatory home intravenous hyperalimentation. Canc Bull 1982;34:218–20.
18. Copeland EM, MacFadyen BV Jr, Lanzotti V, et al. Intravenous hyperalimentation as an adjunct to cancer chemotherapy. Am J Surg 1975;129:167–73.
19. Copeland EM, Souchon EA, MacFadyen BV Jr, et al. Intravenous hyperalimentation as an adjunct to radiation therapy. Cancer 1977;39:609–16.
20. Hasenberg T, Essenbreis A, Herold A, et al. Early supplementation of parenteral nutrition is capable of improving quality of life, chemotherapy-related toxicity and body composition in patients with advanced colorectal carcinoma undergoing palliative treatment: results from a prospective, randomized clinical trial. (The Association of Coloproctology of Great Britain and Ireland). Colorectal Dis 2010;12:e190–9.
21. Burnette B, Jatoi A. Parenteral nutrition in patients with cancer: recent guidelines and a need for further study. Curr Opin Support Palliat Care 2010;4:1–4.

22. Samuels ML, Selig DE, Ogden S, et al. IV hyperalimentation and chemotherapy for stage III testicular cancer: a randomized study. Cancer Treat Rep 1981;65: 615–28.

23. Lanzotti VC, Copeland EM, George SL, et al. Cancer chemotherapeutic response and intravenous hyperalimentation. Canc Chemother Rep 1975;59:437–9.

24. Issell BV, Valdivieso M, Zaren HA, et al. Protection against chemotherapy toxicity by IV hyperalimentation. Cancer Treat Rep 1978;62:1139–43.

25. Muller JM, Dienst C, Brenner U, et al. Perioperative TPN in patients with upper gastrointestinal malignancies. Lancet 1981;1:68–71.

26. Bozzetti F, Gavazzi C, Miceli R, et al. Perioperative total parenteral nutrition in malnourished, gastrointestinal cancer patients: a randomized, clinical trial. JPEN J Parenter Enteral Nutr 2000;24:7–14.

27. Neumeyer LA, Smout RJ, Horn HG, et al. Early and sufficient feeding reduces length of stay and charges in surgical patients. J Surg Res 2001;95:73–7.

28. Brennan MF, Pisters PW, Posner M, et al. A prospective randomized trial of total parenteral nutrition after major pancreatic resection for malignancy. Ann Surg 1994;220:436–40.

29. Fan ST, Lo CM, Lai EC, et al. Perioperative nutritional support in patients undergoing hepatectomy for hepatocellular carcinoma. N Engl J Med 1994;331: 1547–52.

30. Heys SD, Walker LG, Smith I, et al. Enteral nutritional supplementation with key nutrients in patients with critical illness and cancer: a meta-analysis of randomized controlled trials. Ann Surg 1999;229:467–77.

31. The Veterans Affairs Total Parenteral Nutrition Cooperative Study Group. Perioperative total parenteral nutrition in surgical patients. N Engl J Med 1991;325: 525–32.

32. Smale BF, Mullen JL, Buzby GP, et al. The efficacy of nutritional assessment and support in cancer surgery. Cancer 1981;47:2375–81.

33. Klein S, Kinney J, Jeejeebhoy K, et al. Nutrition support in clinical practice: review of published data and recommendations for future research directions. National Institutes of Health. American Society for Parenteral and Enteral Nutrition and American Society for Clinical Nutrition. JPEN J Parenter Enteral Nutr 1997;21: 133–56.

The Relationships of Nutrients, Routes of Delivery, and Immunocompetence

Senthil Jayarajan, MD[a], John M. Daly, MD[b],*

KEYWORDS

• Nutrition • Immune system • Glutamine • Arginine

The nutritional status of patients has a profound effect on the outcome after surgery or traumatic injury. It is well known that malnutrition increases mortality, morbidity, and the treatment costs of patients undergoing surgery.[1,2] Malnutrition has also been associated with a depressed host immune system, which in turn is associated with an increase in major infections and in organ failure associated with sepsis.[3,4] These increased risks are thought to be caused by increased stress after injury. The stress of a major operation also increases requirements for additional resources for wound healing and clearance of infection and toxins. The immune system, in particular, is susceptible to malnutrition because of the high turnover rates of leukocytes and immunoproteins. These findings have prompted investigations into which nutrients require supplementation and how nutrition can best be delivered to support these functions of the immune system, especially after injury or emergency surgical procedures.

The aim of this commentary is to describe and discuss the key nutrients noted to be beneficial for the immune system, examine the physiologic changes associated with immunosuppression in surgical disease, review the routes of nutrition delivery and their immunomodulatory effects, and evaluate the major clinical trials that have evaluated the use and value of immunonutrition.

SPECIFIC NUTRIENTS AND THEIR EFFECT ON THE IMMUNE SYSTEM

Arginine

Arginine is a conditionally essential amino acid that can be produced from a variety of sources, including glutamine and citrulline. The role of arginine in various important

The authors have nothing to disclose.
[a] Department of Surgery, Temple University School of Medicine, 4th floor, Parkinson Pavilion, 3401 North Broad Street, Philadelphia, PA 19140, USA
[b] Department of Surgery, Temple University School of Medicine and Temple University Hospital, Room 445, Parkinson Pavilion, 3500 North Broad Street, Philadelphia, PA 19140, USA
* Corresponding author.
E-mail address: johndaly@temple.edu

biochemical pathways is complex. Its synthesis is the rate-limiting step of the Krebs or urea cycle, which is vital for the conversion of ammonia into the less toxic substance, urea, in the liver. Arginine is involved in the secretion of anabolic hormones, such as insulin and growth hormone, that affect nitrogen balance; protein synthesis; and the production of polyamines, nitric oxide, collagen, and creatinine (**Fig. 1**).[5,6]

Arginine has direct effects on the immune system that are thought to be related to its role as a key substrate in the production of polyamines and nitric oxide. Polyamines promote cell growth and division, and may have a role in curtailing overexpression of proinflammatory cytokines and T-cell proliferation.[7,8] Nitric oxide has antimicrobial and antitumor activity and also regulates the functional activity and expansion of immune cells.[9] Thus, arginine has important functions affecting wound healing, anabolic processes, and the immune system.

Glutamine

Glutamine is also a conditionally essential amino acid, thought to become essential in stressed situations, such as sepsis and trauma. Glutamine is a predominant source of fuel for enterocytes and inflammatory cells, a supporter of anabolic processes, a key participant in cellular respiration, and a building block for protein synthesis.[10,11]

Glutamine also has direct effects on the immune system. Extracellular levels of glutamine regulate T-cell proliferation, production of interleukin (IL)-2, and B-cell differentiation. Glutamine has also been shown to enhance phagocytosis and superoxide production in neutrophils and macrophages.[12]

Fatty Acids

Lipids perform many functions, including the formation of cell membranes and the regulation of intercellular signaling, cellular transport, and many other cell functions. Omega-3 and omega-6 fatty acids are essential polyunsaturated fatty acids. Omega-3 fatty acids are derived primarily from fish oils, whereas omega-6 fatty acids are derived from vegetable oils. Their derivatives compete for prostaglandin and leukotriene synthesis. When the fatty acid ratio is positive toward omega-3 fatty acids, the products cause less of a systemic inflammatory response syndrome and less stimulation of cytokines and inflammatory markers, including those involved in cell adhesion and chemotaxis.[13] For example, the production of leukotriene B4 is a powerful inducer of leukocyte chemotaxis, and cellular adherence is decreased.[14] These immunomodulatory effects have been shown to have benefit in autoimmune disease, cardiovascular disease, and cancer. The sources and effects of these nutrients are summarized in **Table 1**.

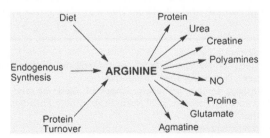

Fig. 1. Sources and metabolic fates of arginine. Note: putrescine, spermine, and spermidine are the polyamines referred to in Fig. 1. NO, nitric oxide. (*From* Morris SM Jr. Arginine: beyond protein. Am J Clin Nutr 2006;83(2):508S–12S; with permission.)

Table 1
Immunonutrients: their sources and their effects

Nutrient	Source	Effect
Arginine	Diet Protein turnover	Via polyamines: promote cell growth, reduce systemic inflammation Via NO: vasodilation, antimicrobial effects, regulate function and growth of immune cells. Build protein Enhances wound healing through promotion of collagen production Key step in urea cycle
Glutamine	Diet Endogenous synthesis	Fuel source for enterocytes and immune cells T-cell proliferation B-cell differentiation Build protein Transport of amino acids Gluconeogenesis/energy balance Anabolic/growth hormone synthesis Cell respiration
Omega-3 fatty acids	Fish oils	Form cell membranes Intercellular signaling Reduce immune cell proliferation Reduce inflammation

IMMUNOSUPPRESSIVE EFFECTS OF DISEASE
Cancer

Cancer and suppression of the immune system have a reciprocal relationship. Malignancy is known to arise in immune-deficient states, such as those that commonly accompany AIDS and patients receiving transplants. Cancer itself has also been shown to cause immune suppression. In 1979, a clinical study demonstrated that approximately 50% impairment of immune status occurred in perioperative patients with breast cancer when compared with immune-competent controls.[15] The study suggested that tumor dissemination might be the cause, instead of the result, of immune suppression.

The immune suppression associated with cancer is thought to occur through several mechanisms. The lymphocytes, macrophages, and the tumor and vascular cells that make up the tumor microenvironment secrete growth factors and cytokines, including vascular endothelial growth factor, transforming growth factor- β, and IL-10, that suppress the activity of dendritic cells and other antigen-presenting cells, as well as cytotoxic T cells.[16,17] This method may be the one used by neoplastic cells to evade immune surveillance, thus allowing increased tumor proliferation. Abnormal processing of antigens by tumor cells and recruitment of inhibitory cells, like regulatory T cells, also contributes to tumor-associated host immunosuppression.[18,19]

Trauma and Major Surgery

Metabolic changes following major trauma follow an *ebb*-and-*flow* pattern.[20] The ebb phase begins in the first minutes after injury and lasts for several hours. It is characterized by decreased body temperature, increased hepatic acute-phase protein response, and immune activation aimed at reducing posttraumatic energy depletion. The flow phase is generally more clinically relevant, and its duration can last for days to weeks. It involves activation of a systemic inflammatory response, a hypermetabolic state (including proteolysis and lipolysis), and immunosuppression.

The immunosuppression associated with major injury or surgery is caused by altered cytokine secretion, especially IL-2, gamma interferon (INF-γ), tumor necrosis factor alpha, and IL-4, which have roles in the activation of T-helper (Th) 1 and Th2 T-helper cells. Major surgery and polytrauma results in a distinct pattern of immune defects with a predominant defect in the T-cell response through T-cell receptor- and CD28 coreceptor-mediated signals.[21] Suppression of cell-mediated immunity may also be caused by other factors, such as excessive activation and uncoordinated recruitment of polymorphonuclear neutrophils, induction of regulatory macrophages with antiinflammatory properties, a shift in the Th1/Th2 balance toward Th2, appearance of regulatory T cells that suppress both the innate and adaptive immune system, and apoptosis of lymphocytes.[22]

Routes of Delivery

Several clinical studies have established that early oral feeding is associated with better outcomes after surgery or multiple traumas than occur in unfed or inadequately fed patients.[23,24] Barriers to the goal of early oral feeding include postoperative ileus, dysphagia, early postoperative bowel obstruction, or other contraindications caused by the nature of the surgery. It is recommended that oral feedings resume within 2 to 3 days, if possible, especially after major trauma.[25] If patients have not been able to eat for 7 days, or have been unable to consume 60% of their daily nutrient requirements, enteral or parenteral nutrition should be initiated, depending on the patients' condition and situation.[26,27]

Enteral Nutrition

Numerous randomized controlled trials have been conducted in postoperative patients undergoing major surgery. Results of enteral feeding have been largely positive regarding early feeding when compared with intravenous isotonic fluids alone, showing improved patient outcomes with fewer complications, better wound healing, and decreased hospital length of stay.[28–33] Others, however, have reported either no difference or negative outcomes, such as decreased respiratory function and impaired mobility, in those receiving early enteral nutrition compared with nonfed controls.[34–36]

Total Parenteral Nutrition

Total parenteral nutrition (TPN) has proven to be a viable option when oral and enteral feedings are contraindicated or inadequate. However, its long-term use has been associated with serious complications, such as catheter-related infections. In a large meta-analysis comprising 2211 hospitalized patients, TPN with different formulations was compared with standard of care, usually oral intake and intravenous dextrose. Overall, there was not a significant difference in mortality, but there was a trend toward lower complication rates in patients given lipid-free TPN formulations. However, when the critically ill patients were compared with routine postoperative patients, a significant increase in mortality and complication rates were noted in those receiving TPN.[37]

Implications of Route of Delivery

According to the American Society of Parenteral and Enteral Nutrition and the European Society of Parenteral and Enteral Nutrition, it is generally recommended that feeding via the gastrointestinal tract is preferred to the use of intravenous nutrition when patients are able to tolerate enteral feeding.[26,27] There appears to be a lower incidence of infections and sepsis, fewer complications, and decreased hospital costs in patients receiving enteral nutrition. Enteral feeding also confers several immunologic advantages over parenteral nutrition as it is currently practiced.

Efficacy

In 2001, a large multicenter, randomized controlled trial was conducted in malnourished patients undergoing resections of gastrointestinal cancers to determine if enteral or parenteral nutrition improved patient outcomes.[38] Postoperative complications were significantly less in the enteral nutrition group (34%) compared with results in the parenteral nutrition group (49%). Enteral feeding was associated with increased incidence of abdominal distention, diarrhea, and vomiting, requiring crossover to parenteral nutrition in 10% of patients. In this study, mortality, hospital length of stay, and the occurrence of major complications and complications requiring surgical intervention were similar between the two groups.[39]

A meta-analysis conducted by the American Gastrointestinal Association showed no clinical difference in mortality and complications between enteral and parenteral feeding.[40] An intention-to-treat meta-analysis did demonstrate a mortality benefit in favor of total parenteral nutrition attributed to an a priori group, in which enteral feeding was started later than total parenteral nutrition (after 24 hours vs within 24 hours after surgery).[41] In a randomized clinical trial studying costs associated with postoperative nutritional support, it was found that parenteral nutrition was nearly 4 times more expensive than enteral nutrition.[42] Thus, even though enteral nutrition might not be as well tolerated, it should be the first choice for feeding, because it is less expensive and demonstrates, perhaps, a slight protective effect in the setting of infection and sepsis over parenteral nutrition. However, parenteral nutrition should be started proactively and as early as feasible if patients are unable to tolerate enteral nutrition.

Effects on Organ Systems

TPN, if used inappropriately, may have several adverse effects on the functions of the liver, kidneys, intestine, and the immune system.[43] TPN may cause hepatic steatosis, cholestasis, and delayed recovery from acute tubular necrosis. TPN may also cause impaired neutrophil, macrophage, and lymphocyte functions, which are not ordinarily caused by enteral feeding.[44] In high-risk surgical patients or in those who have sustained severe burns or trauma, enteral nutrition appears to have a protective effect in the setting of infection and sepsis.[45–47]

Enteral nutrition is thought to boost the immunity of the intestinal tract by preserving the mucosal lining and preventing atrophy, and stimulating the immune cells located in Peyer patches. In animal studies, parenteral nutrition has been associated with reducing sensitized CD4 T-cell and B-cell responses by reducing concentrations of IL-4 and IL-10 in the mucosa-associated lymphoid tissue of the intestinal and respiratory tract. Additionally, there is a corresponding reduction of mucosal immunoglobulin A production mediated by a higher concentration of INF-γ, thereby suppressing important immune functions in the intestines and lungs.[48–50] These effects were found to be reversible in the animals with oral feeding.[51]

These anatomic, physiologic, and immunologic changes were originally thought to occur because of the intravenous nutrient administration bypassing the usual physiologic first pass through the gastrointestinal and hepatic system. It has been shown that by bypassing the intestinal tract, the cells are placed in starvation mode, causing atrophy and decreased gastric, pancreatic, and intestinal secretions, which has been confirmed in animal and human studies.[43,52–55] In animal models, increased intestinal permeability and bacterial translocation occur with parenteral nutrition, but this has not been proven clinically.[56–58] In fact, Sedman and colleagues[59] concluded that bacterial translocation occurred in 5% of patients spontaneously, and that there was no increase in intestinal atrophy or bacterial translocation in patients receiving parenteral nutrition compared with those receiving enteral nutrition. Additionally, it has been shown by Moore and colleagues[46] that in 132 patients with sepsis after trauma, only 7 had septicemia related to gut flora. Thus, it is the current expert opinion that there is little clinical evidence to show that parenteral nutrition is associated with bacterial translocations from the intestine.[60,61]

Hyperglycemia and insulin resistance are more common in patients receiving total parenteral nutrition as shown in a meta-analysis by Moore and colleagues,[46] in which the blood glucose in the parenteral nutrition group was nearly 100 dL/mol greater than that in the enteral group. However, tight glycemic control using intensive insulin therapy has been shown to improve mortality and morbidity in critically ill patients, particularly in those with multiorgan failure associated with sepsis.[62] It has also been shown that control of hyperglycemia is associated with few blood-borne infections, reduction of dialysis requirement for acute renal failure, as well as decreases in the length of stay in the intensive care unit (ICU) and mechanical ventilation. In a recent review of 4 retrospective studies of critically ill patients receiving TPN, there was a significant increase in mortality and a suggestion of a higher complication rate when the blood glucose level was greater than 180 dL/mol.[63] Collectively, these findings suggest that the adverse effects of TPN with respect to infection and the immune system could be caused, in part, by the use of omega-6 fatty acid emulsions, which have been previously shown to have immunosuppressive effects, and poorly controlled iatrogenic hyperglycemia during administration of parenteral nutrition infusion.

CLINICAL EVIDENCE OF USE OF IMMUNONUTRITION
Postoperative Administration

In 1992, Daly and colleagues[64] conducted the first prospective, randomized controlled trial on the effects of immunonutrition in postoperative patients (**Table 2**). In 85 postoperative patients following resection of upper gastrointestinal cancers, a formulation

Table 2		
Summary of clinical trials in immunonutrition		
Scenario	**Nutrient**	**Effects**
Elective surgery Pre/peri/ postoperative	Arginine, omega-3 fatty acids, nucleotides, glutamine	Reduction in infectious complications Enhanced wound healing Reduced length of stay, but difference in mortality
Trauma/critical care: All patients	Glutamine Arginine, omega-3 fatty acids, nucleotides	Reduced infection and sepsis Trend toward reduced infections Possible reduced length of stay Possible increase or no difference in mortality
Sepsis	Glutamine, antioxidants	Faster recovery from organ failure
Severe sepsis	Arginine	Increased ICU mortality
ARDS	Omega-3 fatty acids	Reduce ventilator time and ICU stay Improved oxygenation

Abbreviation: ARDS, acute respiratory distress syndrome.

supplemented with arginine, dietary nucleotides, and omega-3 fatty acids was compared with isocaloric, but not isonitrogenous, standard enteral nutrition. The incidence of postoperative infections was 11% in the immunonutrition group compared with 37% in the control group ($P = .02$). The mean length of hospital stay was significantly reduced by 4.2 days in the immunonutrition group ($P = .01$). In a subsequent study by Daly and colleagues, 60 patients undergoing operations for gastric, pancreatic, and esophageal malignancies were randomly assigned to receive either an arginine, nucleotides, and omega-3 fatty acid–supplemented formulation or a standard enteral feeding formulation, beginning on postoperative day 1 and continuing until discharge. The rate of infectious wound complications was significantly lower in the immunonutrition group (10% vs 43%, $P<.05$). The mean length of stay was also reduced in the immunonutrition group (16 vs 22 days, $P<.05$) compared with the control group.

Sixty patients undergoing gastric or pancreatic resections were enrolled in a randomized controlled trial that compared immune-enhanced enteral feeding, standard enteral feeding, and TPN.[65] More rapid return to baseline of nutritional and immunologic markers occurred in the immune-enriched feeding group, but no significant differences were detected in infection rates among the groups. This finding might have been because of the small number of patients in each group, as well as to the fact that both enterally fed groups received TPN containing omega-6 fatty acids in the immediate postoperative phase. Another trial of 154 patients undergoing operations for upper-gastrointestinal malignancies compared immune-enhanced enteral nutrition with an isocaloric, isonitrogenous formula. The results demonstrated a trend toward reduced length of stay, associated with a statistically significant reduction in late infectious complications, and an overall reduction of 32% in treatment costs in the immune-enhanced group.[66] In a prospective, randomized trial involving patients undergoing gastric resections, immunonutrition improved wound healing, as shown by higher local levels of hydroxyproline in the wound ($P = .0018$) and reduced surgical wound complications ($P = .005$) compared with results in the group fed with standard formula.

Similar results have been noted in populations not undergoing surgery for esophageal and upper-gastrointestinal malignancies. When an immune-enriched formula was compared with a standard formula and intravenous administration of glucose and fats in patients undergoing surgery for any abdominal malignancy, Schilling and colleagues[67] found that return to baseline of postoperative inflammation occurred earlier in the immune-enhanced group as defined by reduction of C-reactive protein levels by postoperative day 4. Although there was a trend to reduced infectious complications in the immune enhanced group, the difference from the control group was not statistically significant. In patients undergoing head and neck resections, fewer wound complications occurred, and length of hospital stay was reduced in malnourished patients receiving an immune-enhanced diet.[68,69]

These patient outcome benefits are not restricted to arginine and omega-3 fatty acid supplementation alone. Glutamine supplementation with TPN has been shown to reduce length of stay in postoperative patients.[70,71] It has also been shown to promote better nitrogen balance and intestinal permeability. TPN does not contain glutamine, and in stressed situations, supplementation with glutamine in the postoperative patient might be beneficial for increased protein synthesis and better healing.

In contrast to the results of these studies, Heslin and colleagues compared immunonutrition with intravenous fluids alone in patients undergoing resection of abdominal cancers. There was no difference in terms of mortality, complication rates, and length of stay. However, the 2 groups were not similar to each other or to those in prior trials.

The operative time, blood loss, and blood products needed were higher in the experimental group. There was also a trend in the experimental group toward having more patients undergoing preoperative chemotherapy. These factors imply that the patients in the experimental group were, in fact, sicker, which might have predisposed them to the negative results.

Immunonutrition, although not having an effect on mortality, has demonstrable benefits in terms of reduced infectious complications, improved cost-effectiveness of therapy, and possibly better wound healing in multiple postoperative settings. These effects may be caused by the rapid normalization of the immune system as a reaction to the stress of surgery, thereby diminishing the potentially deleterious effect of an uncontrolled or unmodulated systemic inflammatory response.

Preoperative and Perioperative Administration

Perioperative administration of immunonutrition has also been studied and appears to have similar results to postoperative feeding alone. A randomized controlled trial by Braga and colleagues[72] compared well-nourished and malnourished patients receiving an immune-enhanced supplement with a group of patients receiving isocaloric formula for 5 days before surgery and resumed at 6 hours after the operation. The results of the study showed that infectious complications were reduced by one-half ($P = .02$), and the length of stay was reduced by 2 days in the immune-supplemented group ($P = .01$) compared with controls. These results were similar in a trial by Senkal and colleagues,[66] in which the number of complications were significantly higher in the control group. They also showed that providing perioperative immune-enhanced feeding might lead to cost savings. The cost of treating each patient with an immune-enhanced formula is nearly 7 times that of the cost of the control formula. However, when factoring in the costs of treating the complications in each group, a net savings of $856 per patient was shown in the immune-enhanced formula group.

Patients who received only preoperative feeding also shared similar benefits. In 2001, Braga and colleagues[42] reported the results of an intention-to-treat randomized control trial involving 200 patients undergoing resections of colon cancers, in an attempt to test whether preoperative immunonutrition was as effective as perioperative therapy, and if it is superior to conventional therapy in its ability to affect infectious complications and mortality. Four groups of 50 patients were studied. The first group received an enteral formula rich in arginine and omega-3 fatty acids for 5 days preoperatively, whereas the second group received the same enteral formula in the 5-day preoperative and postoperative periods. The control group received an isocaloric, isonitrogenous formula in both the preoperative and postoperative periods, whereas the conventional group did not receive any supplementation. All groups were allowed to consume regular food as usual in the preoperative period. The preoperative and perioperative immune-enhanced feeding groups demonstrated better gut oxygenation and microperfusion as measured intraoperatively, and better controlled systemic inflammatory response, as shown by improved macrophage phagocytosis and a rapid return to baseline of T-cell activation and IL-6 production. Both groups receiving immune-enhanced feeding were found to have a statistically significant decrease in length of stay and approximately one-third the number of infectious complications. No differences were noted among the 4 groups in terms of mortality and anastomotic leaks. This well-conducted, randomized controlled trial shows that preoperative and perioperative immunonutrition had a pronounced effect on decreasing infectious morbidity. A cost-effectiveness study was conducted comparing preoperative immune-enhanced feeding with no supplementation, taking into consideration the costs of hospital stay and the treatment costs of complications.[73] Individual patient nutrition costs were nearly 5 times higher in the preoperative supplemented group. A net benefit of approximately €3000 (US \$4454.7) was shown in the preoperative supplemented group, reflecting reduced costs of treating infectious complications and an average of 3 fewer hospital days.

Thus, preoperative immune-enhanced feeding starting 5 to 7 days before surgery appears to be beneficial, but there might not be an added benefit to perioperative feeding. This result may be caused by the priming of the immune system and modulation of the systemic inflammatory response that occur after surgery.

Trauma

Nutrition is recognized to be a vital, but often elusive, component of the care of trauma patients. Enteral feeding has been shown to be beneficial and superior to parenteral nutrition in the trauma population.[46] This superiority is most pronounced in mortality related to sepsis, regardless of the type of trauma. Immunonutrition is postulated to be beneficial to trauma patients because of its role in normalizing the immune system after a systemic inflammatory response secondary to the trauma, and is expected to reduce progression to sepsis after a second hit occurs.[74] Results from several randomized controlled trials have not been uniform in their recommendation of adding immunonutrition to the therapeutic armamentarium for trauma patients.

Two clinical studies used the same base formula, one of which was enriched by arginine, beta-carotene, and omega-3 fatty acids to investigate the efficacy of immunonutrition versus standard enteral formulae in trauma patients.[75,76] Both were small trials involving 37 and 23 patients, and both studies succeeded in showing a trend toward more rapid normalization of the immune system after stress. Brown and colleagues[76] showed a significant reduction in infectious complications in the immune-enriched formula group (3/19 vs 10/18, $P<.05$), but showed no difference in length of stay or mortality. Mendez and colleagues[75] showed a trend toward longer ICU days and overall length of stay, along with more infectious complications in the immune-enriched diet group. These differences may be attributable to the small numbers of patients in each group. In the Brown trial, investigators were unblinded, and the control group started their diet later and received fewer calories, which might imply that the control group (with increased rate of infections) was malnourished in comparison with the immune-enriched group. In the second trial, investigators were blinded and efforts were made to design formulas similar in calories and nitrogen. However, the immune-enhanced group had more patients who were sicker than the control group, as shown by the larger number of patients with acute respiratory distress syndrome (ARDS).

Trials using other immune-enriched formulas have shown advantages in terms of promoting improved immune markers and reduced rates of septic complications and associated multiple organ failure.[77,78] A multicenter, randomized control trial involving 98 patients compared the effects of immunonutrition with an isocaloric, but not isonitrogenous, standard enteral formula in patients with torso trauma.[79] There were fewer total complications, as well as fewer complications related to sepsis, including multiorgan failure. Although there were no differences in wound healing or pneumonia, intra-abdominal abscesses and multiorgan failure only occurred in the control group. This finding cannot be readily explained by the use of immunonutrition and has not been demonstrated in other trials.

Arginine and fatty-acid supplementation has not been the only form of immunonutrition studied in trauma patients. Houdijk and colleagues[80] studied 80 patients with polytrauma and an Injury Severity Score greater than 20, who were randomized into

2 groups: enteral feeding with a glutamine-enriched formula or with a standard, isocaloric, isonitrogenous formula, with which 60 patients were successfully fed for at least 5 days. Glutamine supplementation led to a lower incidence of pneumonia (17% vs 45%, $P<.02$), bacteremia (7% vs 42%, $P<.02$), and sepsis (3% vs 26%, $P<.02$). These results were similar when an intention-to-treat analysis was done, including all 80 randomized patients.

It is difficult to determine precisely the efficacy of immunonutrition and the role that it might play in trauma patients. The current collection of trials has not established the preferred immune-modulating components and the doses that are most effective, nor have the patient populations been defined or standardized. Clinical trials have demonstrated that immunonutrition enhances immune system function and plays an important role in curtailing the systemic inflammatory response. However, this has not translated uniformly to the outcomes that are thought to be modifiable, namely mortality, morbidity, and reduced complications. This finding might be related to the disparate formulas used in each of the studies and issues with patient selection. Therefore, at this time, further clinical trials must be performed before routine adoption of immunonutrition in the care of trauma patients.

Critical Illness

Four trials have explored the use of arginine and omega-3 fatty acid supplementation compared with isocaloric standard therapy in ICU patients.[81] Bower and colleagues[81] showed that immune-enhanced nutrition resulted in the greatest reduction in length of stay in patients with sepsis who received the optimal formula dose, but there was a trend toward increased mortality in the patients with sepsis who were underfed. The second study by Galban and colleagues[82] showed that the mortality benefit of immunonutrition appeared greatest in the population who were less critically ill with Acute Physiology and Chronic Health Evaluation (APACHE) scores less than 15. Atkinson and colleagues[83] showed that mean ventilation time (6.0 vs 10.5 days, $P = .007$) and mean ICU length of stay (15.5 vs 20.0 days, $P = .03$) were reduced in the immune nutrition group, but there was a trend toward greater mortality compared with controls. The most recent and largest trial by Kieft and colleagues[84] demonstrated no differences in any of the studied outcomes with immune nutrition supplementation. How does this make sense? The populations in each of the trials were not identical. The severity of illness and the admitting diagnosis were not standardized in the studies. The Bower study consisted primarily of trauma patients, whereas the Kieft study consisted primarily of postoperative patients. Also, the Kieft study did not have an even distribution of diagnoses, with heart surgery and craniotomies being more common in the control group, wheras the experimental group had more polytrauma and abdominal procedures. All studies, but the most recent trial conducted by Kieft and colleagues, showed decreases in rates of infection in the immune-supplemented group. Atkinson had the highest mortality at 45%, whereas Bower and colleagues and Kieft and colleagues had mortality rates of 11% and 33%, respectively. This finding could mean that using arginine and omega-3 fatty acids liberally in all critically ill patients may not be beneficial at all.

The effect of glutamine supplementation has also been studied in this trauma population. In a prospective cohort study by Schulman and colleagues,[85] 185 surgical and trauma ICU patients were sequentially allocated over a 3-year period to 1 of the 3 groups: standard formula, standard formula supplemented with glutamine, or an immune-enriched formula with glutamine supplementation. The groups were noted to be fairly congruent in patient characteristics, other than the group receiving immune-enriched formula that was found to have a slightly higher APACHE II score than the control group. The results showed no statistical difference in in-hospital mortality, infections, ICU length of stay, or total hospital length of stay.

Thus, immunonutrition formulations might have a benefit in certain critically ill patients. However, it appears that in sicker populations, there is no clear benefit of their use, and harm may ensue. Further study is needed to elucidate which populations are adversely affected by immunonutrition and which of the supplemented immunonutrients is the culprit. In other words, targeted clinical application of immunonutrients appears to be indicated.

Sepsis

A study conducted in 33 ICUs in Italy investigated the efficacy of an arginine-enriched enteral formula compared with total parenteral nutrition in severe sepsis.[86] It showed that in the 39 patients with severe sepsis or septic shock, the 21 patients receiving the arginine-enhanced enteral diet had a higher ICU mortality than those who received TPN (44% vs 14%, $P = .039$). This finding confirms the findings of previous studies that critically ill patients receiving these supplements did poorly. Because of this unanticipated poor outcome found on interim analysis, recruitment of patients with severe sepsis into a larger study was stopped. This adverse occurrence might be caused by the increased production of NO with arginine supplementation, which has been shown to have a harmful effect in sepsis.[87] Based on this study, combined with the results of other studies, arginine supplementation should be withheld from patients with severe sepsis.

Beal and colleagues[88] studied the efficacy of immunonutrition formulas not including arginine in a largely medical ICU patient population with sepsis in England. Patients were selected if they showed at least 2 signs of systemic inflammatory response syndrome, suspected or confirmed infection, and evidence of at least 1 organ failure. Patients were assigned randomly to 10 days of either standard enteral therapy or an immune-enriched enteral therapy containing glutamine, antioxidants, and tributyrate, a novel lipid that breaks down to butyrate. Butyrate is an important substrate for the small and large intestine and also has some antiinflammatory effects. The patients were followed for 6 months after hospital discharge. The trial was originally designed to consist of 344 patients, but was discontinued after statistically significant outcomes were noted during planned interim analysis of 50 enrolled patients. System Organ Failure Assessment (SOFA) is a standardized scale that relates descriptive organ failure scores with mortality and morbidity. The daily changes in mean SOFA scores for each group was plotted, and the slopes showed a faster decline in the immune-enriched group. The differences in regression coefficients of the slopes were statistically significant (on intention-to-treat analysis: -0.32 vs -0.14, $P<.0001$). This finding implies that formulas enriched with glutamine, butyrate, and antioxidants might have had a dramatic effect in reducing organ injury and failure in sepsis.

Acute Respiratory Distress Syndrome

A recent meta-analysis pooled the results of 3 randomized controlled trials studying the effect of omega-3 fatty acid supplementation on outcomes in patients with ARDS.[89] Among the nearly 300 patients followed, the 28-day in-hospital mortality was reduced by 60% in the groups receiving omega-3 fatty acid supplementation ($P = .001$). On intention-to-treat analysis, patients had a 49% reduction in 28-day all-cause mortality ($P = .002$). The investigators also showed significant reductions in mean 28-day ICU-free days (4.3 days, $P<.001$) and in mean 28-day ventilator-free days (4.9, $P<.0001$). They also demonstrated a trend toward improved oxygenation by treatment day 4. From data encompassing 3 clinical trials and roughly 300 patients, it appears that there is considerable evidence to suggest that omega-3 fatty acids have a benefit in treating patients with ARDS.

Meta-Analyses

Multiple meta-analyses have been conducted since 2001, pooling data from all randomized controlled trials, despite the disparate nature of their study designs. The analyses have come to similar conclusions.

In 2001, Heyland and colleagues[90] reviewed 22 randomized trials consisting of 2419 patients in whom the use of immunonutrition was compared with standard therapy. The immunonutrition mostly consisted of arginine and omega-3 fatty acid supplementation, with 2 trials investigating glutamine in ICU patients. There was no mortality benefit with immunonutrition (relative risk [RR] = 1.10, 95% confidence interval [CI]: 0.93–1.31); however, there was a significant reduction in infectious complications with immunonutrition (RR = 0.66, 95% CI: 0.54–0.80). These advantages were most marked with high-arginine supplementation compared with other formulations. Patients undergoing elective major surgery were more likely to benefit from immunonutrition than those who were critically ill, in whom there was a trend toward higher mortality, and no difference in infection rates with immunonutrition.

Avenell[91] conducted a systematic review of all glutamine supplemented trials and pooled data from 15 trials. There was a trend toward a beneficial effect with glutamine supplementation via either enteral or parenteral feeding in terms of mortality (RR = 0.81, 95% CI: 0.66–1.02). However, an overall benefit was shown in terms of reduction of infections (RR = 0.76, 95% CI: 0.64–0.90). This result was most pronounced in the postoperative patients who received glutamine intravenously as well as enteral supplementation in critically ill patients. Using a funnel plot, publication bias was suggested, implying that trials with lowered rates of infection were more likely to be published ($P = .03$). This meta-analysis demonstrates that glutamine supplementation has benefits in the postoperative patient as well as in critically ill patients, but may be dependent on route of administration.

SUMMARY

Nutrition has major effects on the immune system, which are not completely understood. Key nutrients having immunomodulatory effects, such as arginine, glutamine, and omega-3 fatty acids, demonstrated in laboratory studies, are difficult to apply and study precisely in the clinical setting. The route of delivery of these nutrients is also important. Currently, the enteral nutrition route of delivery appears to be superior to the parenteral nutrition route in terms of lower costs and possible reductions in infectious complications. Although not uniform, clinical studies tend to show reductions in infectious complications, ICU and hospital lengths of stay, and costs with immune supplementation. However, interpretation of these results is limited by the variations in study design and patient populations. Until now, immunonutrition has been treated as a supplement to nutrition. This approach may not be the best approach. These nutrients should be directed specifically like pharmacologic agents. Large-scale clinical trials will need to be conducted to identify which nutrients, in which conditions and in which relative dosages, can provide the greatest benefits in specific clinical scenarios.

Immunonutrition may prove to be the most productive and exciting controversy regarding the relationship between specific, directed nutrition regimens and major operations or trauma in the coming years.

REFERENCES

1. Dempsey D, Mullen J, Buzby G. The link between nutritional status and clinical outcome: can nutritional intervention modify it? Am J Clin Nutr 1988;47(2): 352–6.
2. Correia MI, Waitzberg DL. The impact of malnutrition on morbidity, mortality, length of hospital stay and costs evaluated through a multivariate model analysis. Clin Nutr 2003;22(3):235–9.
3. Mullen JL, Gertner MH, Buzby GP, et al. Implications of malnutrition in the surgical patient. Arch Surg 1979;114(2):121–5.
4. Lewis R, Klein H. Risk factors in postoperative sepsis: significance of preoperative lymphocytopenia. J Surg Res 1979;26(4):365–71.
5. Evoy D, Lieberman MD, Fahey TJ III, et al. Immunonutrition: the role of arginine. Nutrition 1998;14(7–8):611–7.
6. Morris SM Jr. Recent advances in arginine metabolism: roles and regulation of the arginases. Br J Pharmacol 2009;157(6):922–30.
7. Williams K. Interactions of polyamines with ion channels. Biochem J 1997; 325(Pt 2):289–97.
8. Zhang M, Caragine T, Wang H, et al. Spermine inhibits proinflammatory cytokine synthesis in human mononuclear cells: a counterregulatory mechanism that restrains the immune response. J Exp Med 1997;185(10):1759–68.
9. Tripathi P, Tripathi P, Kashyap L, et al. The role of nitric oxide in inflammatory reactions. FEMS Immunol Med Microbiol 2007;51(3):443–52.
10. Wilmore DW, Shabert JK. Role of glutamine in immunologic responses. Nutrition 1998;14(7–8):618–26.
11. Amin P. Immunonutrition: current status. Crit Care 2004;7(2):77.
12. Newsholme P. Why is L-glutamine metabolism important to cells of the immune system in health, postinjury, surgery or infection? J Nutr 2001;131(9): 2515S–22S.
13. Alexander JW. Immunonutrition: the role of [omega]-3 fatty acids. Nutrition 1998; 14(7–8):627–33.
14. Simopoulos AP. Omega-3 fatty acids in inflammation and autoimmune diseases. J Am Coll Nutr 2002;21(6):495–505.
15. Stein JA, Adler A, Efraim SB, et al. Immunocompetence, immunosuppression, and human breast cancer. I. An analysis of their relationship by known parameters of cell-mediated immunity in well-defined clinical stages of disease. Cancer 1976;38(3):1171–87.
16. Kusmartsev S, Nefedova Y, Yoder D, et al. Antigen-specific inhibition of CD8+ T cell response by immature myeloid cells in cancer is mediated by reactive oxygen species. J Immunol 2004;172(2):989–99.
17. Pinzon-Charry A, Maxwell T, Lopez JA. Dendritic cell dysfunction in cancer: a mechanism for immunosuppression. Immunol Cell Biol 2005;83(5):451–61.
18. Maeurer MJ, Martin DM, Castelli C, et al. Host immune response in renal cell cancer: interleukin-4 (IL-4) and IL-10 mRNA are frequently detected in freshly collected tumor-infiltrating lymphocytes. Cancer Immunol Immunother 1995; 41(2):111–21.
19. Woo EY, Yeh H, Chu CS, et al. Cutting edge: regulatory T cells from lung cancer patients directly inhibit autologous T cell proliferation. J Immunol 2002;168(9): 4272–6.
20. Hasenboehler E, Williams A, Leinhase I, et al. Metabolic changes after polytrauma: an imperative for early nutritional support. World J Emerg Surg 2006;1(1):29.

21. Hensler T, Hecker H, Heeg K, et al. Distinct mechanisms of immunosuppression as a consequence of major surgery. Infect Immun 1997;65(6):2283–91.
22. Kimura F, Shimizu H, Yoshidome H, et al. Immunosuppression following surgical and traumatic injury. Surg Today 2010;40(9):793–808.
23. Bisgaard T, Kehlet H. Early oral feeding after elective abdominal surgery–what are the issues? Nutrition 2002;18(11–12):944–8.
24. Lewis SJ, Egger M, Sylvester PA, et al. Early enteral feeding versus "nil by mouth" after gastrointestinal surgery: systematic review and meta-analysis of controlled trials. BMJ 2001;323(7316):773.
25. Jacobs DG, Jacobs DO, Kudsk KA, et al. Practice management guidelines for nutritional support of the trauma patient. J Trauma 2004;57(3):660.
26. Braga M, Ljungqvist O, Soeters P, et al. ESPEN guidelines on parenteral nutrition: surgery. Clin Nutr 2009;28(4):378–86.
27. Bankhead R, Boullata J, Brantley S, et al. Enteral nutrition practice recommendations. JPEN J Parenter Enteral Nutr 2009;33(2):122–67.
28. Carr CS, Ling KD, Boulos P, et al. Randomised trial of safety and efficacy of immediate postoperative enteral feeding in patients undergoing gastrointestinal resection. BMJ 1996;312(7035):869–71.
29. Ryan JA Jr, Page CP, Babcock L. Early postoperative jejunal feeding of elemental diet in gastrointestinal surgery. Am Surg 1981;47(9):393.
30. Sagar S, Harland P, Shields R. Early postoperative feeding with elemental diet. Br Med J 1979;1(6159):293.
31. Schroeder D, Gillanders L, Mahr K, et al. Effects of immediate postoperative enteral nutrition on body composition, muscle function, and wound healing. JPEN J Parenter Enteral Nutr 1991;15(4):376.
32. Singh G, Ram RP, Khanna SK. Early postoperative enteral feeding in patients with nontraumatic intestinal perforation and peritonitis. J Am Coll Surg 1998;187(2):142–6.
33. Smith RC, Hartemink RJ, Hollinshead JW, et al. Fine bore jejunostomy feeding following major abdominal surgery: a controlled randomized clinical trial. Br J Surg 1985;72(6):458–61.
34. Beier-Holgersen R, Boesby S. Influence of postoperative enteral nutrition on postsurgical infections. Gut 1996;39(6):833.
35. Heslin MJ, Latkany L, Leung D, et al. A prospective, randomized trial of early enteral feeding after resection of upper gastrointestinal malignancy. Ann Surg 1997;226(4):567.
36. Watters JM, Kirkpatrick SM, Norris SB, et al. Immediate postoperative enteral feeding results in impaired respiratory mechanics and decreased mobility. Ann Surg 1997;226(3):369.
37. Heyland DK, MacDonald S, Keefe L, et al. Total parenteral nutrition in the critically ill patient: a meta-analysis. JAMA 1998;280(23):2013–9.
38. Bozzetti F, Braga M, Gianotti L, et al. Postoperative enteral versus parenteral nutrition in malnourished patients with gastrointestinal cancer: a randomised multicentre trial. Lancet 2001;358(9292):1487–92.
39. Pacelli F, Bossola M, Papa V, et al. Postoperative enteral versus parenteral nutrition. Lancet 2002;359(9318):1697–8.
40. Koretz RL, Lipman TO, Klein S. AGA technical review on parenteral nutrition. Gastroenterology 2001;121(4):970.
41. Simpson F, Doig GS. Parenteral vs. enteral nutrition in the critically ill patient: a meta-analysis of trials using the intention to treat principle. Intensive Care Med 2004;31(1):12–23.

42. Braga M, Gianotti L, Gentilini O, et al. Early postoperative enteral nutrition improves gut oxygenation and reduces costs compared with total parenteral nutrition. Crit Care Med 2001;29(2):242.
43. Zaloga GP. Parenteral nutrition in adult inpatients with functioning gastrointestinal tracts: assessment of outcomes. Lancet 2006;367(9516):1101–11.
44. Marik PE. Maximizing efficacy from parenteral nutrition in critical care: appropriate patient populations, supplemental parenteral nutrition, glucose control, parenteral glutamine, and alternative fat sources. Curr Gastroenterol Rep 2007; 9(4):345–53.
45. Moore EE, Jones TN. Benefits of immediate jejunostomy feeding after major abdominal trauma-a prospective, randomized study. J Trauma 1986;26(10):874.
46. Moore FA, Feliciano DV, Andrassy RJ, et al. Early enteral feeding, compared with parenteral, reduces postoperative septic complications. The results of a meta-analysis. Ann Surg 1992;216(2):172–83.
47. Alexander JW, MacMillan BG, Stinnett JD, et al. Beneficial effects of aggressive protein feeding in severely burned children. Ann Surg 1980;192(4):505.
48. Kudsk KA, Li J, Renegar KB. Loss of upper respiratory tract immunity with parenteral feeding. Ann Surg 1996;223(6):629.
49. King BK, Li J, Kudsk KA. A temporal study of TPN-induced changes in gut-associated lymphoid tissue and mucosal immunity. Arch Surg 1997;132(12): 1303–9.
50. Wu Y, Kudsk KA, DeWitt RC, et al. Route and type of nutrition influence IgA-mediating intestinal cytokines. Ann Surg 1999;229(5):662.
51. Janu P, Li J, Renegar KB, et al. Recovery of gut-associated lymphoid tissue and upper respiratory tract immunity after parenteral nutrition. Ann Surg 1997;225(6):707.
52. Yang H, Kiristioglu I, Fan Y, et al. Interferon-gamma expression by intraepithelial lymphocytes results in a loss of epithelial barrier function in a mouse model of total parenteral nutrition. Ann Surg 2002;236(2):226–34.
53. Wildhaber BE, Lynn KN, Yang H, et al. Total parenteral nutrition-induced apoptosis in mouse intestinal epithelium: regulation by the Bcl-2 protein family. Pediatr Surg Int 2002;18(7):570–5.
54. Buchman AL, Moukarzel AA, Bhuta S, et al. Parenteral nutrition is associated with intestinal morphologic and functional changes in humans. JPEN J Parenter Enteral Nutr 1995;19(6):453.
55. Guedon C, Schmitz J, Lerebours E, et al. Decreased brush border hydrolase activities without gross morphologic changes in human intestinal mucosa after prolonged total parenteral nutrition of adults. Gastroenterology 1986;90(2):373.
56. Deitch EA, Xu D, Naruhn MB, et al. Elemental diet and IV-TPN-induced bacterial translocation is associated with loss of intestinal mucosal barrier function against bacteria. Ann Surg 1995;221(3):299–307.
57. Shou J, Lappin J, Minnard EA, et al. Total parenteral nutrition, bacterial translocation, and host immune function. Am J Surg 1994;167(1):145–50.
58. Spaeth G, Gottwald T, Specian RD, et al. Secretory immunoglobulin A, intestinal mucin, and mucosal permeability in nutritionally induced bacterial translocation in rats. Ann Surg 1994;220(6):798.
59. Sedman PC, Macfie J, Sagar P, et al. The prevalence of gut translocation in humans. Gastroenterology 1994;107(3):643–9.
60. Jeejeebhoy KN. Total parenteral nutrition: potion or poison? Am J Clin Nutr 2001; 74(2):160–3.
61. Lipman TO. Grains or veins: is enteral nutrition really better than parenteral nutrition? A look at the evidence. JPEN J Parenter Enteral Nutr 1998;22(3):167–82.

62. Van den Berghe G, Wouters P, Weekers F, et al. Intensive insulin therapy in critically ill patients. N Engl J Med 2001;345(19):1359.
63. Kumar PR, Crotty P, Raman M. Hyperglycemia in hospitalized patients receiving parental nutrition is associated with increased morbidity and mortality: a review. Gastroenterol Res Pract 2011;2011. pii:760720.
64. Daly JM, Lieberman MD, Goldfine J, et al. Enteral nutrition with supplemental arginine, RNA, and omega-3 fatty acids in patients after operation: immunologic, metabolic, and clinical outcome. Surgery 1992;112(1):56–67.
65. Braga M, Vignali A, Gianotti L, et al. Immune and nutritional effects of early enteral nutrition after major abdominal operations. Eur J Surg 1996;162(2):105–12.
66. Senkal M, Zumtobel V, Bauer K, et al. Outcome and cost-effectiveness of perioperative enteral immunonutrition in patients undergoing elective upper gastrointestinal tract surgery: a prospective randomized study. Arch Surg 1999; 134(12):1309–16.
67. Schilling J, Vranjes N, Fierz W, et al. Clinical outcome and immunology of postoperative arginine, [omega]-3 fatty acids, and nucleotide-enriched enteral feeding: a randomized prospective comparison with standard enteral and low calorie/low fat IV solutions. Nutrition 1996;12(6):423–9.
68. de Luis DA, Izaola O, Cuellar L, et al. Clinical and biochemical outcomes after a randomized trial with a high dose of enteral arginine formula in postsurgical head and neck cancer patients. Eur J Clin Nutr 2006;61(2):200–4.
69. Riso S, Aluffi P, Brugnani M, et al. Postoperative enteral immunonutrition in head and neck cancer patients. Clin Nutr 2000;19(6):407–12.
70. Mertes N, Schulzki C, Goeters C, et al. Cost containment through L-alanyl-L-glutamine supplemented total parenteral nutrition after major abdominal surgery: a prospective randomized double-blind controlled study. Clin Nutr 2000;19(6): 395–401.
71. Jian ZM, Cao JD, Zhu XG, et al. The impact of alanyl-glutamine on clinical safety, nitrogen balance, intestinal permeability, and clinical outcome in postoperative patients: a randomized, double-blind, controlled study of 120 patients. JPEN J Parenter Enteral Nutr 1999;23(Suppl 5):S62–6.
72. Braga M, Gianotti L, Radaelli G, et al. Perioperative immunonutrition in patients undergoing cancer surgery: results of a randomized double-blind phase 3 trial. Arch Surg 1999;134(4):428–33.
73. Braga M, Gianotti L. Preoperative immunonutrition: cost-benefit analysis. JPEN J Parenter Enteral Nutr 2005;29(Suppl 1):S57–61.
74. Moore FA, Moore EE. The evolving rationale for early enteral nutrition based on paradigms of multiple organ failure: a personal journey. Nutr Clin Pract 2009; 24(3):297–304.
75. Mendez C, Jurkovich GJ, Garcia I, et al. Effects of an immune-enhancing diet in critically injured patients. J Trauma 1997;42(5):933–40 [discussion: 940–1].
76. Brown RO, Hunt H, Mowatt-Larssen CA, et al. Comparison of specialized and standard enteral formulas in trauma patients. Pharmacotherapy 1994;14(3): 314–20.
77. Kudsk KA, Minard G, Croce MA, et al. A randomized trial of isonitrogenous enteral diets after severe trauma. An immune-enhancing diet reduces septic complications. Ann Surg 1996;224(4):531–43.
78. Weimann A, Bastian L, Bischoff WE, et al. Influence of arginine, omega-3 fatty acids and nucleotide-supplemented enteral support on systemic inflammatory response syndrome and multiple organ failure in patients after severe trauma. Nutrition 1998;14(2):165–72.

79. Moore FA, Moore EE, Kudsk KA, et al. Clinical benefits of an immune-enhancing diet for early postinjury enteral feeding. J Trauma 1994;37(4):607–15.
80. Houdijk AP, Rijnsburger ER, Jansen J, et al. Randomised trial of glutamine-enriched enteral nutrition on infectious morbidity in patients with multiple trauma. Lancet 1998;352(9130):772–6.
81. Bower RH, Cerra FB, Bershadsky B, et al. Early enteral administration of a formula (Impact) supplemented with arginine, nucleotides, and fish oil in intensive care unit patients: results of a multicenter, prospective, randomized, clinical trial. Crit Care Med 1995;23(3):436–49.
82. Galbán C, Montejo JC, Mesejo A, et al. An immune-enhancing enteral diet reduces mortality rate and episodes of bacteremia in septic intensive care unit patients. Crit Care Med 2000;28(3):643–8.
83. Atkinson S, Sieffert E, Bihari D. A prospective, randomized, double-blind, controlled clinical trial of enteral immunonutrition in the critically ill. Guy's Hospital Intensive Care Group. Crit Care Med 1998;26(7):1164–72.
84. Kieft H, Roos AN, Drunen JDE, et al. Clinical outcome of immunonutrition in a heterogeneous intensive care population. Intensive Care Med 2005;31(4): 524–32.
85. Schulman AS, Willcutts KF, Claridge JA, et al. Does the addition of glutamine to enteral feeds affect patient mortality?*. Crit Care Med 2005;33(11):2501–6.
86. Bertolini G, Iapichino G, Radrizzani D, et al. Early enteral immunonutrition in patients with severe sepsis: results of an interim analysis of a randomized multi-centre clinical trial. Intensive Care Med 2003;29(5):834–40.
87. Heyland DK, Samis A. Does immunonutrition in patients with sepsis do more harm than good? Intensive Care Med 2003;29:669–71.
88. Beale RJ, Sherry T, Lei K, et al. Early enteral supplementation with key pharma-conutrients improves sequential organ failure assessment score in critically ill patients with sepsis: outcome of a randomized, controlled, double-blind trial*. Crit Care Med 2008;36(1):131–44.
89. Pontes-Arruda A, Demichele S, Seth A, et al. The use of an inflammation-modulating diet in patients with acute lung injury or acute respiratory distress syndrome: a meta-analysis of outcome data. JPEN J Parenter Enteral Nutr 2008;32(6):596–605.
90. Heyland DK, Novak F, Drover JW, et al. Should immunonutrition become routine in critically ill patients? A systematic review of the evidence. JAMA 2001;286(8): 944–53.
91. Avenell A. Glutamine in critical care: current evidence from systematic reviews. Proc Nutr Soc 2006;65(3):236–41.

Nutrition and Gut Immunity

Kazuhiko Fukatsu, MD, PhD[a], Kenneth A. Kudsk, MD[b,c],*

KEYWORDS

- Phospholipase A2 • Gut-associated lymphoid tissue
- Immunoglobulin A • Glutamine • Mucosal immunity
- Enteral nutrition • Parenteral nutrition

The human intestine contains huge amounts of nonpathologic bacteria surviving in an environment that is beneficial to both the host and the bacterial populations. In the normal healthy individual, adequate nutrient intake and a normal environment provide a nonthreatening environment for the bacteria that live in a symbiotic relationship in very close proximity to the intestinal mucosa. Several barriers effectively keep the bacteria from entry into the systemic circulation. These barriers include mucus produced as a result of goblet cell secretion as well as the presence of microbicidal and antiviral agents such as α-defensins, cryptdins, lysozymes, and secretory phospholipase A2 ($sPLA_2$). These barriers work together with the adaptive immune system that produces secretory IgA (sIgA), which provides a specific immune defense against the intraluminal bacteria. Although minor alterations in this symbiotic relationship may occur during minor stress, when short pauses in oral intake occur with minimal alterations in the mucosa-microbial interface, critical illness, with its attendant acidosis, prolonged gastrointestinal tract starvation, exogenous antibiotics, and breakdown in mucosal defenses, renders the host vulnerable to bacterial challenge and also threatens the survival of the bacteria. Under these conditions, the bacteria face weakened host defenses while attempting to survive, rendering them hostile to the host. This review examines the altered innate and adaptive immunologic host defenses that occur as a result of altered oral or enteral intake and/or injury.

[a] Department of Surgery, Surgical Center, The University of Tokyo Hospital, 7-3-1 Hongo, Bunkyo-Ku, Tokyo 1138655, Japan
[b] Veterans Administration Surgical Services, William S. Middleton Memorial Veterans Hospital, Madison, WI, USA
[c] Department of Surgery, University of Wisconsin School of Medicine and Public Health, 600 Highland Avenue, G5/341, Madison, WI 53792, USA
* Corresponding author. Department of Surgery, University of Wisconsin School of Medicine and Public Health, 600 Highland Avenue, G5/341, Madison, WI 53792.
E-mail address: kudsk@surgery.wisc.edu

Surg Clin N Am 91 (2011) 755–770
doi:10.1016/j.suc.2011.04.007
0039-6109/11/$ – see front matter © 2011 Elsevier Inc. All rights reserved.

surgical.theclinics.com

INTACT DEFENSES UNDER NORMAL CONDITIONS
Physical Barriers

A first line of defense against bacteria is the physical barrier, which separates the bacteria from the systemic circulation. The intestinal epithelium consists of a single layer of columnar cells starting at the gastroesophageal junction and extending to the squamous epithelium of the anal canal. This physical barrier is selectively permeable and capable of preventing transmigration of pathologic luminal substances from the external environment, that is, the lumen, to the internal environment. The mucosal cells are closely bound to one another with filaments at both the basal and apical portions of the cell to maintain normal polarity and tight junctions. Cell turnover occurs in an orderly manner approximately every 5 to 7 days under the control of various factors, including epidermal growth factor, intestinal trefoil factor, and so forth. The mucosa is covered by microproteins in the form of mucin, which coats its surface to create a physical barrier to the bacteria. The mucin contains high concentrations of defensins and other antibacterial molecules such as lactoferrin, lysozymes, and sPLA$_2$.[1] sPLA$_2$ destroys the integrity of the bacterial cell wall, whereas lactoferrin impairs the ability of bacteria to adhere to epithelial cells.[1,2] Under conditions of severe stress and with alterations in normal oral intake, reductions in the mucin layer, impairment of the antimicrobial peptides in the mucin layer, and increased mucosal permeability to weaken this intrinsic defense and render it vulnerable to bacterial invasion occur.

Acquired Immunity

The mucosal immune system constitutes approximately 50% to 60% of the body's total immunity, producing about 7% of the antibody made by the body.[3] This system produces specific antibodies against intraluminal bacteria antibody in the form of sIgA, which does not function through inflammation but rather through adhesion and bacterial exclusion. Under normal conditions, antigen is sampled from the lumen after entry through specialized microvilli cells, which cover the Peyer patches (**Fig. 1**). Dendritic cells within the Peyer patches process the antigens and sensitize naive T and B cells to these antigens.[4] The sensitized T and B cells then migrate to the mesenteric lymph nodes to mature and/or proliferate before their release into the thoracic duct. There these cells enter the systemic circulation to be distributed to submucosal sites in the upper and lower respiratory tracts as well as the small and large intestines. In these sites, the influence of helper T cell subtype 2 (T$_H$2) cytokines, such as interleukin (IL) 4, IL-5, IL-6, IL-10, and probably others, stimulate antibody production and transform the B cells into plasma cells capable of producing IgM and IgA for transport across the mucosa via a specialized transport mechanism.[5] After release of dimeric IgA from the plasma cells, the IgA binds to molecules of polyimmune globulin receptor (pIgR) located on the basal surfaces of the mucosal cell. The mucosal cell transports this pIgR-IgA complex to the luminal surface where the IgA is released into the lumen.[6,7] A small segment of pIgR (secretory component) remains attached to the IgA, identifying it as sIgA. Within the lumen, sIgA does not activate the complement system but functions by binding to bacterial surface antigens to prevent or inhibit attachment of the bacteria to the mucosa. Preventing attachment precludes invasion by the bacteria. In both experimental and clinical works, alterations in diet and injury dramatically affect this coordinated system of acquired immunity in the respiratory and gastrointestinal tracts.

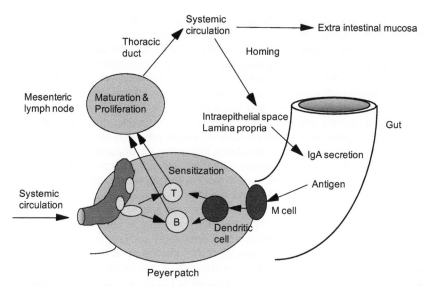

Fig. 1. Gut-associated lymphoid tissue (GALT) and systemic mucosal immunity. GALT is a center of systemic mucosal immunity. Naive lymphocytes are sensitized at Peyer patches, migrate to mesenteric lymph nodes, enter into systemic circulation via thoracic duct, and home to mucosal sites.

THE CLINICAL CORRELATES

In the 1960s and 1970s, a rapid growth in the use of parenteral nutrition occurred because it provided clinicians an avenue and method to provide adequate amounts of protein, carbohydrate, fat, electrolytes, trace elements, and so forth to patients who otherwise starved because of loss of gut function. In the late 1970s, experimental work suggested that benefits were gained when nutrients were delivered via the gastrointestinal tract, which did not occur with intravenous feeding exclusively, when the gut was completely bypassed.[8,9] Clinically, early studies of trauma patients noted that patients randomized either to starvation or to parenteral feeding had significant increases in rates of pneumonia and intra-abdominal abscess compared with patients who were fed directly into the intestine via jejunostomy.[10–12] Subsequent studies on diverse patient populations confirmed this clinical effect. Several hypotheses, including the gut origin sepsis theory and the common mucosal immune hypothesis, have provided experimental data, which provide cogent explanations for how enteral feeding maintains normal gut barrier function.

MUCOSAL IMMUNE CHANGES WITH SPECIALIZED NUTRITION SUPPORT

The common mucosal immune hypothesis provides a framework for mucosal immune maintenance, repopulation, and function. Specifically, T and B cells, "educated" or sensitized at a specific mucosal site are distributed to other mucosal sites, providing protection throughout the entire mucosal immune system.[13] This process occurs through a coordinated system of sensitization and distribution dependent on cytokines, chemokines, adhesion molecules, and ligands to those adhesion molecules.

Approximately 80% of circulating human and murine lymphocytes express $\alpha_4\beta_7$ and L-selectin, 2 molecules that identify these cells as destined for the mucosal immune system.[14] As a result of eating, increased gastrointestinal tract blood flow stimulated by the dietary intake carries the naive $\alpha_4\beta_7{}^+$ L-selectin$^+$ cells to their sites of sensitization, the Peyer patches. In both the lamina propria and Peyer patches, cells express mucosal addressin adhesion molecule 1 (MAdCAM-1), a molecule that interacts with $\alpha_4\beta_7$ and L-selectin. In the Peyer patches, MAdCAM-1 expressed in a modified form on the high endothelial venules interacts vigorously with the cells expressing L-selectin, the predominating adhesion molecule expressed on naive T and B cells.[15] After attachment, chemokines cause arrest and diapedesis of the T and B cells into the Peyer patches. Chemokines are very small, soluble, tissue-specific proteins that activate cell signaling systems and increase integrin–cellular adhesion molecule binding.[16,17] Overall, chemokines stimulate chemotaxis. Within the Peyer patches, the chemokine CCL21 regulates T cell entry, whereas CXCL13 regulates B cell entry. Both chemokines play important roles in cell migration into the Peyer patches, where the naive T and B cells become sensitized to antigens processed by the dendritic cells. This sensitization alters the cell surface molecule expression, which reduces expression of L-selectin but increases expression of $\alpha_4\beta_7$. This alteration renders the cells more attractive to unmodified MAdCAM-1, which attracts the sensitized T and B cells to sites of function within the submucosa in the lamina propria of the intestine as well as the lung and nasal passages. The B cells, under the influence of the sensitized T cells, switch into a plasma cell. The sensitized T cells release IgA-stimulating T_H2 cytokines, which stimulate IgA production for eventual transport by pIgR into the lumen.[18]

This entire process seems integrated with stimulation of the gastrointestinal tract during enteral feeding.[19] The gateway molecule for naive B and T cells is MAdCAM-1, expressed on the high endothelial venules of the Peyer patches.[15] The administration of parenteral feeding (which relatively starves the gastrointestinal tract but prevents malnutrition of the animals) results in a rapid downregulation of MAdCAM-1 expression to approximately 50% of normal levels and obstructs entry of naive B and T cells into the mucosal immune system (**Fig. 2**).[20] The role of MAdCAM-1 in this process is clearly demonstrated by administration of a blocking anti-MAdCAM antibody; blockade of MAdCAM-1 reproduces the effect of parenteral feeding.[21] The proportion of T and B cells within the Peyer patches remains unchanged, but total cell numbers are reduced to approximately 40% to 50% of the normal by 3 days. Simultaneously, cell levels decrease in both the lung and intestinal lamina propria. MAdCAM-1 expression is stimulated by normal levels of IL-4 and stimulation of lymphotoxin β receptor (LTβR) through interaction with activated T cells.[22,23] Absence of enteral stimulation results in a significant decrease in LTβR levels in the Peyer patches. Without activation of LTβR, levels of both MAdCAM-1 and IL-4 decrease because of impaired intracellular nuclear factor κB (NF-κB) activation.

In addition to the MAdCAM-1–related lymphocyte-homing mechanism, gut immunity is controlled by mitogen-activated protein kinase pathways, which play significant roles in mediating signals triggered by cytokines, growth factors, and environmental stress and are involved in cell proliferation, cell differentiation, and cell death. Gut starvation blunts extracellular-regulated kinase (ERK) phosphorylation in effector sites of gut immunity, that is, lamina propria and intraepithelial lymphocytes, in response to phorbol 12-myristate 13-acetate (PMA) in vitro stimulation, whereas increased phosphorylation with PMA is observed in enteral feeding groups.[24] In association with this change, lamina propria cell proliferation with PMA is reduced after parenteral feeding.

Within the lamina propria, significant changes occur in both IgA production and transport when the gut is starved. The lack of enteral feeding reduces levels of T regulatory cells, resulting in significant reductions in IL-4 and IL-10 levels, 2 important IgA-stimulating cytokines necessary for IgA production.[18] Gut starvation also impairs IgA

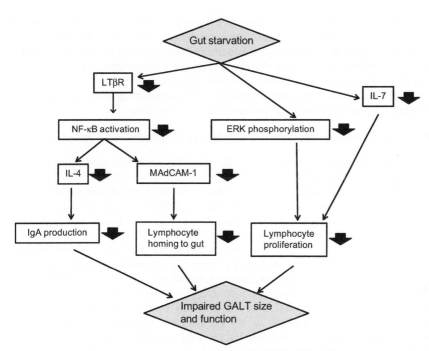

Fig. 2. Mechanisms underlying impaired immunity during gut starvation. Impairment of gut immunity as a result of gut starvation is related to reduced lymphotoxin β receptor (LTβR) expression, extracellular-regulated kinase (ERK) phosphorylation, IL-7 production, and other factors. GALT, gut-associated lymphoid tissue; NF-κB, nuclear factor κB.

transport mechanisms through inhibition of the JAK-STAT signaling system, which maintains normal levels of pIgR. The combination of these changes results in impaired intestinal IgA production, reduced transport of IgA into the lumen, and impairment of this defense mechanism. Surprisingly, lung pIgR levels are not affected during gut starvation and remain capable of transporting IgA produced by the underlying T and B cells.[25] However, lung mechanisms are not completely intact because gut starvation reduces the absolute number of T and B cells within the lung, thus impairing mucosal immune function.

These changes impair both antiviral and antibacterial defenses. Experimentally, murine defense against the H1N1 virus in the APR-8 mouse resides within IgA-mediated immunity.[26] If the H1N1 virus is administered intranasally to naive mice, the mice continue to shed virus from their nasal passages for 9 to 10 days until generation of adequate levels of IgA eliminate the infection. Immune mice then rapidly clear any subsequent doses of virus and sterilize the nasal passages if immunity remains intact. Animals fed via the gastrointestinal tract maintain this immunity; however, animals fed parenterally lose this established immunity if challenged a second time with the virus.[27] This impairment is functional and not because of loss of immunologic memory because 2 days of enteral feeding completely restores antiviral immunity. A similar observation has been made in antibacterial defense against *Pseudomonas* in a murine pneumonia model.[28] Prior immunization with *Pseudomonas* antigen administered in liposomes reduces a 90% lethal model of intratracheal *Pseudomonas* to 10% mortality in enterally fed mice. However, the challenge is lethal to immunized animals fed parenterally for 5 days.

Gut starvation also impairs the ability of animals to generate new immunity, a condition analogous to critically ill patients exposed to new bacterial challenge in intensive care units.[29] Normally, immunocytes specifically programmed to produce anti-H1N1 antibody begin to appear 6 days after naive mice are initially exposed to the virus. Antiviral cell numbers peak around day 13. If the gut is starved during this time while the animals are fed parenterally, this process of cell programming and proliferation does not occur, and animals fail to generate immunity to the virus.

THE EFFECT OF ROUTE AND TYPE OF NUTRITION ON INNATE IMMUNE DEFENSE

Unlike adaptive immunity, innate immunity recognizes and responds to organisms in a nonspecific system of defense. Paneth cells located at the base of crypts in the intestinal mucosa produce and release granules containing antimicrobial proteins and peptides into the lumen. These peptides, which include lysozymes, $sPLA_2$, and defensins, are conserved components of innate immune responses found at all evolutionary levels of plants and animals. For example, $sPLA_2$ is an enzyme that is expressed in many cell types and in various body fluids. $sPLA_2$ functions as a proinflammatory enzyme in tissues to activate neutrophils within the circulatory system, but it serves an antibacterial function within the lumen of the intestine by binding to the bacterial cell wall and killing the microbe via phospholipolytic enzyme activity.[1] Gut starvation during parenteral nutrition influences the innate system, resulting in significant decreases in the levels of $sPLA_2$ within the intestinal secretions. The $sPLA_2$ that is present in parenterally fed mice is less bactericidal than $sPLA_2$ obtained from enterally fed mice at equal molar concentrations.

THE EFFECTS OF NUTRITION ON RESPONSE TO INJURY

Critically ill patients requiring nutrition support have sustained injury whether it is trauma related or related to the stress and injury of surgery. Experimentally, the route of nutrition affects the inflammatory response generated by both the innate and adaptive immunities.

Effects of Injury on Systemic Inflammation

Disproportionate splanchnic hypoperfusion, a common feature of shock and trauma, is considered to be an important factor in multiple organ failure (MOF). Gut hypoxia directly injures gut morphologic structure, rendering gut barrier function compromised and allowing translocation of bacteria and toxins in gut lumen.

Alterations in cytokines caused by gut starvation affect both the mucosal immune system and systemic inflammatory responses. The lamina propria contains large numbers of blood vessels, which respond to the changes in cytokines and alter endothelial adhesion molecule expression.[30] As discussed earlier, IL-4 and IL-10 levels decrease in the lamina propria during gut starvation and parenteral feeding; no changes occur in the helper T cell subtype 1 (T_H1) cytokine, interferon-γ (IFN-γ).[11,31] These 3 cytokines influence expression of vascular endothelial molecules. Normal levels of IL-4 and IL-10 suppress expression of intracellular adhesion molecule 1 (ICAM-1), a molecule that attracts neutrophils to the vascular endothelium, leading to their attachment.[30] IFN-γ, however, stimulates expression of ICAM-1. Normally, the opposing influences of the T_H1 and T_H2 cytokines maintain homeostasis and controlled activation of neutrophils. However, because gut starvation reduces IL-4 and II-10 levels, endothelial ICAM-1 expression increases within the small intestine and neutrophils accumulate in the tissues. This occurrence is significant because the gut is capable of priming neutrophils to subsequent injury.[32] This priming occurs through interaction between tissue priming signals, such as sPLA$_2$ and the accumulated neutrophils, which then are released from the gut and distributed to other sites, such as the lung and liver. In these sites, the primed neutrophils generate an exaggerated inflammatory response to subsequent injury. Gut starvation with parenteral nutrition increases ICAM-1 levels, and neutrophils accumulate within the small intestine and are primed. The priming of neutrophils is evident because relatively short episodes of gut ischemia and reperfusion produce an intense inflammatory response in the lung and liver in association with increased expression of CD11B and CD18 on circulating and tissue-bound cells, respectively.[32] The ultimate result is an increase in the mortality rate of parenterally fed mice after gut ischemia and reperfusion with increases in both permeability and edema of the liver and lung.[33] A kinetic study of gut immunity after severe gut ischemia/reperfusion in mice clarified an important mechanism for poor outcome after injury. Gut ischemia/reperfusion caused rapid and prolonged reduction of gut-associated lymphoid tissue (GALT) cell lymphocytes, particularly in intraepithelial space and lamina propria. The administration of an oral intake of diet after gut ischemia/reperfusion, normally a potent stimulant for gut immunity recovery, resulted in marked GALT atrophy as long as day 7 after injury.

The relevance of this augmented response to critically injured patients is just now becoming evident. Studies of trauma patients undergoing bronchoalveolar lavage (BAL) show acute increases in airway IgA along with the increased levels of tumor necrosis factor (TNF) α, IL-1β, and IL-6 within BAL specimens.[34,35] A similar response occurs in the airways of mice 8 hours after a controlled surgical injury; IgA levels increase in concert with elevated TNF-α, IL-1β, and IL-6 levels in BAL specimens. Clearly, these cytokines are involved because administration of anti-TNF or anti–IL-1β monoclonal antibodies eliminates the airway IgA response in the mice.[36] This IgA response to injury is also eliminated after gut starvation and parenteral nutrition.

Effects of Diet on Innate Immune Responses to Injury

sPLA$_2$ seems to be the factor that primes neutrophils after their attachment to the gut wall during hemorrhagic shock or parenteral nutrition. sPLA$_2$ activity within the lumen is bactericidal. sPLA$_2$ is a family of lipolytic enzymes that hydrolyze phospholipids to release long-chain fatty acids from bacterial membranes. In vitro, sPLA$_2$-IIa kills gram-positive and some gram-negative bacterial species[37–40]; over expression of sPLA$_2$-IIa in transgenic mice reduces their susceptibility to sepsis during bacterial challenge.[41] Parenteral nutrition with gut starvation reduces the activity of sPLA$_2$ in intestinal fluid. This reduction is associated with an impaired bactericidal activity as a result of reduced absolute amounts of sPLA$_2$ in the fluid as well as production of a less active form of the enzyme. Surprisingly, injury reduces levels of sPLA$_2$ to levels comparable to parenterally fed animals, which may be a protective mechanism because high levels of luminal sPLA$_2$ can attack not only the bacteria but also the mucosa in the presence of increased mucosal permeability. However, levels of intestinal IgA increased in enterally fed animals in response to the injury, which may serve to neutralize bacteria within the lumen. Gut starvation with parenteral feeding does not increase intestinal (or lung) IgA, denoting a failure in both innate and acquired mucosal immunities.[42]

EXOGENOUS SUPPORT OF DIET-RELATED IMPAIRMENT OF GUT IMMUNITY
Neuropeptides

The intestine is infiltrated with approximately 3 m of nerve for every cubic millimeter of tissue, with most on these nervous tissues located in and around the GALT (**Table 1**). These fibers release several neuropeptides, including gastrin-releasing peptide (GRP),

Table 1
Exogenous support of gut immunity during gut starvation

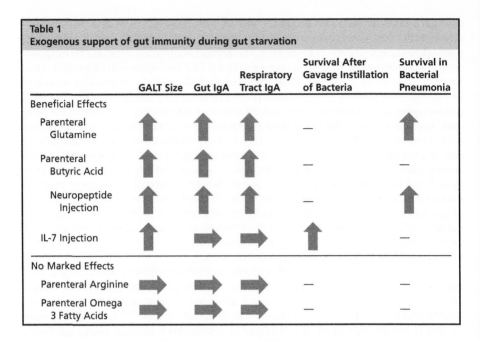

	GALT Size	Gut IgA	Respiratory Tract IgA	Survival After Gavage Instillation of Bacteria	Survival in Bacterial Pneumonia
Beneficial Effects					
Parenteral Glutamine	↑	↑	↑	—	↑
Parenteral Butyric Acid	↑	↑	↑	—	—
Neuropeptide Injection	↑	↑	↑	—	↑
IL-7 Injection	↑	→	→	↑	—
No Marked Effects					
Parenteral Arginine	→	→	→	—	—
Parenteral Omega 3 Fatty Acids	→	→	→	—	—

neurotensin, cholecystokinin, and so forth. GRP is one of the first peptides released during eating, and it stimulates the release of other neuropeptides throughout the intestine, including gastrin.[43] Experimentally, the peptide bombesin (BBS) has been used to study GRP effects because both share the same 7–amino acid sequence, which provides their function. Parenteral feeding supplemented with BBS prevents the reduced cell numbers within the Peyer patches and the lamina propria, normalizes the T_H2 cytokine levels, maintains both respiratory and intestinal IgA levels, and reverses the defect in antibacterial and antiviral defenses noted in parenterally fed mice.[43–46] BBS has no effect on MAdCAM-1 and probably works via direct cell effects. This peptide provides no protective effect after gut ischemia with reperfusion. However, BBS warrants further investigation as a tool to improve respiratory immunity in patients who are unable to be fed via the gastrointestinal tract.

Glutamine

Glutamine is the most abundant free amino acid within the body, and because it can be synthesized by the body, glutamine is not considered an essential amino acid in health. However, during prolonged severe stress, production in tissues fails to meet the systemic demands, and glutamine becomes conditionally essential. Glutamine is not a usual component of commercial amino acid components of parenteral nutrition because heat sterilization converts the molecule into pyroglutamate, a toxic substance. However, glutamine can be added to parenteral nutrition before filter sterilization. Glutamine supplementation improves mucosal immunity by increasing the number of lymphocytes in the Peyer patches and the lamina propria, partially normalizes tissue T_H2 cytokine levels, and improves respiratory and intestinal IgA levels, but not to levels maintained in chow-fed mice.[47–49] Glutamine also improves, but does not normalize, the antibacterial and antiviral defenses.[47,50] This amino acid completely reverses the increase in mortality of parenterally fed mice after gut ischemia and reperfusion.[51]

Glutamine does not work through MAdCAM-1, which remains unchanged from parenteral levels.[52] At present, several clinical studies suggest an improvement in infectious complications with glutamine-supplemented parenteral nutrition, and larger clinical trials are underway.

Butyric Acid

Dietary carbohydrates escaping digestion/absorption in the small intestine and prebiotics undergo fermentation in the colon to give rise to short-chain fatty acids (SCFAs).[53] Butyric acid, an SCFA, provides a significant source of calories, exerting trophic effects on both the small and large intestines.[54,55] Parenteral administration of butyric acid reportedly reverses parenteral nutrition–induced gut atrophy.[56] Partial replacement of acetic acid (which is added for pH adjustment to parenteral nutrition solution) by butyric acid moderately improved Peyer patch lymphocyte number and IgA levels in small intestine and bronchoalveolar washings of parenterally fed animals, but the mechanism underlying the immune changes remains unclear.[57]

IL-7

The immune processes in the GALT are mediated by various cytokine receptor pathways. IL-7 produced by intestinal epithelial cells seems particularly important because of its pleiotropic functions.[58] Epithelial cell–derived IL-7 and its receptor contribute to the development and activation of intraepithelial $\gamma\delta$ T cells and prevents spontaneous apoptosis of $\gamma\delta$ and $\alpha\beta$ intraepithelial lymphocytes by inhibiting caspase-dependent and caspase-independent pathways.[59] IL-7 also plays a role in the proliferation and function of intraepithelial, lamina propia, and Peyer patches lymphocytes.[60] Parenteral nutrition decreases intestinal epithelial cell–derived IL-7 mRNA expression, whereas exogenous IL-7 during parenteral nutrition restores lymphocyte numbers in the Peyer patches, intraepithelial space, and lamina propria but has no effect on IgA levels.[61–63] Exogenous IL-7 administration also improved survival in a gut-derived sepsis model induced by gavage administration of live *Pseudomonas*.

INFLUENCES OF CHEMOTHERAPY INSULTS ON GUT IMMUNITY

Chemotherapy-induced intestinal injury induces morphologic changes in the gastrointestinal tract while certain anticancer drugs impair gut immunity. Continuous infusion of 5-fluorouracil, a fluorinated pyrimidine, reduces GALT mass and sIgA levels in a murine model without reducing oral intake or creating other gastrointestinal symptoms.[64] Concomitant enteral infusion of fish oil as a source of omega 3 fatty acids restored intraepithelial and lamina propria lymphocyte numbers and bronchoalveolar IgA levels in control group levels, whereas fish oil added to parenteral nutrition had no beneficial effects on parenteral nutrition–induced atrophy of GALT.[65,66] Because omega 3 fatty acids reportedly have the property to enhance sensitivity of certain tumor cells to chemotherapy,[67] combination therapy using anticancer drugs and omega 3 fatty acids could provide a therapeutic tool to enhance anticancer effects and decrease infectious complications.

PERITONEAL DEFENSES

Clinical studies of trauma patients demonstrated that parenteral feeding resulted in significant increases in intra-abdominal abscess compared with enteral feeding.[10–12] Experimental work demonstrates that gut starvation affects peritoneal host defense against bacterial contamination as well as gut and respiratory mucosal immunities.

Several host defense mechanisms come into play early after bacterial contamination of the peritoneal cavity.[68] Peritonitis activates peritoneal resident macrophages to produce proinflammatory cytokines and chemokines. These macrophages phagocytize and kill bacteria, while secreted mediators stimulate massive influx of neutrophils into the peritoneal cavity. The exudative neutrophils eliminate microbes by releasing oxygen products and enzymes. In addition, diaphragmatic lymphatics clear bacteria from the peritoneal cavity. This appropriate activation of peritoneal resident and exudative leukocytes in response to peritoneal contamination seems to be essential for preventing intra-abdominal abscess.

NF-κB is a key ubiquitous transcription factor increasing gene expressions of proinflammatory cytokines, growth factors, chemokines, and adhesion molecules.[69] NF-κB resides in the cytoplasm in an inactive form as a heterodimer consisting of p50 and RelA subunits complexed to the inhibitory molecule IκB. Degradation of IκB allows NF-κB to translocate to the nucleus and bind to its specific DNA site. Work using laser scanning cytometer clarified that gut starvation inhibits NF-κB translocation in peritoneal resident macrophages and exudative neutrophils even when the animals receive sufficient nutrients parenterally (**Fig. 3**).[70,71] The blunted NF-κB activation in parenterally fed animals resulted in delayed increases in the levels of peritoneal proinflammatory and antiinflammatory cytokines as well as the levels of the chemokine macrophage inflammatory protein 2. An impaired peritoneal defense was confirmed using a cecal ligation and puncture (CLP)-induced peritonitis model to mimic clinical peritonitis caused by bacterial contamination and necrotic tissue. The absence of enteral feeding significantly reduced survival time compared with enterally feeding the animals.

Specialized parenteral formulas designed to maintain peritoneal host defense have been investigated. An arginine-enriched (1% arginine) parenteral formula restored NF-κB activation in peritoneal resident and exudative leukocytes as well as the intraperitoneal cytokine response, leading to improved survival after CLP compared with standard parenteral formulas containing 0.3% arginine.[72] An alanyl-glutamine–supplemented parenteral formula also enhanced TNF-α levels in peritoneal cavity as well as liver and splenic IFN-γ levels after intraperitoneal injection of live *Escherichia*

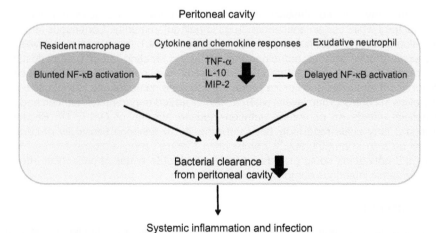

Fig. 3. Influence of gut starvation on peritoneal host defense. Gut starvation blunts NF-κB activation in peritoneal resident macrophages and exudative neutrophils, impairing peritoneal host defense against bacterial contamination. MIP-2, macrophage inflammatory protein.

coli.[73] The formula also reduced IL-8 levels and the number of bacteria isolated from systemic blood samples. This finding suggests that glutamine augments peritoneal defenses to minimize bacterial dissemination into the systemic circulation. This action does not seem to be because of normalization of NF-κB activation.

HEPATIC IMMUNITY

Parenteral nutrition induces hepatic steatosis, decreases bile flow and hepatic secretory function, and impairs albumin synthesis and drug conjugation. Gut starvation also influences hepatic immunity.

The liver plays an important role in the innate immune response, providing a first line of defense against intestinal microbes and toxins crossing the intestinal barrier. The liver contains a significant number of mononuclear cells (MNCs), including Kupffer cells, resident hepatic macrophages (which constantly clear bacteria and toxins from the peripheral circulation), resident and liver-infiltrating natural killer cells, and T and B cells.[74] When activated with bacterial endotoxin, Kupffer cells produce proinflammatory cytokines and clear pathogens by phagocytosis. Therefore, the liver plays a central role in immunity, responding to, and eliminating, pathogenic microorganisms and toxins.

Gut starvation reduces hepatic MNC number to approximately 50% of chow-fed levels.[75] Parenterally fed mice express lower levels of the lipopolysaccharide (LPS) receptors CD14 and toll-like receptor 4 on cell membrane compared with enteral feeding, leading to a lower ERK phosphorylation response to LPS stimulation. Hepatic MNCs after parenteral feeding do not increase TNF-α, IFN-γ, or IL-10 production when cultured in vitro with LPS, whereas hepatic MNCs after enteral feeding remain capable of dose-dependent increases in cytokine production following LPS. Deranged function of the hepatic MNC system during gut starvation may allow systemic dissemination of bacteria and toxins, which have crossed the gut barrier and enter the portal circulation. Parenteral feeding significantly worsens survival after injection of *Pseudomonas aeruginosa* into the portal vein.

Dietary alteration in hepatic immunity may be partly explained through changes in portal blood flow.[76,77] Twelve hours of chow feeding almost completely restores gut starvation–induced reduction in hepatic MNC numbers to normal levels in mice. Simultaneously, blood flow in the small intestine and portal vein fully recovers to normal levels. A positive correlation exists between portal vein blood flow and hepatic MNC number. Intravenous administration of prostaglandin E_1, a potent enhancer of portal vein blood flow, significantly restores hepatic MNC number during fasting, confirming that an increase in portal blood flow is important for maintenance of hepatic immunity.

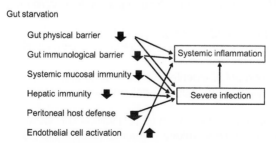

Fig. 4. Influences of gut starvation on host immunity and inflammation. Gut starvation impairs various host defense systems while causing inappropriate activation of endothelial cells.

SUMMARY

Gut starvation impairs intestinal and extraintestinal mucosal immunity via changes in mucosa-associated lymphoid tissue mass and function. Gut starvation also affects extraintestinal nonmucosal immunity, including peritoneal host defense and hepatic MNCs (**Fig. 4**). Key features of these changes are: (1) reduction of immune cells in local sites and (2) hyporesponsiveness of immune cells to stimulation. Excessive inflammatory response after severe insults has been discussed with special emphasis on mechanisms underlying tissue injury and MOF. Preventing excessive inflammation is one goal when treating severely injured and/or critically ill patients. Nutrition, particularly route and quality of nutrient delivery, affects the integrity of the entire host defense system.

ACKNOWLEDGMENTS

This research is supported by National Institute of Health (NIH) Grant R01 GM53439. This material is also based upon work supported in part by the Department of Veterans Affairs, Veterans Health Administration, Office of Research and Development, Biomedical Laboratory Research and Development Service. The contents of the article do not represent the views of the Department of Veterans Affairs or the United States Government.

REFERENCES

1. Beers SA, Buckland AG, Koduri RS, et al. The antibacterial properties of secreted phospholipase A2: a major physiological role for the group IIA enzyme that depends on the very high pI of the enzyme to allow penetration of the bacterial cell wall. J Biol Chem 2002;277:1788–93.
2. Koduri RS, Gronroos JO, Laine VJ, et al. Bactericidal properties of human and murine groups I, II, V, X, and XII secreted phospholipases A2. J Biol Chem 2002; 277:5849–57.
3. McGhee JR, Mestecky J, Dertzbaugh MT, et al. The mucosal immune system: from fundamental concepts to vaccine development. Vaccine 1992;10:75–88.
4. Guy-Grand D, Griscelli C, Vassalli P. The gut-associated lymphoid system: nature and properties of the large dividing cells. Eur J Immunol 1974;4:435–43.
5. Roux ME, McWilliams M, Phillips-Quagliata JM, et al. Differentiation pathway of Peyer's patch precursors of IgA plasma cells in the secretory immune system. Cell Immunol 1981;61:141–53.
6. Kaetzel CS. The polymeric immunoglobulin receptor: bridging innate and adaptive immune responses at mucosal surfaces. Immunol Rev 2005;206:83–99.
7. Mostov KE, Friedlander M, Blobel G. The receptor for transepithelial transport of IgA and IgM contains multiple immunoglobulin-like domains. Nature 1984;308: 37–43.
8. Kudsk KA, Carpenter BS, Peterson S, et al. Effect of enteral and parenteral feeding in malnourished rats with E. coli-hemoglobin adjuvant peritonitis. J Surg Res 1981; 31:105–10.
9. Kudsk KA, Stone JM, Carpenter BA, et al. Enteral and parenteral feeding influences mortality after hemoglobin-E. coli peritonitis in normal rats. J Trauma 1983; 23:605–9.
10. Moore FA, Moore EE, Jones TN, et al. TEN versus TPN following major abdominal trauma-reduced septic morbidity. J Trauma 1989;29:916–23.
11. Moore EE, Jones TN. Benefits of immediate jejunostomy feeding after major abdominal trauma—a prospective, randomized study. J Trauma 1986;26:874–81.

12. Kudsk KA, Croce MA, Fabian TC, et al. Enteral vs. parenteral feeding: effects on septic morbidity following blunt and penetrating abdominal trauma. Ann Surg 1992;215(5):503–13.

13. Czerkinsky C, Prince SJ, Michalek SM, et al. IgA antibody-producing cells in peripheral blood after antigen ingestion: evidence for a common mucosal immune system in humans. Proc Natl Acad Sci U S A 1987;84:2449–53.

14. Bargatze RF, Jutila MA, Butcher EC. Distinct roles of L-selectin and integrins alpha 4 beta 7 and LFA-1 in lymphocyte homing to Peyer's patch-HEV in situ: the multistep model confirmed and refined. Immunity 1995;3:99–108.

15. Sikorski EE, Hallmann R, Berg EL, et al. The Peyer's patch high endothelial receptor for lymphocytes, the mucosal vascular addressin, is induced on a murine endothelial cell line by tumor necrosis factor-α and IL-1. J Immunol 1993;151: 5239–50.

16. Campbell JJ, Hedrick J, Zlotnik A, et al. Chemokines and the arrest of lymphocytes rolling under flow conditions. Science 1998;279:381–4.

17. Laudanna C, Kim JY, Constantin G, et al. Rapid leukocyte integrin activation by chemokines. Immunol Rev 2002;186:37–46.

18. Wu Y, Kudsk KA, DeWitt RC, et al. Route and type of nutrition influence IgA-mediated intestinal cytokines. Ann Surg 1999;229:662–8.

19. Kudsk KA. Jonathan E Rhoads lecture: of mice and men… and a few hundred rats. JPEN J Parenter Enteral Nutr 2008;32(4):460–73.

20. Zarzaur BL, Fukatsu K, Johnson CJ, et al. A temporal study of diet-induced changes in Peyer patch MAdCAM-1 expression. Surg Forum 2001;52:194–6.

21. Ikeda S, Kudsk KA, Fukatsu K, et al. Enteral feeding preserves mucosal immunity despite in vivo MAdCAM-1 blockage of lymphocyte homing. Ann Surg 2003; 237(5):677–85.

22. Kang W, Gomez EF, Lan J, et al. Parenteral nutrition (PN) impairs gut-associated lymphoid tissue (GALT) and mucosal immunity by reducing lymphotoxin β receptor (LTβR) expression. Ann Surg 2006;244(3):392–9.

23. Kang W, Kudsk KA, Sano Y, et al. Effects of lymphotoxin β receptor blockade on intestinal mucosal immunity. JPEN J Parenter Enteral Nutr 2007;31(5):358–65.

24. Maeshima Y, Fukatsu K, Kang W, et al. Lack of enteral nutrition blunts extracellular regulated kinase phosphorylation in gut-associated lymphoid tissue. Shock 2007;27(3):320–5.

25. Kudsk KA, Gomez FE, Kang W, et al. Enteral feeding of a chemically-defined diet preserves pulmonary immunity but not intestinal immunity: the role of lymphotoxin beta receptor (LTβR). JPEN J Parenter Enteral Nutr 2007;31(6): 477–81.

26. Renegar KB, Johnson C, DeWitt RC, et al. Impairment of mucosal immunity by total parenteral nutrition (TPN): requirement for IgA in murine nasotracheal anti-influenza immunity. J Immunol 2001;166:819–25.

27. Kudsk KA, Li J, Renegar KB. Loss of upper respiratory tract immunity with parenteral feeding. Ann Surg 1996;223(6):629–38.

28. King BK, Kudsk KA, Li J, et al. Route and type of nutrition influence mucosal immunity to bacterial pneumonia. Ann Surg 1999;229(2):272–8.

29. Johnson CD, Kudsk KA, Fukatsu K, et al. Route of nutrition influences generation of antibody-forming cells (AFCs) and initial defense to an active viral infection in the upper respiratory tract. Ann Surg 2003;4:565–73.

30. Fukatsu K, Lundberg AH, Hanna MK, et al. Route of nutrition influences intercellular adhesion molecule-1 expression and neutrophil accumulation in intestine. Arch Surg 1999;134:1055–60.

31. Fukatsu K, Kudsk KA, Wu Y, et al. TPN decreases IL-4 and IL-10 mRNA expression in lamina propria cells but glutamine supplementation preserves the expression. Shock 2001;15(4):318–22.
32. Fukatsu K, Kudsk KA, Zarzaur BL, et al. Increased ICAM-1 and β2 integrin expression in parenterally fed mice after a gut ischemic insult. Shock 2002;18(2):119–24.
33. Fukatsu K, Zarzaur BL, Johnson CD, et al. Enteral nutrition prevents remote organ injury and mortality following a gut ischemic insult. Ann Surg 2001; 233(5):660–8.
34. Kudsk KA, Hermsen JL, Genton L, et al. Injury stimulates an innate respiratory IgA immune response in humans. J Trauma 2008;64(2):316–25.
35. Jonker MA, Hermsen JL, Gomez FE, et al. Injury induces localized airway increases in pro-inflammatory cytokines in humans and mice. Surg Infect (Larchmt) 2011; 12(1):49–56.
36. Hermsen JL, Sano Y, Gomez FE, et al. Parenteral nutrition inhibits a tumor necrosis factor-α mediated IgA response to injury. Surg Infect (Larchmt) 2008;9(1):33–40.
37. Weinrauch Y, Elsbach P, Madsen LM, et al. The potent anti-Staphylococcus aureus activity of a sterile rabbit inflammatory fluid is due to a 14-kD phospholipase A2. J Clin Invest 1996;97(1):250–7.
38. Weinrauch Y, Abad C, Liang NS, et al. Mobilization of potent plasma bactericidal activity during systemic bacterial challenge. Role of group IIA phospholipase A2. J Clin Invest 1998;102(3):633–8.
39. Harwig SS, Tan L, Qu XD, et al. Bactericidal properties of murine intestinal phospholipase A2. J Clin Invest 1995;95(2):603–10.
40. Weiss J, Inada M, Elsbach P, et al. Structural determinants of the action against Escherichia coli of a human inflammatory fluid phospholipase A2 in concert with polymorphonuclear leukocytes. Biol Chem 1994;269(42):26331–7.
41. Laine VJ, Grass DS, Nevalainen TJ. Protection by Group II phospholipase A2 against Staphylococcus aureus. J Immunol 1999;162:7402–8.
42. Sano Y, Hermsen JL, Kang K, et al. Parenteral nutrition maintains pulmonary IgA antibody transport capacity, but not active transport, following injury. Am J Surg 2009;198(1):105–9.
43. Li J, Kudsk KA, Hamidian M, et al. Bombesin affects mucosal immunity and gut-associated lymphoid tissue in IV-fed mice. Arch Surg 1995;130:1164–70.
44. Janu P, Kudsk KA, Li J, et al. Effect of bombesin on impairment of upper respiratory tract immunity induced by total parenteral nutrition. Arch Surg 1997;132: 89–93.
45. DeWitt RC, Wu Y, Renegar KB, et al. Bombesin recovers gut-associated lymphoid tissue (GALT) and preserves immunity to bacterial pneumonia in TPN-fed mice. Ann Surg 2000;231(1):1–8.
46. Hanna MK, Zarzaur BL, Fukatsu K, et al. Individual neuropeptides regulate gut-associated lymphoid tissue integrity, intestinal IgA levels, and respiratory antibacterial immunity. JPEN J Parenter Enteral Nutr 2000;24(5):261–9.
47. Li J, Kudsk KA, Janu P, et al. Effect of glutamine-enriched TPN on small intestine gut-associated lymphoid tissue (GALT) and upper respiratory tract immunity. Surgery 1997;121(5):542–9.
48. Li J, King KA, Janu PG, et al. Glycyl-L-glutamine-enriched total parenteral nutrition maintains small intestine gut-associated lymphoid tissue and upper respiratory tract immunity. JPEN J Parenter Enteral Nutr 1998;22(1):31–6.
49. Kudsk KA, Wu Y, Fukatsu K, et al. Glutamine-enriched total parenteral nutrition maintains intestinal interleukin-4 and mucosal immunoglobulin A levels. JPEN J Parenter Enteral Nutr 2000;24(5):270–5.

50. DeWitt RC, Wu Y, Renegar KB, et al. Glutamine-enriched TPN preserves respiratory immunity and improves survival to a Pseudomonas pneumonia. J Surg Res 1999;84:13–8.
51. Ikeda S, Zarzaur BL, Johnson CD, et al. Total parenteral nutrition supplementation with glutamine improves survival after gut ischemia/reperfusion. JPEN J Parenter Enteral Nutr 2002;26(3):169–73.
52. Zarzaur BL, Ikeda S, Johnson CD, et al. Mucosal immunity preservation with bombesin or glutamine is not dependent on mucosal addressin cell adhesion molecule-1 (MAdCAM-1) expression. JPEN J Parenter Enteral Nutr 2002;26(5):265–70.
53. Roy CC, Kien CL, Bouthillier L, et al. Short-chain fatty acids: ready for prime time. Nutr Clin Pract 2006;21:351–66.
54. Topping DL, Clifton PM. Short-chain fatty acids and human colonic function: roles of resistant starch and non starch polysaccharides. Physiol Rev 2001;81:1031–64.
55. Tungland BC, Meyer D. Nondigestible oligo-and polysaccharides (dietary fiber): their physiology and role in human health and food. Comprehensive Review in Food Science and Food Safety 2002;1:90–109.
56. McAndrew HF, Lloyd DA, Rintala R, et al. Intravenous glutamine or short-chain fatty acids reduce central venous catheter infection in a model of total parenteral nutrition. J Pediatr Surg 1999;34:281–5.
57. Murakoshi S, Fukatsu K, Omata J, et al. Effects of adding butyric acid to total parenteral nutrition on gut-associated lymphoid tissue and mucosal immunoglobulin A levels. JPEN J Parenter Enteral Nutr 2011. [Epub ahead of print].
58. Fujihashi K, Ernst PB. A mucosal internet. In: Ogra PL, Mestecky J, Lamm ME, et al, editors. Mucosal immunology. San Diego (CA): Academic Press; 1999. p. 619–30.
59. Yada S, Nukina H, Kishihara K, et al. IL-7 prevents both caspase-dependent and -independent pathways that lead to the spontaneous apoptosis of i-IEL. Cell Immunol 2001;208(2):88–95.
60. Watanabe M, Ueno Y, Yajima T, et al. Interleukin 7 is produced by human intestinal epithelial cells and regulates the proliferation of intestinal mucosal lymphocytes. J Clin Invest 1995;95(6):2945–53.
61. Yang H, Sun X, Haxhija EQ, et al. Intestinal epithelial cell-derived interleukin-7: a mechanism for the alteration of intraepithelial lymphocytes in a mouse model of total parenteral nutrition. Am J Physiol Gastrointest Liver Physiol 2007;292(1): G84–91.
62. Fukatsu K, Moriya T, Maeshima Y, et al. Exogenous IL-7 affects gut associated lymphoid tissue in mice receiving total parenteral nutrition. Shock 2005;24(6):541–6.
63. Fukatsu K, Moriya T, Ikezawa F, et al. Interleukin-7 dose dependently restores parenteral nutrition-induced gut associated lymphoid tissue cell loss. JPEN J Parenter Enteral Nutr 2006;30(5):388–93.
64. Nagayoshi H, Fukatsu K, Ueno C, et al. 5-fluorouracil infusion reduces gut-associated lymphoid tissue cell number and mucosal IgA levels. JPEN J Parenter Enteral Nutr 2005;29(6):395–400.
65. Fukatsu K, Nagayoshi H, Maeshima Y, et al. Fish oil infusion reverses 5-fluorouracil-induced impairments in mucosal immunity in mice. Clin Nutr 2008;27(2):269–75.
66. Maeshima Y, Fukatsu K, Moriya T, et al. Influence of adding fish oil to parenteral nutrition on gut-associated lymphoid tissue. JPEN J Parenter Enteral Nutr 2007; 31(5):416–22.
67. Hering J, Garrean S, Dekoj TR, et al. Inhibition of proliferation by omega-3 fatty acids in chemoresistant pancreatic cancer cells. Ann Surg Oncol 2007;14(12):3620–8.
68. Maddaus MA, Ahrenholz D, Simmons RL. The biology of peritonitis and implications for treatment. Surg Clin North Am 1988;68:431–43.

69. Barnes PJ, Karlin M. NFκB—a pivotal transcription factor in chronic inflammatory diseases. N Engl J Med 1997;336:1066–71.
70. Ueno C, Fukatsu K, Kang WD, et al. Route and type of nutrition influence nuclear factor kappaB activation in peritoneal resident cells. Shock 2005;24(4):382–7.
71. Ueno C, Fukatsu K, Kang W, et al. Lack of enteral nutrition delays nuclear factor kappa B activation in peritoneal exudative cells in a murine glycogen-induced peritonitis model. JPEN J Parenter Enteral Nutr 2006;30(3):179–85.
72. Ueno C, Fukatsu K, Maeshima Y, et al. Arginine-enriched total parenteral nutrition improves survival in peritonitis by normalizing NFkappaB activation in peritoneal resident and exudative leukocytes. Ann Surg 2010;251(5):959–65.
73. Lin MT, Saito H, Furukawa S, et al. Alanyl-glutamine enriched total parenteral nutrition improves local, systemic, and remote organ responses to intraperitoneal bacterial challenge. JPEN J Parenter Enteral Nutr 2001;25(6):346–51.
74. Mackay IR. Hepatoimmunology: a perspective. Immunol Cell Biol 2002;80:36–44.
75. Moriya T, Fukatsu K, Maeshima Y, et al. Nutritional route affects ERK phosphorylation and cytokine production in hepatic mononuclear cells. Ann Surg 2007;245(4):642–50.
76. Omata J, Fukatsu K, Maeshima Y, et al. Enteral nutrition rapidly reverses total parenteral nutrition-induced impairment of hepatic immunity in a murine model. Clin Nutr 2009;28(6):668–73.
77. Omata J, Fukatsu K, Murakoshi S, et al. Enteral re-feeding rapidly restores parenteral nutrition-induced reduction of hepatic mononuclear cell number through recovery of small intestine and portal vein blood flows. JPEN J Parenter Enteral Nutr 2009;33(6):618–25.

Contributions of Intestinal Bacteria to Nutrition and Metabolism in the Critically Ill

Michael J. Morowitz, MD[a], Erica M. Carlisle, MD[b],
John C. Alverdy, MD[c],*

KEYWORDS

• Gut bacteria • Microbiome • Nutrition • Obesity • Critical care

MICROBES AND NUTRITION DURING CRITICAL ILLNESS

It has been known for decades that intestinal bacteria make important contributions to human metabolism and physiology. Perhaps the example best known to clinicians is the microbial synthesis of the essential nutrient vitamin B_{12}; the enzymes required for B_{12} synthesis are possessed by bacteria but not by plants or animals.[1] However, research from the past decade has conclusively established that the host-microbe relationship in humans is more complex than previously appreciated. The implications of this research for assessing and meeting the nutritional needs of critically ill patients are substantial.

The goals of this review are: (1) to offer a broad overview of the importance of the host-microbe relationship, (2) to detail what is known about the host-microbe relationship with regard to nutrition and metabolism in the healthy host, (3) to review the scarce existing literature about how microbial ecology changes during critical illness,

---

This work was supported by Grant No. GM62344-11 (JCA) from the National Institutes of Health.
The authors have nothing to disclose.
[a] Division of Pediatric General and Thoracic Surgery, University of Pittsburgh School of Medicine, Children's Hospital of Pittsburgh of UPMC, Faculty Pavilion 7th Floor, 4401 Penn Avenue, Pittsburgh, PA 15224, USA
[b] Department of Surgery, University of Chicago Pritzker School of Medicine, 5841 South Maryland Avenue, Chicago, IL 60637, USA
[c] Department of Surgery, University of Chicago Pritzker School of Medicine, University of Chicago Medical Center, 5841 South Maryland Avenue, MC 6090, Chicago, IL 60637, USA
* Corresponding author.
E-mail address: jalverdy@surgery.bsd.uchicago.edu

Surg Clin N Am 91 (2011) 771–785
doi:10.1016/j.suc.2011.05.001
0039-6109/11/$ – see front matter © 2011 Elsevier Inc. All rights reserved.

and (4) to discuss specific interventions that have been used to manipulate the gut flora to improve patient nutrition and outcomes in the intensive care unit (ICU).

REVOLUTIONARY ADVANCES IN UNDERSTANDING THE HUMAN MICROBIOME

An understanding of the complex relationship between humans and our microbes dates back at least to Pasteur. However, until recently, the ability of microbiologists and clinicians to characterize and dissect this relationship was hampered by the reality that only some of the microbes on the planet (and in the human body) can be cultured, isolated, and systematically studied in the laboratory.[2] As a result, most clinical focus on bacteria and viruses has been directed toward the statistical minority of organisms that cause clinical disease and can be easily isolated in culture.

More than 25 years ago, microbial ecologists conclusively showed that bacterial DNA can be used to identify which organisms are present in a complex biologic sample without dependence on cultivating those organisms in the laboratory.[3] Until recently, these culture-independent techniques to characterize microbial diversity were relatively restricted to studies of ocean and soil samples. Over the past decade, concerted efforts have been made to use these techniques to undertake comprehensive molecular surveys of the organisms associated with humans. These efforts have benefited from remarkable advances in DNA sequencing technologies, as well as from well-funded initiatives such as the National Institutes of Health Human Microbiome Project[4,5] and its European counterpart MetaHIT.[6]

Perhaps the foremost lesson of these recent efforts has been that all humans, both healthy and critically ill, are intimately associated with a vast population of microbial organisms. Uncertainty remains regarding the precise number of bacteria in the human body, but it is generally agreed that there at least 10 bacterial cells for every 1 human cell.[7] This belief has led authorities in the field to describe humans as superorganisms composed of both human and microbial cells.[8] Although clinicians have not historically thought about their patients in this way, it is easy to recognize the evolutionary logic of a symbiotic relationship between humans and microbes. By supporting lifelong colonization by organisms that possess a diverse set of metabolic capabilities, the host effectively augments its own genome; this is a more efficient arrangement than waiting for humans to evolve new metabolic capacities on their own.[9] In return for their contributions, microbes associated with the body are rewarded with a relatively safe, predictable, and nutrient-rich niche for colonization. As is discussed in subsequent sections, the impact of critical illness on this symbiotic relationship remains poorly understood.

All epithelial surfaces that interface with the external world harbor microbes, but the most dense microbial communities are those in the distal intestinal tract. Recent estimates suggest that 10 to 100 trillion microbes (including up to 1000 species) reside in this location.[8,10] Although more than 70 bacterial divisions (deep evolutionary lineages) are known to exist on the planet, human gut microbial communities are dominated by just 4 lineages. Two dominant divisions, the Bacteroidetes and the Firmicutes, comprise more than 95% of the total community; most of these organisms are strict anaerobes such as the *Bacteroides* and *Clostridium* species.[11] The remainder of human gut microbes are often from 2 other divisions: Actinobacteria (eg, *Bifidobacterium* species) and Proteobacteria. The phylum Proteobacteria contains the gram-negative enterics that despite being well known to clinicians, represent only a fraction of the gut microbial community.[11] The dominance of these 4 bacterial phyla and the relative absence of all other phyla suggests that, under normal circumstances, the human-microbe relationship is highly selective and highly stable. Throughout most of a person's life, this relationship is either symbiotic (mutually beneficial) or commensal (providing benefit to 1 member without harming the other); pathogenic host-microbe interactions are the exception rather than the rule.[9]

There is enormous interest in characterizing the clinical relevance of the human microbiome (defined as the collective set of microbial genomes associated with the human body). In addition to the gastrointestinal (GI) tract, important sites of colonization also under study include the skin, oropharynx, respiratory tract, and genitourinary tract. A primary objective of current research is to better define the basic features of the human microbiome (eg, how do microbial communities change over time in a given individual and how much interindividual variability is observed in various microbial communities?). An equally important objective is to identify associations between the microbiome and human health and disease.[12]

SPECIFIC CONTRIBUTIONS OF THE GUT MICROBIOTA TO HUMAN METABOLISM

A particularly compelling example of the importance of the gut microbiota to host metabolism is provided by comparing the nutritional status of germ-free (GF) and conventionally raised laboratory animals. Numerous investigators have reported that conventionally raised animals require up to 30% less caloric intake to maintain their body weight.[9] This observation is not only surprising, it is also counterintuitive because one might reasonably expect that bacteria and their human host may compete for a limited supply of ingested nutrients. This section summarizes what is known about how microbes directly affect human nutrition.

Microbiota and Carbohydrates

The sophisticated relationship that has evolved between the human GI tract and gut microbiota allows for efficient use of dietary carbohydrates. In the proximal GI tract, simple sugars such as glucose are absorbed, and disaccharides (eg, lactose) are hydrolyzed into their corresponding monosaccharide components such that they too can be absorbed.[9] However, a significant portion of dietary carbohydrates, including complex plant-derived polysaccharides and unhydrolyzed starch, normally passes undigested through to the distal GI tract.[13] Here, dense microbial populations (up to 10^{11} cells per gram of colonic matter) are present that are well equipped to hydrolyze complex carbohydrates. Many of the enzymes required to use these dietary substrates are not encoded in the human genome; by contrast, the microbiome, which contains approximately 100 times more genes than the human genome, is highly enriched in such enzymes.[9]

Use of complex polysaccharides via fermentation by anaerobic bacteria in the large intestine results in the accumulation of short chain fatty acids (SCFAs).[14] The principal SCFAs seen in the colon (acetate, propionate, and butyrate) have inherent nutritional value but also affect gut epithelial physiology in other ways. They are absorbed by passive diffusion across the colonic epithelium, and are subsequently used by different organs. Acetate, the SCFA produced in highest concentration, is used by skeletal and cardiac muscle and can be used by adipocytes for lipogenesis. Butyrate is metabolized primarily in the gut epithelium to yield ketone bodies or CO_2.[9] The colonic epithelium derives up to 70% of its energy needs directly from butyrate. Propionate metabolism is poorly understood but seems to involve transport to the liver by the portal circulation. It is believed that SCFAs also affect water absorption, local blood flow, and epithelial proliferation in the large intestine.[9]

Genomic analysis of gut bacteria offers vivid examples of the role of microbes in nutrient use. For example, in 2003, Xu and colleagues[10] published the complete genome sequence of the gram-negative anaerobe *Bacteroides thetaiotaomicron*, a prominent member of the normal intestinal microbiota. Annotation and analysis of the genome revealed a sophisticated apparatus for acquiring and digesting otherwise unusable dietary polysaccharides. This apparatus, including a complex, multicomponent, multi-enzyme complex starch use system, consists of more than 230 glycoside hydrolase and 15 polysaccharide lyase genes.[15] The genomic analysis showed that B thetaiotao-micron has evolved the remarkable capacity to sense the availability of carbohydrates in its microenvironment, and that it also has the ability to forage and use host-derived glycans (eg, mucin and heparin). Mechanistic studies in gnotobiotic animals further showed that, when B thetaiotaomicron senses a scarcity of fucose in the intestinal lumen, it induces the gut epithelium to upregulate expression of fucosylated glycans that can be used by the bacteria as an energy source without harming the host.[16] This body of work illustrates how the remarkable host-microbe symbiosis can be teased apart by pairing genomic sequencing efforts with creative in vivo laboratory studies.

Microbiota and Protein Metabolism

In contrast to carbohydrates, little attention has been paid to the relationship between the intestinal microbiota and nitrogen balance in humans. This situation is partly because conventional wisdom states that all essential amino acid requirements in humans must be supplied by the diet;[17] however, emerging evidence indicates that gut microbes can affect nitrogen balance by de novo synthesis of amino acids and intestinal urea recycling. These contributions are most pronounced in ruminant animals, which can live on a protein-free diet because their microbiota is capable of synthesizing most or all amino acids required for survival.

Microbial synthesis of essential amino acids has been notoriously difficult to measure in humans, but studies with radiolabeled tracers (eg, ^{13}C and ^{15}N) indicate that the intestinal microbiota makes a measurable contribution to the pool of essential amino acids. A series of experiments involving labeled inorganic nitrogen suggests that up to 20% of circulating lysine and threonine in nonruminant mammals, including adult humans, is synthesized by gut microbes.[18,19] Similarly, Raj and colleagues[17] showed that gut microbial synthesis of leucine in adult men was approximately 20% of the dietary amount. Another study showed that several substrates required for microbial synthesis of essential amino acids are derived from dietary carbohydrates.[20] Taken together, these studies provide compelling evidence that gut microbes contribute to the circulating pool of essential amino acids. More work is needed to define these contributions in both healthy and undernourished humans.

The intestinal microbiota also contributes to nitrogen balance by participating in urea nitrogen salvaging (UNS).[21,22] Increased urease expression in gut microbes results in metabolism of urea in the GI tract into ammonia and carbon dioxide. Some of the ammonia can be used for microbial synthesis of amino acids. Perhaps more importantly, the nitrogen generated during this process (urea nitrogen) can reenter the host circulation and serve as a substrate for synthetic processes.[21] Reduced urea recycling has been reported in GF animals[23] and in humans receiving antibiotic therapy.[24] Furthermore, several reports indicate that regulation of UNS is important in settings of low N intake and high N demand (eg, during pregnancy and during periods of rapid somatic growth in infancy).[25–27] Although still relatively preliminary, these studies underscore the relationship between gut microbes and protein metabolism that will likely be further described through ongoing characterization of the human microbiome.

Microbiota and Lipid Metabolism

Until recently, few studies of the association between lipid metabolism and the micro-biome existed. However, important research by Jeffrey Gordon, Fredrick Backhed and colleagues[28] suggests that the body's supply of triglycerides, a prominent source of energy during critical illness, is tightly linked to the intestinal microbiota. These findings have enormous potential relevance for research in a wide range of disease states, including metabolic disorders such as obesity (see later discussion) and cardiovascular disease.

This line of inquiry began with comparisons of lipid metabolism in GF and conventionally raised adult mice. By use of x-ray absorptiometry and epididymal fat pad weight analysis, it was shown that wild-type (WT) animals contained 42% more total body fat than GF animals, despite a higher metabolic rate and a reduced daily consumption of standard chow.[28] To mechanistically evaluate this finding, the investigators transferred the microbiota of WT animals to GF animals. A rapid increase (within 10 days) of total body fat content and epididymal fat weight was noted despite no significant difference in total body weight. Colonization of GF mice with just a single gut microbe (B thetaiotaocmicron, discussed later) also yielded a significant increase in total body fat content, although the increase in fat content was less than that seen with transfer of the complete mouse microbiota. Further work in this model suggested that the microbiota stimulates increased hepatic triglyceride production and promotes storage of adipocyte triglycerides by suppressing the activity of a circulating inhibitor of lipoprotein lipase.[28]

These pioneering studies have led to a sustained effort to understand the relationship between the microbiota and adiposity. In one experiment, GF mice were colonized with gut bacteria from humans fed with a typical Western diet (high fat, high carbohydrate), and a similar increase in adiposity was seen in the GF mice.[29] Other experiments that analyzed the lipids present in the serum and adipose tissue of WT and GF mice show that WT animals had increased levels of 18 phosphatidylcholine species and decreased levels of 9 triglyceride species relative to GF animals.[30] Alternatively, in the adipose tissue the concentration of most phosphatidylcholine compounds was similar between the 2 groups, but an increased concentration of triglycerides was detected in WT animals. Even more between-group differences were detected in the liver lipid profiles. For example, in addition to numerous differences in cholesteryl ester and phosphatidylcholine species, WT mice had a significant increase in 95 types of liver triglycerides. The translational relevance of these findings must still be defined, but these results provide clues to the role of microbes in lipid metabolism.

Vitamins

Most human diets provide a robust supply of vitamins, the essential human nutrients that must be obtained from exogenous sources. However, it has long been recognized that gut microbes also contribute to vitamin synthesis. The magnitude of this contribution in healthy and unhealthy patients is poorly understood.

It has been known for nearly a century that ruminants have no dietary requirement for water-soluble vitamins as a consequence of the dense microbial populations in the rumen, and that GF laboratory animals require dietary supplements of vitamins that are not needed by their WT counterparts.[31] Several bacterial genera that are common in the distal intestine (eg, Bacteroides, Bifidobacterium, and Enterococcus) are known to synthesize vitamins. Thiamine, folate, biotin, riboflavin, and panthothenic acid are water-soluble vitamins that are plentiful in the diet, but that are also synthesized by gut bacteria. Likewise, it has been estimated that up to half of the daily vitamin K requirement is provided by gut bacteria.[31] The molecular structure of bacterially synthesized vitamins is not always identical to the dietary forms of the vitamins. Several specialized epithelial transporters have been recognized to participate specifically in the absorption of vitamins derived from gut bacteria.[32] Perhaps the relative ease in replenishing vitamin stores in patients in the ICU has minimized enthusiasm for aggressive investigation of how bacterial vitamin biosynthesis is altered in hospitalized patients.

LESSONS LEARNED FROM STUDIES OF NUTRIENT EXCESS AND DEPRIVATION

Studying the relationship between the gut microbiota and energy balance in the extreme states of obesity and starvation may improve our ability to assess and satisfy nutritional needs in the ICU.

Obesity

Studies of energy balance in conventional and GF animals led to the hypothesis that the microbial ecology of the GI tract contributes to the pathogenesis of obesity.[33] Although it is widely acknowledged that excessive caloric intake is the root cause of obesity, it is reasonable to question whether an individual's metabolic response to caloric excess might vary according to the gut microbiota. Much of the work in this area has relied on a rodent model of obesity in which animals homozygous for a mutation in the leptin gene (ob/ob) harbor a fully penetrant obese phenotype.[34] Early studies using 16S ribosomal RNA-based genetic sequencing identified that obese animals have a markedly decreased abundance of Bacteroidetes organisms (such as B thetaiotaomicron) and a corresponding increase in Firmicutes.[34] Obese mice also possessed an abundance of methanogenic organisms from the domain Archaea, and it is believed that these organisms can aid in bacterial fermentation in the gut via removal of H_2.[35] The microbial differences observed in these experiments were division wide (ie, not skewed by the presence or absence of a single species). Further, the differences could not be explained by differences in food consumption. Corresponding studies have shown similar features of the gut microbes in obese humans.[36,37]

Why would a microbial community enriched in Firmicutes promote obesity? Recent work has suggested that the microbiota of obese individuals has an increased capacity to harvest energy from the diet.[33] Landmark articles, using high-throughput metagenomic sequencing platforms to identify as many genes as possible from all members of a mixed population of bacteria, from Gordon, Turnbaugh, Ley and colleagues,[35] have conclusively shown that the metabolic potential of the gut microbiome varies according to the microbial community composition. Molecular analysis of the microbiota of lean and obese mice showed that the obese microbiome is markedly enriched in genes enabling breakdown of dietary polysaccharides (eg, glucosidases, galactosidases, and amylases) and genes encoding proteins that transport and metabolize the products of polysaccharide metabolism. Biochemical and bomb calorimetry analyses in the same experiments showed increased concentrations of SCFAs (indicating a higher degree of bacterial fermentation) and significantly less energy remaining in the feces of obese mice relative to their lean counterparts.[35] These phenotypic traits were transmissible; colonization of GF animals with the microbiota of obese animals led to higher weight gain than colonization with microbiota from lean WT mice.

Turnbaugh and colleagues[29] have advanced these ideas even further by showing that the microbiome associated with diet-induced obesity (DIO) (in contrast to the ob/ob mutant model) is also rich in Firmicutes species and is similarly efficient at extracting energy from the diet. This set of experiments used a mouse model of DIO in which conversion to a high-fat/high-sugar (Western) diet reliably produces increased total body weight and increased epididymal fat content. The investigators showed that DIO alters gut microbial ecology by supporting the growth of Firmicutes species, and, in this case, they detected a specific association between obesity and the abundance of a class of organisms (Mollicutes) from the Firmicutes division that has also been identified in humans. Transplantation of cecal contents from DIO mice, similar to experiments with the ob/ob mice, yielded higher increases in body weight and fat than when cecal contents were transplanted from lean, WT animals. Here, again, metagenomic analyses were used to prove that the gut microbiome of animals fed a Western diet is enriched in genes encoding proteins related to energy harvest, including phosphotransferase proteins that enable the transport of simple sugars such as glucose and fructose.

A critical lesson from this body of work is that alterations in the microbiome of obese individuals are reversible. Early on, Ley and colleagues[37] showed that the ratio of Firmicutes to Bacteroidetes species decreases over time in humans on either a fat-restricted or carbohydrate-restricted diet. This finding was subsequently supported by Turnbaugh's findings that the bloom in Mollicutes seen in DIO was reversible with dietary manipulation.[29] Additional studies monitoring changes in the microbiota after surgical and nonsurgical weight loss interventions have produced similar findings.[38–40]

Fasting

Because caloric excess and obesity are associated with an altered gut microbiota, a corollary hypothesis is that the mirror-image pattern of alterations would be observed during periods of nutrient deprivation. This question is central to the issue of whether the host-microbe relationship might be exploited to improve the nutritional status of critically ill patients. Little is known about the impact of short-term and long-term fasting on the gut microbiota.

In 1968, Tennant and colleagues[41] showed that GF mice do not survive as long as WT mice during starvation despite similar patterns of starvation-induced weight loss. However, this group did not characterize the microbiota of the WT animals. In 1974, Tannock and Savage[42] used a culture-based approach to characterize the intestinal bacteria of mice exposed to a stress model that included deprivation of food, water, and bedding for 48 hours. These investigators concluded that stressed animals had a reduction in *Lactobacilli* and total mucosal-associated bacteria relative to control animals, but maintained a similar number of colonic anaerobes. In 1987, Deitch and colleagues[43] similarly reported that starvation induced a decrease in *Lactobacilli* in the murine GI tract; however, they noted a bloom of gram-negative enteric organisms. Subsequently, several studies have contrasted gut microbes in newborn animals receiving either enteral or parenteral nutrition.[43] These studies suggest that animals fed with total parenteral nutrition have an increased relative abundance of potential pathogens, such as *Clostridium perfringens*, that can forage on glycans lining the gut epithelium.[44,45] However, it is not known if these findings can be extended to critically ill adults who have shifted abruptly from the fed to the fasting state.

Two recent studies harnessed the power of high-throughput DNA sequencing to profile changes in microbial ecology during fasting in animal models. Crawford and colleagues[46] performed a fascinating study of myocardial ketone body metabolism by the intestinal microbiota during nutrient deprivation. After a 24-hour fast, the investigators observed a significant increase in the abundance of Bacteroidetes species and a corresponding decrease in Firmicutes; this is the converse of what was observed in models of caloric excess. The investigators proceeded to provide convincing evidence that the microbiota plays an integral role in fasting-induced hepatic ketogenesis, an important energy source during stress and starvation. In GF animals, ketogenesis was markedly reduced, and it was shown that myocardial metabolism was redirected toward glucose use. To understand further how microbial ecology is altered during fasting, Costello and colleagues[47] performed an innovative study in which they studied the Burmese python, a vertebrate that consumes large meals between long intervals of fasting. These investigators also showed an abundance of Bacteroidetes during fasting that shifted toward a postprandial abundance of Firmicutes. Species that were enriched in the postprandial state included *Clostridium* and *Lactobacillus*. These innovative studies serve as a foundation to study gut microbes in hospitalized patients who are not candidates for enteral nutrition.

WHAT HAPPENS TO THE MICROBIOME DURING CRITICAL ILLNESS?

High-throughput culture-independent techniques have not yet been widely applied to study how the human microbiome changes during critical illness. However, several clinical trials have evaluated strategies to manipulate the gut flora without thoroughly assessing the microbiome before or after therapy. Given the emerging evidence that the microbiota contributes to normal physiology, therapeutic attempts to eradicate pathogens might be coupled with attempts to restore the normal microbiota. For example, the earlier discussion suggests that optimizing the balance between Bacteroidetes and Firmicutes is a promising, but untested, strategy to improve energy balance among the critically ill.

Evaluations of the microbial ecology of the ICU have largely been restricted to culture-based studies. Studies frequently report that patients admitted to the ICU are rapidly colonized with opportunistic pathogens.[48–51] It has also been shown that pathogens detected by routine surveillance of the airways or the GI tract can serve as harbingers of an ensuing clinical infection by that organism.[52,53] Frequently encountered organisms in skin, oropharyngeal, endotracheal, and fecal samples from critically ill patients include the gram-negative enterics as well as species of *Candida*, *Pseudomonas*, and *Staphylococcus*. However, the fate of commensal organisms, many of which serve beneficial purposes, in the ICU is poorly understood. For this reason, a trial with prospective monitoring of the microbiome in patients in the ICU with comprehensive culture-independent techniques is needed.

Although we lack a comprehensive molecular readout of gut microbes in the ICU, several human and animal studies provide clues about how the microbiota is altered by common ICU exposures. Several excellent studies have reported that the pervasive, site-specific, and drug-specific effects of antibiotic therapy on the microbiota can be long lasting.[54–56] Multiple host factors relevant to the critically ill, including epithelial inflammation and hypoxia, are also known to perturb the microbiota and encourage the overgrowth of pathogens.[57,58] Some of the most commonly used pharmaceutical agents in the ICU, including acid suppression therapies, vasopressors, and opioids, are known to affect the human microbiota.[59,60] Our group was the first to report that the use of total parenteral nutrition or enteral nutrition with processed liquid diets dramatically alters the intestinal microbiota such that bacterial translocation to extraintestinal sites is promoted. As the effects of artificial nutrition, polypharmacy, and the selective pressures of extreme physiologic stress and injury accumulate over the course of critical illness, their impact on the ecologic health of the intestinal microbiota is likely to have a major untoward effect on recovery. Clinical interventions that can preserve gut microbial communities such that a benefit in overall recovery is realized require more in-depth analysis of the direct impact of these interventions on the gut flora.

SELECTIVE MANIPULATION OF THE GUT MICROBIOTA IN THE ICU

If one accepts that a healthy intestinal microbiota serves important biologic functions, then it is reasonable to hypothesize that gut microbial communities can be manipulated or optimized during critical illness to increase the chances of achieving desired clinical outcomes. In theory, manipulation of the gut microbiota could be used to improve energy balance and decrease the incidence of infectious complications. A fundamental problem with clinical application of this theory has been that we lack a detailed understanding of if and how the microbiome is altered during critical illness. As a result, interventions in this field have been introduced with a limited scientific foundation. Nonetheless, several strategies to optimize the microbiome have now been evaluated clinically. Some, such as the recent description of fecal transplantation for *Clostridium difficile* colitis,[61] are not discussed here. Others with obvious relevance to nutrition are discussed.

Gut Decontamination

Over the past 2 decades, several clinical trials have documented that selective decontamination of the GI tract or the oropharynx improves outcomes in critically ill patients and simultaneously promotes the growth of antibiotic-resistant bacteria.[62] Accepted approaches to decontamination consist of administering a regimen of broad-spectrum nonabsorbable antibiotics that theoretically spares the colonic anaerobes, and instead targets yeast, gram-negative pathogens (eg, the Enterobacteriaceae and *Pseudomonas aeruginosa*), and gram-positive pathogens (eg, *Staphylococcus aureus*) in the oral cavity or the GI tract. These protocols drastically alter the ICU microbiota,[62] and by extension decrease both mortality and the incidence of infectious complications such as ventilator-associated pneumonia.[50,63,64] Although these landmark studies serve as proof of principle that the intestinal microbiota can be manipulated in the ICU to achieve desirable outcomes, no studies used molecular techniques to profile the ICU microbiome before, during, or after decontamination. As a result, a precise understanding of how decontamination protocols work is lacking. Nevertheless, enthusiasm for decontamination protocols has diminished because of unacceptable increases in drug-resistant bacterial strains within the ICU.

Probiotics

The administration of probiotics and prebiotics represents an increasingly popular alternative to gut decontamination protocols. Probiotics are defined as live microorganisms that confer health benefits on humans and animals that ingest them in adequate amounts;[65] prebiotics are nondigestible food ingredients that confer health benefits by selectively inducing the growth of probiotic species.[66] Commonly, probiotics and prebiotics are administered together as a food or dietary supplement known as a synbiotic.[66] Although trials in a wide range of clinical settings have shown promise regarding the safety and efficacy of these supplements,[66] many critical issues pertaining to their use remain unresolved. Although they are often used to treat patients with disease, probiotics and prebiotics are viewed by regulatory agencies as nutritional supplements rather than as pharmaceutical agents or biohazards. This definition has allowed for lax oversight, which has resulted in the commercial use of the terms probiotics and prebiotics even when scientific criteria for the terms have not been met.[66]

The practice of administering live microbes with putative health benefits to unhealthy patients dates back to the early twentieth century. Much of the early work in the field was performed at the Pasteur Institute in Paris, where Nobel laureate Eli Metchnikoff and others advanced the notion of a differential gut microbiota in health and disease.[67] These scientists hypothesized that the protective effects of specific diets in some regions of Europe could be attributed to the diet-induced growth of beneficial microbes. This hypothesis led almost instantly to commercial attempts to capitalize on these ideas, hence the development of probiotics. The most commonly used probiotic species are nonpathogenic yeasts and organisms from the genera *Lactobacillus* and *Bifidobacterium*.[68] The most commonly used prebiotics are the naturally occurring oligosaccharides known as fructans that are normally found in foods such as garlic, artichokes, and bananas.[66] Another well-studied class of prebiotics is resistant starches, such as those found in unripe bananas and raw potatoes. As knowledge of the intestinal microbiome expands, it is likely that many more potential probiotic species and prebiotic supplements will be identified.

The long list of clinical diagnoses that have been treated with probiotics or prebiotics ranges from intestinal infections (eg, rotavirus infection) to extraintestinal infections (eg, urinary infections)[56] to allergic disorders (eg, asthma); in other cases, these agents have been used prophylactically (eg, to prevent colon cancer).[65] The strongest clinical data come from trials of probiotics and prebiotics in the treatment of intestinal infections, inflammatory bowel disease, and irritable bowel syndrome.[68] Despite their widespread use, knowledge of the putative mechanism of action of probiotics and prebiotics is limited. Most mechanistic studies in this area have centered on production of antimicrobial substances to inhibit colonization by pathogens, enhance the mucosal barrier function, and downregulate mucosal inflammation.[68] Despite the growing awareness of how gut microbes contribute to energy balance and despite the administration of probiotics/prebiotics as nutritional supplements, little research on this topic has focused on how these agents specifically affect nutrition, metabolism, or energy balance.

Several studies have been conducted to test the hypothesis that outcomes in critically ill patients can be improved by administering probiotics and prebiotics. These studies, including a randomized trial comparing the effects of early enteral nutrition with and without prebiotic supplementation, indicate that the incidence of sepsis and multiorgan dysfunction syndrome among patients with severe pancreatitis is lower after treatment with probiotics/prebiotics.[69] However, in 2008, the Dutch Acute Pancreatitis Study Group[70] released results of a well-publicized multicenter, randomized, controlled study reporting increased mortality among patients with severe acute pancreatitis who received probiotic prophylaxis. The increased mortality was attributed to a high incidence of intestinal ischemia, although a direct link between the probiotic and bowel ischemia was not proved. A subsequent meta-analysis concluded that probiotics do not influence mortality in the treatment of acute pancreatitis,[71] however, the results of the Dutch study have raised important questions about whether and how probiotics should be administered to vulnerable populations. Nonetheless, several other studies conducted in surgical and medical ICUs document improved outcomes after probiotic administration after trauma, liver transplant, and ICU admission for severe sepsis.[72]

As noted, data regarding the safety and efficacy of probiotic and prebiotic administration are limited. Potential safety issues involved with manipulation of the microbiota with probiotics/prebiotics include probiotic-induced disease and antibiotic resistance.[72] Even if questions remain about efficacy and optimal route of delivery, it is generally accepted that probiotic administration in healthy individuals is safe. However, there is little understanding of how to approach these issues in the ICU. Although probiotics have been safely administered to vulnerable hospitalized populations such as neonates and transplant recipients, the significance of the results of the Dutch pancreatitis study cannot be overemphasized. They serve as a powerful reminder of the seemingly obvious fact that administering live microbial organisms to unhealthy patients might be dangerous, particularly when so little is known about the putative mechanism of action. The importance of exercising caution is further underscored by the scant federal regulation of commercial interests in this area.

Modulating the Local Gut Microenvironment

Another possible approach to improve outcomes for critically ill patients is to manipulate the intestinal microenvironment to maintain the local microbial ecology of the GI tract indirectly. It is well established that the use of vasoactive pressors, antibiotics, and highly processed nutrients changes not only the local microbiota but also pH, oxygen tension, SCFA production, and various critical micronutrients that maintain the health of normal intestinal microbes. Our group and others have shown that maintenance of a more acidic intestinal pH through the course of surgical injury and administration of oral pH solutions enhance local intestinal immunity and prevent lethal gut-derived sepsis.[73] Most recently we have shown that surgical injury causes a rapid depletion of mucus phosphate, thereby inducing certain strains of pathogenic bacteria to upregulate their virulence against the intestinal epithelial barrier.[74] Most bacteria that cause serious infections in ICU patients are equipped with exquisite sensory mechanisms to detect the level of local phosphate concentration. Phosphate concentration is a key trigger by which bacteria activate their virulence machinery to, in some cases, cause lethal sepsis. When phosphate levels are high at sites of local microbial colonization, such as the intestinal mucus, microbes use the PhoB phosphosensory/phosphoregulatory system to repress virulence activation. However, during phosphate depletion, the PhoB system is derepressed and virulence is activated even to the point of tissue invasion, immune activation, and organ failure.[74] The PhoB and analogous systems are highly conserved among microbes and offer an opportunity for clinicians to understand the precise host signals that trigger microbes to transform from indolent colonizers to lethal pathogens. We have shown in animal studies that maintenance of local phosphate concentration can suppress virulence activation among highly pathogenic bacteria such as *P aeruginosa* even during periods of severe physiologic stress.[73] This situation also seems to be the case for other pathogens such as *Candida albicans* and *Enterococcus faecalis* (unpublished observations). Therefore, providing therapies at the microenvironmental level could be a novel approach to create molecular diplomacy between pathogen and host through the course of severe physiologic stress such as occurs during human critical illness.

SUMMARY

The intersection between the microbiome, nutrition, and critical illness will undoubtedly grow in interest in the coming years. Although the studies discussed in this article provide clear evidence that gut microbes contribute to human nutrition and metabolism, it is too early to know if this information will be translated into meaningful improvements in current practice patterns. However, it is easy to identify clinical scenarios in critical care that are likely to be affected by this growing field of study; these topics include achieving positive nitrogen balance, managing hyperglycemia and cholestasis, and reducing the incidence of infectious complications during critical illness.

At present, a few concluding points can be safely made. First, it is apparent that future evaluations of human nutritional status during critical illness should include consideration of the gut microbiota. Second, it is important to conduct the necessary studies to understand how the microbial ecology of the human body is altered during critical illness. Third, opportunities to manipulate the gut microbes in hospitalized patients are already presenting themselves, and the efficacy of such interventions must be rigorously evaluated by multidisciplinary teams of clinicians and scientists with a solid understanding of microbial behavior.

REFERENCES

1. Martens J, Barg H, Warren MJ, et al. Microbial production of vitamin B12. Appl Microbiol Biotechnol 2002;58:275–85.
2. Zoetendal EG, RajilicStojanovic M, de Vos WM. High-throughput diversity and functionality analysis of the gastrointestinal tract microbiota. Gut 2008;57(11): 1605–15.
3. Pace N. The universal nature of biochemistry. Proc Natl Acad Sci U S A 2000;98(3): 805–8.
4. Peterson J, Garges S, Giovanni M, et al, NIH HMP Working Group. The NIH human microbiome project. Genome Res 2009;19(12):2317–23.
5. The Human Microbiome Jumpstart Reference Strains Consortium. A catalog of reference genomes from the human microbiome. Science 2010;328(5981):994–9.
6. Qin J, Li R, Raes J, et al. A human gut microbial gene catalogue established by metagenomic sequencing. Nature 2010;464(7285):59–65.
7. Ley RE, Peterson DA, Gordon JI. Ecological and evolutionary forces shaping microbial diversity in the human intestine. Cell 2006;124(4):837–48.
8. Gill SR, Pop M, Deboy RT, et al. Metagenomic analysis of the human distal gut microbiome. Science 2006;312(5778):1355–9.
9. Hooper LV, Midtvedt T, Gordon JI. How host-microbial interactions shape the nutrient environment of the mammalian intestine. Annu Rev Nutr 2002;22:283–307.
10. Xu J, Bjursell MK, Himrod J, et al. A genomic view of the human-bacteroides thetaiotaomicron symbiosis. Science 2003;299(5615):2074–6.
11. Manson JM, Rauch M, Gilmore MS. The commensal microbiology of the gastrointestinal tract. Adv Exp Med Biol 2008;635:15–28.
12. Turnbaugh PJ, Ley RE, Hamady M, et al. The human microbiome project. Nature 2007;449(7164):804–10.
13. Wong JM, de Souza R, Kendall CW, et al. Colonic health: fermentation and short chain fatty acids. J Clin Gastroenterol 2006;40(3):235–43.
14. Macfarlane S, Macfarlane GT. Regulation of short-chain fatty acid production. Proc Nutr Soc 2003;62(1):67–72.
15. Flint HJ, Bayer EA, Rincon MT, et al. Polysaccharide utilization by gut bacteria: potential for new insights from genomic analysis. Nat Rev Microbiol 2008;6(2): 121–31.
16. Hooper LV, Xu J, Falk PG, et al. A molecular sensor that allows a gut commensal to control its nutrient foundation in a competitive ecosystem. Proc Natl Acad Sci U S A 1999;96(17):9833–8.
17. Raj T, Dileep U, Vaz M, et al. Intestinal microbial contribution to metabolic leucine input in adult men. J Nutr 2008;138(11):2217–21.
18. Metges CC. Contribution of microbial amino acids to amino acid homeostasis of the host. J Nutr 2000;130(7):1857S–64S.
19. Metges CC, Petzke KJ. Utilization of essential amino acids synthesized in the intestinal microbiota of monogastric mammals. Br J Nutr 2005;94(5):621–2.
20. Torrallardona D, Harris CI, Fuller MF. Pigs' gastrointestinal microflora provide them with essential amino acids. J Nutr 2003;133(4):1127–31.
21. Stewart GS, Smith CP. Urea nitrogen salvage mechanisms and their relevance to ruminants, non-ruminants and man. Nutr Res Rev 2005;18(1):49–62.
22. Bergen WG, Wu G. Intestinal nitrogen recycling and utilization in health and disease. J Nutr 2009;139(5):821–5.
23. Levenson SM, Crowley LV, Horowitz RE, et al. The metabolism of carbon-labeled urea in the germ free rat. J Biol Chem 1959;234(8):2061–2.

24. Walser M, Bodenlos LJ. Urea metabolism in man. J Clin Invest 1959;38:1617–26.
25. Waterlow JC. The mysteries of nitrogen balance. Nutr Res Rev 1999;12(1):25–54.
26. Steinbrecher HA, Griffiths DM, Jackson AA. Urea production in normal breast-fed infants measured with primed/intermittent oral doses of [15N, 15N]urea. Acta Paediatr 1996;85(6):656–62.
27. Forrester T, Badaloo AV, Persaud C, et al. Urea production and salvage during pregnancy in normal Jamaican women. Am J Clin Nutr 1994;60(3):341–6.
28. Backhed F, Ding H, Wang T, et al. The gut microbiota as an environmental factor that regulates fat storage. Proc Natl Acad Sci U S A 2004;101(44):15718–23.
29. Turnbaugh PJ, Backhed F, Fulton L, et al. Diet-induced obesity is linked to marked but reversible alterations in the mouse distal gut microbiome. Cell Host Microbe 2008;3(4):213–23.
30. Velagapudi VR, Hezaveh R, Reigstad CS, et al. The gut microbiota modulates host energy and lipid metabolism in mice. J Lipid Res 2010;51(5):1101–12.
31. Hill MJ. Intestinal flora and endogenous vitamin synthesis. Eur J Cancer Prev 1997;6(Suppl 1):S43–5.
32. Said HM, Mohammed ZM. Intestinal absorption of water-soluble vitamins: an update. Curr Opin Gastroenterol 2006;22(2):140–6.
33. Tilg H, Moschen AR, Kaser A. Obesity and the microbiota. Gastroenterology 2009;136(5):1476–83.
34. Ley RE, Backhed F, Turnbaugh P, et al. Obesity alters gut microbial ecology. Proc Natl Acad Sci U S A 2005;102(31):11070–5.
35. Turnbaugh PJ, Ley RE, Mahowald MA, et al. An obesity-associated gut microbiome with increased capacity for energy harvest. Nature 2006;444(7122):1027–31.
36. Turnbaugh PJ, Hamady M, Yatsunenko T, et al. A core gut microbiome in obese and lean twins. Nature 2009;457(7228):480–4.
37. Ley RE, Turnbaugh PJ, Klein S, et al. Microbial ecology: human gut microbes associated with obesity. Nature 2006;444(7122):1022–3.
38. Nadal I, Santacruz A, Marcos A, et al. Shifts in clostridia, bacteroides and immunoglobulin-coating fecal bacteria associated with weight loss in obese adolescents. Int J Obes 2008;33(7):758–67.
39. Zhang H, DiBaise JK, Zuccolo A, et al. Human gut microbiota in obesity and after gastric bypass. Proc Natl Acad Sci U S A 2009;106(7):2365–70.
40. Walker AW, Ince J, Duncan SH, et al. Dominant and diet-responsive groups of bacteria within the human colonic microbiota. ISME J 2011;5(2):220–30.
41. Tennant B, Malm OJ, Horowitz RE, et al. Response of germfree, conventional, conventionalized and *E. coli* monocontaminated mice to starvation. J Nutr 1968;94(2):151–60.
42. Tannock GW, Savage DC. Influences of dietary and environmental stress on microbial populations in the murine gastrointestinal tract. Infect Immun 1974;9(3):591–8.
43. Dietch EA, Winterton J, Berg R. Effect of starvation, malnutrition, and trauma on the gastrointestinal tract flora and bacterial translocation. Arch Surg 1987;122(9):1019–24.
44. Bjornvad CR, Thymann T, Deutz NE, et al. Enteral feeding induces diet-dependent mucosal dysfunction, bacterial proliferation, and necrotizing enterocolitis in preterm pigs on parenteral nutrition. Am J Physiol Gastrointest Liver Physiol 2008;295(5):G1092–103.
45. Deplancke B, Vidal O, Ganessunker D, et al. Selective growth of mucolytic bacteria including *Clostridium perfringens* in a neonatal piglet model of total parenteral nutrition. Am J Clin Nutr 2002;76(5):1117–25.

46. Crawford PA, Crowley JR, Sambandam N, et al. Regulation of myocardial ketone body metabolism by the gut microbiota during nutrient deprivation. Proc Natl Acad Sci U S A 2009;106(27):11276–81.
47. Costello E, Gordon JI, Secor SM, et al. Postprandial remodeling of the gut microbiota in Burmese pythons. ISME J 2010;4(11):1375–85.
48. Shimizu K, Ogura H, Goto M, et al. Altered gut flora and environment in patients with severe SIRS. J Trauma 2006;60(1):126–33.
49. Heyland D, Mandell LA. Gastric colonization by gram-negative bacilli and nosocomial pneumonia in the intensive care unit patient. Evidence for causation. Chest 1992;101(1):187–93.
50. Kerver AJ, Rommes JH, Mevissen-Verhage E, et al. Prevention of colonization and infection in critically ill patients: a prospective randomized study. Crit Care Med 1988;16(11):1087–93.
51. Kerver A, Rommes JH, Mevissen-Verhage E. Colonization and infection in surgical intensive care patients: a prospective study. Intensive Care Med 1987; 13(5):347–51.
52. Ubeda C, Taur Y, Jenq RR, et al. Vancomycin-resistant Enterococcus domination of intestinal microbiota is enabled by antibiotic treatment in mice and precedes bloodstream invasion in humans. J Clin Invest 2010;120(12):4332–41.
53. Marshall JC, Christou NV, Meakins JL. The gastrointestinal tract. the "undrained abscess" of multiple organ failure. Ann Surg 1993;218(2):111–9.
54. Dethlefsen L, Huse S, Sogin ML, et al. The pervasive effects of an antibiotic on the human gut microbiota, as revealed by deep 16S rRNA sequencing. PLoS Biol 2008;6(11):e280.
55. Croswell A, Amir E, Teggatz P, et al. Prolonged impact of antibiotics on intestinal microbial ecology and susceptibility to enteric Salmonella infection. Infect Immun 2009;77(7):2741–53.
56. Antonopoulos DA, Huse SM, Morrison HG, et al. Reproducible community dynamics of the gastrointestinal microbiota following antibiotic perturbation. Infect Immun 2009;77(6):2367–75.
57. Lupp C, Robertson ML, Wickham ME, et al. Host-mediated inflammation disrupts the intestinal microbiota and promotes the overgrowth of Enterobacteriaceae. Cell Host Microbe 2007;2(3):204.
58. Kohler JE, Zaborina O, Wu L, et al. Components of intestinal epithelial hypoxia activate the virulence circuitry of Pseudomonas. Am J Physiol Gastrointest Liver Physiol 2005;288(5):G1048–54.
59. Canani RB, Terrin G. Gastric acidity inhibitors and the risk of intestinal infections. Curr Opin Gastroenterol 2010;26(1):31–5.
60. Alverdy J, Zaborina O, Wu L. The impact of stress and nutrition on bacterial-host interactions at the intestinal epithelial surface. Curr Opin Clin Nutr Metab Care 2005;8(2):205–9.
61. Khoruts A, Sadowsky MJ. Therapeutic transplantation of the distal gut microbiota. Mucosal Immunol 2011;4(1):4–7.
62. Oostdijk EA, de Smet A, Blok HE, et al. Ecological effects of selective decontamination on resistant gram-negative bacterial colonization. Am J Respir Crit Care Med 2010;181(5):452–7.
63. de Smet A, Kluytmans JA, Cooper BS, et al. Decontamination of the digestive tract and oropharynx in ICU patients. N Engl J Med 2009;360(1):20–31.
64. Stoutenbeek CP, van Saene H, Little RA, et al. The effect of selective decontamination of the digestive tract on mortality in multiple trauma patients: a multicenter randomized controlled trial. Intensive Care Med 2007;33(2):261–70.

65. Santosa S, Farnworth E, Jones PJ. Probiotics and their potential health claims. Nutr Rev 2006;64(6):265–74.
66. Douglas LC, Sanders ME. Probiotics and prebiotics in dietetics practice. J Am Diet Assoc 2008;108(3):510–21.
67. Fooks LJ, Gibson GR. Probiotics as modulators of the gut flora. Br J Nutr 2002; 88(Suppl 1):S39–49.
68. Quigley EM. Prebiotics and probiotics; modifying and mining the microbiota. Pharmacol Res 2010;61(3):213–8.
69. Manzanares W, Hardy G. The role of prebiotics and synbiotics in critically ill patients. Curr Opin Clin Nutr Metab Care 2008;11(6):782–9.
70. Besselink MG, van Santvoort HC, Buskens E, et al. Probiotic prophylaxis in predicted severe acute pancreatitis: a randomised, double-blind, placebo-controlled trial. Lancet 2008;371(9613):651–9.
71. Sun S, Yang K, He X, et al. Probiotics in patients with severe acute pancreatitis: a meta-analysis. Arch Surg 2009;394(1):171–7.
72. Morrow LE. Probiotics in the intensive care unit. Curr Opin Crit Care 2009;15(2): 144–8.
73. Zaborina O, Zaborin A, Romanowski K, et al. Host stress and virulence expression in intestinal pathogens: development of therapeutic strategies using mice and *C. elegans*. Curr Pharm Des 2011 April 6. [Epub ahead of print].
74. Long J, Zaborina O, Holbrook C, et al. Depletion of intestinal phosphate after operative injury activates the virulence of *P aeruginosa* causing lethal gut-derived sepsis. Surgery 2008;144(2):189–97.

Nutritional Support of Surgical Patients with Inflammatory Bowel Disease

I. Janelle Wagner, MD*, John L. Rombeau, MD

KEYWORDS

- Inflammatory bowel disease • Nutrition • Crohn disease
- Ulcerative colitis

Surgical patients with inflammatory bowel disease (IBD), especially those with Crohn disease (CD), are often malnourished. Approximately 25% and 50% of CD patients will require surgery within the first 5 and 10 years of diagnosis, respectively.[1,2] Among ulcerative colitis (UC) patients, 15% to 40% will require surgery within the first 10 to 20 years after diagnosis.[2] IBD patients in need of surgery are particularly vulnerable to nutritionally associated postoperative complications, due to the chronicity of disease, the need for potent medications, and the presence of malnutrition preoperatively. This review addresses nutritional-metabolic assessment and treatment of patients with IBD who require surgery.

DEFINITION OF MALNUTRITION IN IBD

Defining malnutrition is deceptively challenging. There are no clinical or laboratory measurements exclusively specific to nutritional status, particularly in patients with IBD. As recently as 2010, a literature review revealed that no consensus could be reached among nutritionists for a gold-standard test of malnutrition.[3] Thus, today's frequently used tests to measure malnutrition are often surrogate measures and can result in part from other clinical abnormalities (**Table 1**). For clinical relevance in perioperative patients, the authors arbitrarily define malnutrition as serum albumin levels of less than 3.5 g/dL and/or nonvolitional weight loss of 15% of the patient's usual weight over 3 to 4 months.

Serum albumin levels are frequently used to determine nutritional status; however, there are limitations to the clinical applications of this measure. Hypoalbuminemia is

The authors have nothing to disclose.

Department of Surgery, Temple University School of Medicine, 3401 North Broad Street, Parkinson Pavilion, Suite 400, Philadelphia, PA 19140, USA

* Corresponding author.

E-mail address: janellewagner@gmail.com

doi:10.1016/j.suc.2011.04.013
0039-6109/11/$ – see front matter © 2011 Elsevier Inc. All rights reserved.

surgical.theclinics.com

Table 1
Surrogate serum nutritional markers

	Half-Life (days)	Levels Reflect	Synthesis	Function	Levels Subject To
Albumin	18–20	Chronic protein repletion	Liver	• Maintenance of colloidal oncotic pressure • Ion binding/ transport	• Volume status • Liver function • Renal loss
Prealbumin	2–3	Acute protein repletion	Liver	Ion binding/ transport	• Liver function • Renal loss
Transferrin	7–10	Acute protein repletion	Liver	Iron ion delivery/ transport	• Alcohol use • Serum iron levels • Liver function • Renal loss

not a specific marker for malnutrition, and is most often a surrogate marker for chronic disease. Moreover, serum albumin level cannot be used reliably as an index of nutritional repletion, given its long half-life (18–20 days). Because serum albumin levels vary with the blood volume status of the patient, comparison of albumin levels obtained at different points in the course of fluid resuscitation may inaccurately reflect changes in nutritional status. Therefore, to increase clinical relevance, measurements should be obtained when a patient is in a stable, euvolemic state.

Serum prealbumin has a shorter half-life (2–3 days) than serum albumin. Levels of prealbumin may reflect nutritional intake as recent as the preceding meal, and can vary unpredictably with carbohydrate load and metabolic stress. Therefore prealbumin is not an accurate laboratory marker for chronic nutritional status, but may be helpful in assessing dynamic responses to protein repletion.

Transferrin is a plasma protein with a half-life of 7 to 10 days. Similar to albumin, low serum levels of transferrin are associated with increased morbidity. However, transferrin levels are affected by iron intake and may not accurately reflect nutritional status in the setting of iron deficiency anemia.

Malnutrition is more prevalent in CD than in UC, possibly due to greater small bowel involvement, with impaired absorption, and loss of nutrients secondary to severe diarrhea and intestinal fistulae.[4] A report using data from the National Inpatient Sample, a national database of inpatient hospital stays, found the prevalence of protein calorie malnutrition to be significantly higher among hospitalized CD and UC patients when compared with a general inpatient population (1.8% vs 6.1% [CD] and 7.2% [UC], P<.0001). After adjustment for age, comorbidities, and socioeconomic factors, the odds ratio for malnutrition among IBD patients compared with non-IBD patients was 5.57 (95% confidence interval [CI]: 5.29–5.86).[5] IBD patients were also more likely than non-IBD patients to receive total parenteral nutrition (TPN) therapy (**Table 2**).

Nutritional Deficiencies in IBD

Body mass index (BMI), fat mass, bone mineral content, lean body mass, and nutrient deficiencies have been documented in CD and UC patients.[4] These indices are affected by both the level of activity and the duration of the disease. For example, fat mass is sharply depleted in active disease and only recovers partially during

Table 2
Prevalence of protein calorie malnutrition (PCM) among inpatients with and without IBD

Inpatient Population	Percentage with PCM (%)	P Value	Percentage Receiving TPN Therapy (%)
Patients without IBD	1.8	—	6
Patients with UC	7.2	<.0001	25
Patients with CD	6.1	<.0001	26

Data from Nguyen GC, Munsell M, Harris ML. Nationwide prevalence and prognostic significance of clinically diagnosable protein-calorie malnutrition in hospitalized inflammatory bowel disease patients. Inflamm Bowel Dis 2008;14:1105–11.

remission.[4] CD patients in remission for 3 months have lower body fat mass than controls.[6] BMI is elevated in patients in remission when compared with patients having active disease.[4] In UC, the duration of disease enhances the depletion of bone mineral content, lean body mass, and fat mass.[7] Bone mineral content and lean body mass are lower in CD than in UC and in controls. Micronutrient deficiencies commonly observed in UC include β-carotene, zinc, selenium, and magnesium, and in CD consist of vitamin B-12, vitamin B-2, copper, and zinc.[8]

A study of 126 patients with IBD evaluated multiple nutrient serologic markers. Forty percent of patients had low hemoglobin levels.[9] Dietary intake of vitamin B-12, folate, and vitamin B-6 correlated with serum levels, independent of disease activity. Low vitamin D levels were observed even in patients in remission. The investigators recommended routine evaluation of serum vitamin B-6 and vitamin D levels in IBD patients.[9]

Etiology of Nutritional Deficiencies in IBD

The etiology of malnutrition in IBD is complex and multifactorial, and includes poor dietary intake, malabsorption of dietary nutrients, and adverse effects of medications.[4]

Insufficient dietary intake

Poor dietary intake secondary to postprandial abdominal pain and diarrhea is the most common cause of malnutrition in IBD.[4,10] This condition is most prevalent during active disease when abdominal pain and anorexia are often relentless.

Paradoxically, patients may avoid certain nutrient dense foods due to their preconceived, incorrect ideas regarding the effects of these foods, even when the disease is quiescent. For example, some patients avoid dairy products for fear of intolerance, which in turn leads to calcium deficiencies.[10] Poor intake of β-carotene, vitamin B-1, vitamin B-6, vitamin C, and magnesium have also been documented in CD patients.[6]

Nutrient malabsorption and systemic inflammation

Nutrient malabsorption and ensuing deficiencies are due, in part, to chronic, longstanding bowel mucosal inflammation and diarrhea, which in turn leads to losses of protein, blood, minerals, electrolytes, and trace elements.[4,10]

Systemic proinflammatory cytokines (interleukin [IL]-1, IL-6, and tumor necrosis factor [TNF]) contribute to nutrient deficiencies in IBD. The inflammatory process enhances protein catabolism and alters normal protein synthesis. When TNF levels are increased, protein synthesis is diverted from nutritional proteins to inflammatory proteins.[11] Cytokines also stimulate osteoclast activity, causing increased bone resorption. Forty to fifty percent of UC and CD patients have osteopenia, while 5% to 36% have osteoporosis.[12–15]

Adverse effects of medications

Many medications used to treat the inflammatory process in IBD are inherently toxic and are associated with extensive side effects. This section discusses gastrointestinal side effects of IBD medications that may potentiate malnutrition (**Table 3**).

Common medications used in treating CD and UC patients include aminosalicylates, steroids, azathioprine, mercaptopurine, and infliximab. All of these medications can cause nausea, vomiting, and diarrhea. Aminosalicylates (mesalamine [Asacol, Lialda, Canasa, Apriso], olsalazine [Dipentum], sulfasalazine [Azulfidine], balsalazide [Colazal]) can cause abdominal pain and cramping.[16] Side effects of steroids include anorexia, weight loss, abdominal pain, gastritis, esophagitis, and protein catabolism.[17] Long-term steroidal therapy can result in osteopenia. Azathioprine (Imuran, Azasan) can cause pancreatitis and negative nitrogen balance.[18] Mercaptopurine (Purinethol) can cause intestinal ulceration.[19] Infliximab (Remicade) use may result in dyspepsia, pancreatitis, and even intestinal perforation.[20]

The Prognostic Inflammatory and Nutritional Index (PINI) measures α1-acid glyco-protein, C-reactive protein, albumin, and prealbumin, and is used as a measure of nutrition status in critically ill patients.[21] Of interest, a study of 7 patients with CD showed that infliximab had positive effects on nutritional status as measured by PINI. The investigators concluded that infliximab improves PINI by reducing inflammation; however, the small sample size and the lack of validation of PINI in CD patients support the need for further studies in this area.[21]

Table 3
Side effects of medications used to treat IBD

	Mechanism	Route of Administration	Gastrointestinal Side Effects
Aminosalicylates	Unknown	Oral Suppository Enema	Abdominal pain Cramping
Corticosteroids	Transactivation and transrepression of nuclear proteins	Oral Intravenous	Anorexia Weight loss Abdominal pain Gastritis Esophagitis Protein catabolism Osteopenia Osteoporosis
Azathioprine	Purine analogue, inhibits DNA synthesis	Oral Intravenous	Pancreatitis Negative nitrogen balance
Mercaptopurine	Alters RNA and DNA function via inhibition of purine synthesis and metabolism	Oral	Intestinal ulceration
Infliximab	Anti–tumor necrosis factor antibody	Intravenous	Dyspepsia Pancreatitis Intestinal perforation

Data from Refs.[16–20]

PREOPERATIVE NUTRITIONAL SUPPORT
Nutritional Assessment

Evaluation of nutritional status is of primary importance when beginning a preoperative workup in IBD patients. Before prescribing nutritional support preoperatively, nutritional status must be assessed and nutritional goals must be defined. As previously mentioned, nutritional status may be evaluated by determining serum albumin levels and changes in body weight.

Preoperative Nutritional Goals

The primary nutritional-metabolic goals for preoperative patients are to improve nutritional status and reduce anastomotic and wound-healing complications.

Anastomotic leak is among the most serious of postoperative complications, and one that may be decreased in incidence with appropriate preoperative nutrition. The association between anastomotic failure and hypoalbuminemia has been well studied.[22–24] Preoperative serum albumin levels below 3.5 g/dL are consistently associated with anastomotic breakdown in elective colorectal surgery patients. A serum albumin level of less than 3.5 g/dL was one of 5 risk factors identified in a case-controlled study of 90 patients with anastomotic leak and 180 patients without anastomotic leak.[25] Suding and colleagues[26] concluded that a baseline serum albumin level of less than 3.5 g/dL was associated with anastomotic leaks in both univariate and multivariate analyses (adjusted odds ratio, 2.56). Mäkelä and colleagues[24] identified 44 patients with anastomotic leak after left colectomy with colorectal anastomosis. When compared with 44 controls matched for age, gender, and operative indication, hypoalbuminemia and weight loss greater than 5 kg were significantly associated with anastomotic leak. Although these studies confirm the association of hypoalbuminemia with anastomotic leak, to the authors' knowledge no prospective studies have conclusively demonstrated that preoperative protein replenishment reduces the risk of anastomotic leak. Further investigation is needed to define specific preoperative protein repletion goals, and the quantity and type of protein required to meet these goals.

At present, there are no evidence-based preoperative nutritional goals for IBD patients. Prospective studies must be performed to define nutritional end points. Despite the lack of established norms for malnutrition, the clinician is still faced with the decision at the bedside as to how and what to feed, how to administer the nutrients, and what end points to use to determine nutritional efficacy.

PREOPERATIVE NUTRITIONAL THERAPY

Nutritional deficiencies may be corrected by either enteral (oral or tube feeding) or parenteral supplementation. Enteral feeding should be prescribed whenever possible: "if the gut works, and can be used safely, use it." When compared with TPN, enteral feeding is less costly, safer, and more physiologic in that it promotes gastrointestinal tract growth and function.[27] Preoperative enteral and parenteral therapies are discussed subsequently. In many instances these feeding modalities are used concurrently, particularly in very ill patients. Thus these routes for feeding are complementary, and not necessarily competitive or mutually exclusive.

Enteral Therapy

Enteral nutrition, when ingested, has the greatest potential to improve preoperative nutritional status in IBD patients. Because most malnutrition in IBD is due to poor nutrient intake, the authors recommend preoperative dietary counseling with a registered dietician (RD). Under the supervision of an RD food avoidance issues may be addressed constructively, and a proper nutrition plan drafted that takes into account individual nutritional deficiencies and offers targeted nutrient supplementation.

Elemental (protein delivered in amino acid form) and polymeric (whole or modified protein) formulae have been studied in CD patients as methods of inducing disease remission.[28] These formulae improve nutritional status and body composition while decreasing levels of proinflammatory cytokines and serum inflammatory markers.[28] A 3-week trial of elemental feeds (Vivonex or Peptamen [Nestle Healthcare Nutrition Inc, Florham Park, NJ]) delivered via nasoduodenal tube increased body weight, fat, and protein.[29] These referenced studies were performed in nonoperative patients. Although disease remission was the primary emphasis and goal of these studies, similar benefits might accrue with preoperative nutritional enhancement.

Total Parenteral Nutrition

Similar to other clinical conditions, TPN is recommended for malnourished IBD patients who cannot be fed effectively by either mouth or enteric tube. Many studies have examined the safety and effectiveness of TPN for preoperative nutritional therapy; however, only a few of these studies have included IBD patients and, to the authors' knowledge, no large, controlled clinical trials have been performed exclusively in this population. The rationale for the use of preoperative TPN in IBD is based on restoration of protein deficits, which in turn leads to improved organ function. The catabolism of the disease produces significant protein losses, with protein requirements increased proportionately more than nonprotein calories.

In one retrospective study, IBD patients who received preoperative TPN had significantly fewer postoperative complications than those who did not receive similar feedings.[30] The investigators recommended a course of 5 days of preoperative TPN therapy in IBD patients with severe protein depletion. Another study showed that preoperative TPN reduced the length of small bowel resected in IBD.[31] Finally, healing of wounds and bowel anastomoses can be improved by the use of TPN.[30]

Reports of the effects of preoperative TPN on the systemic inflammatory response have been conflicting in colorectal surgical patients. Lin and colleagues[32] found that preoperative TPN increased IL-6 and IL-8 levels in patients after colorectal surgery, suggesting that the postoperative inflammatory response was enhanced. Although this study included IBD patients, it did not report specifically the results of the IBD subpopulation. A study by Yao and colleagues[33] found no difference between levels of immunoglobulins A, M, and G and postoperative complications in malnourished CD patients who received pre- and perioperative TPN; however, those who received nutritional supplementation returned to work sooner than those who were not fed similarly. These investigators suggested that perioperative parenteral nutrition ameliorated humoral immune response, reversed malnutrition, and facilitated rehabilitation. In summary, there are few controlled data on the inflammatory sequelae of TPN in IBD patients, so this is an area in need of further investigation.

Preoperative Correction of Nutritional Deficiencies in Patients with Intestinal Fistulae

Enterocutaneous fistula (ECF) and colocutaneous fistula (CCF) are manifestations of CD that are associated with high morbidity and mortality.[34] The mortality rate of untreated colonic fistulae is 16%, with that of small bowel fistulae 54%.[34] Decreased dietary intake, increased nutrient losses, and enhanced nutrient requirements (often secondary to sepsis) collectively contribute to malnutrition in these patients. The incidence of malnutrition in patients who do not receive nutritional support is 20% with colonic fistula, 74% with jejunal or ileal fistula, and 53% with duodenal fistula.[34]

Initial management includes correction of fluid and electrolyte imbalances, control of fistula output, and drainage of intra-abdominal fluid collections. Nutritional therapy is essential in the adjunctive management of these patients.

TPN is indicated when there is high fistula output (>500 mL/d), inability to obtain enteral access, or gastrointestinal intolerance of an oral diet or enteral nutrition. TPN ameliorates the progressive malnutrition in ECF patients and provides bowel and pancreatic rest, which in turn reduces the volume and changes the composition of gastrointestinal secretions.[34] A study of 12 patients showed that fistuloclysis could replace TPN for nutritional maintenance in high-output jejunocutaneous or ileocutaneous fistulae[35]; however, this process was labor intensive and cumbersome. Operative repair is reserved for high-output fistulae that fail to close after at least 3 months of aggressive nutritional therapy.[36]

POSTOPERATIVE NUTRITION

The goal of postoperative nutrition is to provide maintenance nutrient repletion throughout the catabolic period, which in turn helps to minimize posttraumatic tissue breakdown and enhance wound healing. The amount and route of postoperative feeding is based on the patient's preoperative nutritional status, nutrient requirements, and the type and extent of operation. Attention is directed toward correcting nutritional deficits following the resolution of catabolism.

Several operations and postoperative conditions, unique to IBD patients, are described here, including proctocolectomy with ileal pouch-anal anastomosis (IPAA), pouchitis, ileostomy, short bowel syndrome (SBS), and the nutritional risk factors for disease recurrence. Early postoperative enteral feeding and TPN therapy are also discussed.

Ileal Pouch Anal Anastomosis

IPAA is the gold-standard therapy for most UC patients in need of surgery. In malnourished patients, especially those receiving large amounts of steroids (>30 mg prednisone per day), and other immunosuppressants, the total operative approach is often performed in 3 steps: initial total abdominal colectomy with Hartmann closure of rectum and end-ileostomy, proctectomy with pouch formation and neoileostomy, and finally, ileostomy reversal. The 3-stage approach provides the opportunity to correct nutritional deficits before the patient undergoes the pouch procedure.

Patients undergoing the aforementioned procedures have varied nutritional requirements at different operative stages. Of greatest concern is the severity of malnutrition prior to the first operation. At this time the patient is the most severely ill, with an acutely inflamed and sometimes toxic colon, low protein stores, and decreased body weight. After resection of the inflamed colon, the diarrhea and abdominal pain that impair oral intake resolve, allowing improvement of nutritional status, return of appetite, and gain in body weight.

After take-down of the ileostomy and placement of the pouch in intestinal continuity (third operative stage), new nutritional issues arise such as vitamin B-12 and iron deficiencies, fat and bile acid malabsorption, abnormal deficits of trace elements, fluids, and electrolytes, and food intolerance.

Deficiency of vitamin B-12 is a frequent finding in these patients and is caused by decreased absorptive capacity in the distal ileum, inadequate dietary intake, overgrowth of bacteria, which bind vitamin B-12, in the pouch, and pouchitis. Coull and colleagues[37] found low serum vitamin B-12 levels in 25% of 171 patients with J-pouches evaluated postoperatively (after the third operative stage). Malabsorption was ruled out with Schilling tests, but further mechanisms were not investigated. Oral vitamin B-12 supplementation restored the levels to normal over the course of 1 year. By contrast, only 2 of 39 patients with end-ileostomies and J-pouches (second operative stage) had vitamin B-12 deficiencies.[37] Another study evaluated 17 patients for bacterial overgrowth and vitamin B-12 deficiency.[38] Twenty-nine percent had abnormal Schilling tests at 3 months and 35% at 18 months. Fifty-six percent of the patients with abnormal Schilling tests also had impaired bacterial deconjugation.[38] These findings suggest that bacterial overgrowth secondary to pouch stasis plays a role in mediating vitamin B-12 deficiency.[38] Moreover, these results suggest that J-pouch patients may benefit from lifelong vitamin B-12 supplementation.

Iron deficiency is a common sequela in these patients and is caused by impaired absorption, decreased oral intake, increased iron requirements, and blood loss. Seventeen percent of patients have some form of postoperative anemia, and patients with a J-pouch are 5 times more likely than those with an S-pouch to be anemic.[38] In a study of 18 patients with J-pouches, 10 were anemic, all of whom had pouchitis, which in turn was thought to play a causative or compounding role in the anemia.[38]

Fat malabsorption is secondary to interruption of the biliary enterohepatic circulation. Decreased bile absorption occurs in patients with end-ileostomies as well as in patients with pouches in continuity, who in turn absorb less bile acid than those with end-ileostomies. The proposed mechanism for this is threefold: increased bacterial colonization in the pouch leading to biotransformation to secondary bile acids, decreased lipophilicity with subsequent mucosal damage, and malabsorption.[38] A study by Hakala and colleagues[39] found decreased bile acid and cholesterol absorption as well as decreased total and low-density cholesterol levels, presumably due to pouch bacterial overgrowth.

Various studies have noted slight, but not clinically significant, differences in sodium, chloride, and magnesium levels in postoperative patients.[38] Several studies[40–42] have examined the levels of trace elements in IPAA patients. With the possible exception of zinc, trace element levels are not decreased significantly by IPAA.[38]

A study of 105 patients defined and rated the severity of food intolerance after IPAA (**Table 4**).[43] More than 10% were noted to have food intolerance manifested by diarrhea, thirst, and fatigue.[43] Other common symptoms of food intolerance included increased or decreased stool consistency, flatulence, and perianal irritation.[43]

Pouchitis

Pouchitis, inflammation of the ileal pouch, is a phenomenon unique to IPAA patients. Pouchitis was traditionally thought to be caused by bacterial overgrowth. However, all pouches by nature contain large numbers of bacteria and are not necessarily inflamed. In fact, bacterial overgrowth is a necessary step in the maturation of the pouch.[44] After several months of being placed in intestinal continuity, the ileal mucosa of the pouch adjusts to its new role as a neorectum and even undergoes cellular transformation to colonic mucosa.[44] Pouchitis can lead to villous atrophy of this mucosa, causing a reduction in absorptive capacity. A study of 38 patients found that 33% experienced fat malabsorption preoperatively, versus 35% at 12 months and 41% at 36 months postoperatively.[45] These differences were statistically significant. Symptoms of pouchitis include increased frequency of bowel movements, abdominal pain, fever, and bleeding per neorectum.

Table 4
Food intolerances post-IPAA and ileostomy

Food Source	Outcome
IPAA	
Spicy foods Vegetables Fruit Fruit juice	Decreased stool consistency
Potatoes Bread Bananas	Increased stool consistency
Onions Cabbage Leeks	Increased flatulence
Spicy foods	Increased number of daily stools
Spicy foods Citrus fruit Nuts Seeds	Perianal irritation
Cooked meals	Increased urge to defecate
Ileostomy	
Onions Grilled fish	"Intolerance"
Rhubarb Alcohol	"Watery flow"
Peas Onions Beans	Increased flatulence
Onions Pineapples Mushrooms	Abdominal pain

Data from Buckman SA, Heise CP. Nutrition considerations surrounding restorative proctocolectomy. Nutr Clin Pract 2010;25:250–6; and Steenhagen E, de Roos NM, Bouwman CA, et al. Sources and severity of self-reported food intolerance after ileal pouch-anal anastomosis. J Am Diet Assoc 2006;106:1459–62.

The inflammation observed in pouchitis is accompanied by increased bowel pH, decreased fecal butyrate, altered fecal flora, and increased concentrations of bile acids. Inulin, a dietary fiber, is fermented to short-chain fatty acids and reduces bowel pH. One study investigated the effects of enteral inulin supplementation on inflammation of the ileal reservoir.[46] After 3 weeks of supplementation, inulin increased butyrate levels, and decreased pH, *Bacteroides fragilis* levels, and bile acid levels in the pouch lumen. This finding was accompanied by endoscopically and histologically reduced inflammation in the ileal reservoir.[46] Alles and colleagues[44] evaluated the extent to which pouches ferment undigested carbohydrates. The ability of the ileal pouch to ferment dietary carbohydrates is associated with the absence of pouchitis. It is interesting that resistant starches are fermented into butyrate, the primary fuel of the colonic mucosa. Moreover, negative correlation between butyrate levels and pouch mucosa villous atrophy has been previously established.[44] These findings provide sufficient rationale to study the ingestion of resistant starches in IPAA patients to either prevent or treat pouchitis.[44]

Probiotics are live microorganisms that replenish and strengthen the normal intestinal flora, and are effective in preventing and treating pouchitis.[47] *Lactobacillus* and bifidobacteria are the most common probiotic microbes. Four strains of Lactobacillus, 3 strains of *Bifidobacterium*, and 1 strain of *Streptococcus* have been studied for their effects on pouchitis.[38,47–49] In vitro, *Lactobacillus casei* decreased mucosal levels of TNF-α, interferon-γ, IL-2, IL-6, and IL-8, a neutrophil chemoattractant, resulting in a decreased tissue influx of neutrophils.[50] In addition, probiotics controlled release of IL-1β and reinforced intestinal mucosal barrier function.[49] VSL#3, a combination of 8 probiotic microbes (*Streptococcus salivarius*, *L casei*, *Lactobacillus plantarum*, *Lactobacillus acidophilus*, *Lactobacillus delbrueckii*, *Bifidobacterium longum*, *Bifidobacterium infantis*, and *Bifidobacterium breve*) increased the number of intestinal mucosal regulatory T cells in IPAA patients, potentially conferring a beneficial immunoregulatory mechanism.[47] In an uncontrolled study, Laake and colleagues[48] evaluated 51 IPAA patients who took a probiotic supplement for 4 weeks. There were significant decreases in involuntary defecation, abdominal cramps, leaking anal sphincter, mucus production, urge to defecate, bloody stools, and morning fevers.[48] Gionchetti and colleagues[51] observed that patients who took probiotics had a statistically significant decrease in acute pouchitis within the first year, as well as an improved quality of life when compared with a placebo.

In summary, administration of digestion-resistant starches, inulin, and probiotics provide several promising nutritional therapies for both the treatment and prevention of pouchitis.

Ileostomy

Dietary restrictions should be discussed with patients with newly created ileostomies. Both nut and fiber consumption (particularly raw fruits and vegetables) should be reduced in the immediate postoperative period, and slowly reintroduced after the first 6 weeks. To prevent or decrease the risk of ileostomy obstruction in the early postoperative period, fruits and vegetables should be preferentially consumed after removal of peels, seeds, and pits, and should be thoroughly masticated. Ileostomy patients have fewer food intolerances than IPAA patients (see **Table 4**).[38] A study of 952 ileostomy patients found that onions and grilled fish were commonly tolerated poorly.[38] Onions, pineapple, and mushrooms caused abdominal pain, whereas onions, peas, and beans caused flatulence (see **Table 3**).

Ileostomy patients are susceptible to dehydration, and they must be trained to recognize and prevent this sequela. These patients can lose 50 to 80 mmol of sodium per day, thus they should be advised to increase oral sodium intake.[38] In addition, serum cholesterol and α-lipoprotein levels may be decreased and triglycerides may be increased after diverting loop ileostomy.[45] These alterations resolve at 12 months after ileostomy reversal combined with a functioning pouch.[45]

Early Feeding: Enhanced Recovery Protocol

The iconoclastic trend toward early postoperative feeding began in the mid-1990s, when the surgical dogma of nil by mouth until resolution of postoperative ileus was investigatively challenged. Since that time the development of early enteral feeding, or enhanced recovery protocols, in postoperative colorectal patients has been well described.[52] One study of early enteral feeding in CD patients undergoing open ileocolic resections noted that early feeding significantly reduced hospital stay, with low morbidity and readmission rates.[53] The investigators used a previously described postoperative regimen of food and protein drinks (60–80 g/d) starting on postoperative day zero.[52]

Postoperative TPN

Most studies of postoperative TPN are not specific to IBD patients; however, it can be inferred that reasonably similar results probably occur in IBD patients undergoing operations of similar magnitudes. Fasth and colleagues[54] found that TPN, administered after major colorectal surgery, reduced postoperative weight loss even after termination of the nutritional treatment. This finding was thought to be due to preservation of body fat. Patients on postoperative TPN lost less weight than controls, and this difference remained statistically significant for up to 6 months after completion of TPN.[54] An extensive review by the same investigators, which cited 13 studies over 8 years, concluded that postoperative TPN decreased the amount of weight lost and improved nitrogen balance; however, it did not improve morbidity or mortality, and was associated with its own complications.[55]

Recent investigations have involved attempts to decrease intestinal inflammation via manipulation of TPN lipid emulsions. As mentioned previously, the postoperative inflammatory response is mediated in part by leukotrienes. High levels of omega-3 fatty acids along with a high ratio of omega-3 fatty acids to omega-6 fatty acids direct eicosanoid synthesis away from series-4 leukotriene production, thereby reducing inflammation (**Fig. 1**); this is also the supportive principle for fish oil therapy (see section on current therapeutic trends). A prospective study of 40 patients presenting

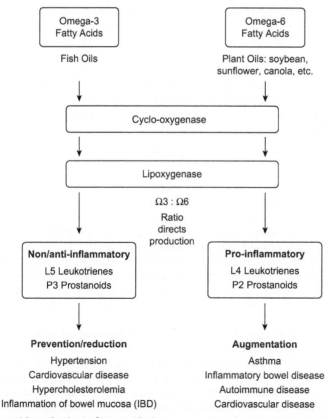

Fig. 1. Eicosanoid synthesis via fatty oxidation: omega-3 and omega-6 competition.

for elective colorectal procedures compared those receiving postoperative TPN containing a standard lipid profile with those receiving TPN containing an omega-3 polyunsaturated fatty acid (PUFA)-supplemented 20% lipid emulsion. The investigators concluded that postoperative administration of TPN supplemented with omega-3 fatty acids was well tolerated and ameliorated the postoperative inflammatory response.[56]

Short Bowel Syndrome

After massive small bowel resection, the intestine adapts to the loss of absorptive surface area; however, in some patients the adaptive process is insufficient, leading to chronically high fecal output and dehydration. In these patients, initial evaluation should include a detailed dietary history to determine the effects of specific foods on fecal output. The goals of nutritional management for patients with SBS are to minimize malabsorption, optimize nutrient absorption, minimize the need for TPN and exogenous fluids, and stimulate intestinal adaptation.[57]

Careful monitoring of fluid balance is essential, as fluid and electrolyte disturbances are common sources of morbidity among SBS patients. Fluid and electrolyte repletion may be implemented by intravenous fluid at a rate of 35 mL/kg/d, or by commercial oral rehydration solution and mineral supplementation.[57] Replacement fluids are administered in response to measured losses, with the goal of maintaining appropriate urine output. Measurements of electrolyte concentrations in stomal aliquots may help to estimate deficits and replacements.

The SBS patient should be given a detailed 1- to 3-week menu. Patients need to be educated as to what to eat and what to avoid. For example, complex carbohydrates are preferred over simple sugars to decrease the osmotic load to the gut. Patients should be instructed to eat small frequent meals, divided throughout the day. Soluble fiber supplements can be used to slow gut transit time.[57] Patients with SBS are likely to have deficiencies in zinc, potassium, magnesium, and vitamins, especially B-12. Vitamin B-12 injections should be administered after surgical resection of greater than 100 cm of terminal ileum, and SBS patients should be maintained on multivitamin supplementation.[57]

Nutrition and Postoperative Recurrence of IBD

Eighty percent of CD patients have early postoperative endoscopic disease recurrence, with 20% to 30% manifesting clinical signs of relapse 1 year after surgery.[58] Preoperative nutritional status has not been identified as a risk factor for relapse. The role of nutrition in prevention of postoperative relapse is under investigation. Probiotics and enteral therapy are two modalities currently being studied.

Two prospective trials of probiotics were performed in 2004 and in 2005 to evaluate the hypothesis that probiotic administration reduced the appearance of new intestinal lesions. Lactobacillus rhamnosus and Lactobacillus johnsonii LA1 had no significant effect on relapse rates of CD postoperatively.[49] It is possible that different strains or doses may ultimately prove effective, therefore further studies must be performed.

Cottone and colleagues[49] studied the effectiveness of enteral nutrition on prevention of postoperative CD recurrence. Enteral nutrition reduced postoperative recurrence to such an extent that the investigators suggested that enteral nutrition may be prophylactic in preventing postoperative recurrence. Limitations of the study included small sample size and the lack of investigator "blindedness" and placebo controls; however, the results emphasized the need for further investigation of enteral nutrition in prevention of CD postoperatively. These findings were further supported in a study by Ikeuchi and colleagues[59] who investigated the combined effects of enteral nutrition with nutritional education in postoperative patients with CD. These investigators concluded that this regimen delayed the timing of a second resection, especially in patients with perforating CD.[59]

CURRENT THERAPEUTIC TRENDS AND FUTURE RESEARCH

New nutritional treatments of UC and CD surgical patients include immunonutrition and fish oil therapy. Although not yet the standard of care, these treatments are undergoing further investigation and are more frequently being used clinically in patients with IBD.

Immunonutrition

Immunonutrition involves the use of nutrients to enhance immune function. Enteral and parenteral immunonutrition formulae may be specifically tailored to modulate the response to metabolic changes induced by the stress of surgery. Although not studied specifically in patients with IBD, enteral preparations modified with glutamine, arginine, and omega-3 fatty acids controlled the immune response and modulated protein synthesis during the acute phase, subsequently reducing morbidity and mortality.[60] Six days of perioperative immunonutrition (in nonmalnourished patients) increased CD4 lymphocyte counts on the day before surgery.[60] Parenteral glutamine supplementation decreased infectious complications postoperatively.[60] It is not known whether supplementing the function of immune cells overstimulates the immune response; therefore, these therapies remain controversial.

Reduction of Bowel Inflammation: Fish Oils

Fish oils are derived from the fatty tissues of fish and contain omega-3 essential fatty acids. Omega-3 fatty acids compete with omega-6 fatty acids in the eicosanoid pathway (see **Fig. 1**). A high ratio of omega-3 to omega-6 fatty acids favors production of noninflammatory or anti-inflammatory eicosanoid products, whereas a low ratio favors production of proinflammatory series-4 leukotrienes and series-2 prostanoids. Omega-3 fatty acids also function as transcription factors, to decrease expression of proinflammatory genes such as those that code for cytokines.[61]

Omega-3 fatty acids, found in fish oil, have recently been evaluated for their effects on reduction of intestinal mucosal inflammation. Preliminary studies have examined the potential of fish oil administration to reduce or eliminate requirements of anti-inflammatory medications in patients with IBD. Prospective studies of patients with UC demonstrated that fish oils decreased steroid requirements.[62] UC patients who received a supplement of fiber, fish oil, and antioxidants had reduced prednisone requirements and were less likely to need mesalamine.[63] In CD patients with high C-reactive protein and erythrocyte sedimentation rate, who received fish oil supplementation, greater proportions of docosahexaenoic acid and eicosapentaenoic acid (omega-3 fatty acids) were incorporated into neutrophils as compared with arachidonic acid (omega-6 fatty acid), and these patients exhibited lower production of both interferon-γ and prostaglandin E2.[64] Despite these metabolic benefits, there was no demonstrable significant effect on disease activity.[64] To the authors' knowledge, the administration of fish oils to reduce bowel inflammation preoperatively in patients with IBD has not been studied; however, it is reasonable to infer that their perioperative administration could benefit IBD patients by controlling inflammation. This issue is an important one for further investigation.

Areas for Future Research

Areas for further research in surgical patients with IBD include the need to identify prognostic nutritional indices, to derive a working definition of malnutrition, and to identify optimal nutrient formulations. At present there are no proven standards to measure nutritional status, and no evidence-based end points to define optimum nutritional state. Further research must be conducted to identify these measures. Preoperative goals for nutritional supplementation need further definition. This task would be made simpler by the use of a systematic set of nutritional parameters. In addition to defining malnutrition quantitatively and qualitatively, further research must be performed to determine causality between preoperative malnutrition and poor postoperative outcome.

Although TPN has been clinically available since 1968, much of the research on perioperative TPN is not specific to the IBD population. Further studies of ameliorating inflammation by giving either parenteral or enteral lipids to perioperative patients with IBD need to be performed.

SUMMARY

IBD patients in need of surgery require individualized preoperative and postoperative nutritional assessment as well as determination of nutrient requirements. Malnutrition remains a clinical diagnosis, as defined by serum albumin levels of less than 3.5 g/dL and/or a nonvolitional weight loss of 15% or more of the patient's usual weight. Preoperative and postoperative TPN should be reserved for severely malnourished patients. There is substantial evidence to support the use of early enteral feeding postoperatively. Special considerations for IPAA patients include dietary changes after ileostomy, vitamin B-12 deficiency after pouch formation, and treatment and prevention of pouchitis. Areas of further investigation in IBD patients include the therapeutic effects of fish oils and probiotics, and the potential efficacy of immunonutrition.

REFERENCES

1. Nakahara T, Yao T, Sakurai T, et al. Long-term prognosis of Crohn's disease. Jpn J Gastroenterol 1991;88:1305–12.
2. Thompson NP, Wakefield AJ, Pounder RE. Prognosis and prognostic factors in inflammatory bowel disease. Saudi J Gastroenterol 1995;1:129–37.
3. Meijers JM, van Bokhorst-de van der Schueren MA, Schols JM, et al. Defining malnutrition: mission or mission impossible? Nutrition 2010;26:432–40.
4. Rocha R, Santana GO, Almeida N, et al. Analysis of fat and muscle mass in patients with inflammatory bowel disease during remission and active phase. Br J Nutr 2009;101:676–9.
5. Nguyen GC, Munsell M, Harris ML. Nationwide prevalence and prognostic significance of clinically diagnosable protein-calorie malnutrition in hospitalized inflammatory bowel disease patients. Inflamm Bowel Dis 2008;14:1105–11.
6. Filippi J, Al-Jaouni R, Wiroth J, et al. Nutritional deficiencies in patients with Crohn's disease in remission. Inflamm Bowel Dis 2006;12:185–91.
7. Jahnsen J, Falch JA, Mowinckel P, et al. Body composition in patients with inflammatory bowel disease: a population based study. Am J Dig Dis 2003;98: 1556–62.
8. Geerling BJ, Badart-Smook A, Stockbrugger RW, et al. Comprehensive nutritional status in recently diagnosed patients with inflammatory bowel disease compared with population controls. Eur J Clin Nutr 2000;54:514–21.

9. Vagianos K, Bector S, McConnell J, et al. Nutrition assessment of patients with inflammatory bowel disease. JPEN J Parenter Enteral Nutr 2007;31:311–9.

10. Razack R, Seidner DL. Nutrition in inflammatory bowel disease. Curr Opin Gastro-enterol 2007;23:400–5.

11. Passos RA, Santana GO, Andrade A, et al. Response to cachexia in Crohn's disease following treatment with anti-TNF: a case report. Rev Bras Nutr Clin 2006;21:333–6.

12. Silvennoinen JA, Karttunen TJ, Niemela SE, et al. A controlled study of bone mineral density in patients with inflammatory bowel disease. Gut 1995;37:71–6.

13. Bernstein CN, Seeger LL, Sayre JW, et al. Decreased bone density in inflamma-tory bowel disease is related to corticosteroid use and not disease diagnosis. J Bone Miner Res 1995;10:250–6.

14. Compston JE, Judd D, Crawley EO, et al. Osteoporosis in patients with inflamma-tory bowel disease. Gut 1987;28:410–5.

15. Bjarnason I, Macpherson A, Mackintosh C, et al. Reduced bone density in patients with inflammatory bowel disease. Gut 1997;40:228–33.

16. Healthwise. WebMd. Available at: http://www.webmd.com/ibd-crohns-disease/aminosalicylates-for-inflammatory-bowel-disease. Updated October 9, 2008. Accessed November 26, 2010.

17. National Center for Biotechnology Information. PubMed Health. Available at: http://www.ncbi.nlm.nih.gov/pubmedhealth/PMH0000091. Updated September 1, 2008. Accessed November 26, 2010.

18. National Center for Biotechnology Information. PubMed Health. Available at: http://www.ncbi.nlm.nih.gov/pubmedhealth/PMH0000602. Updated September 1, 2008. Accessed November 26, 2010.

19. National Institutes of Health. Medline Plus. Available at: http://www.nlm.nih.gov/medlineplus/druginfo/meds/a682653.html. Updated February 1, 2009. Accessed November 26, 2010.

20. Centocor Ortho Biotech. Remicade.com. Available at: http://www.remicade.com/remicade/crohns/crohns_index.html. Updated April 13, 2010. Accessed November 26, 2010.

21. Weise DM, Rivera R, Seidner DL. Is there a role for bowel rest in nutrition manage-ment of Crohn's disease? Nutr Clin Pract 2008;23:309–17.

22. Badia-Tahull MB, Llop-Talaveron J, Fort-Casamartina E, et al. Preoperative albumin as a predictor of outcome in gastrointestinal surgery. E Spen Eur E J Clin Nutr Metab 2009;4:e248–51.

23. Saha AK, Tapping CR, Foley GT. Morbidity and mortality after closure of loop ileostomy. Colorectal Dis 2009;11:866–71.

24. Mäkelä JT, Kiviniemi H, Laitinen S. Risk factors for anastomotic leakage after left sided colorectal resection with rectal anastomosis. Dis Colon Rectum 2003;46: 653–60.

25. Telem DA, Chin EH, Nguyen SQ, et al. Risk factors for anastomotic leak following colorectal surgery: a case-control study. Arch Surg 2010;145:371–6.

26. Suding P, Jensen E, Abramson MA, et al. Definitive risk factors for anastomotic leaks in elective open colorectal resection. Arch Surg 2008;143:907–11.

27. Moyes LH, McKee RF. A review of surgical nutrition. Scott Med J 2008;53:38–43.

28. Hartman C, Eliakim R, Shamir R. Nutritional status and nutritional therapy in inflammatory bowel diseases. World J Gastroenterol 2009;15:2570–8.

29. Royall D, Greenberg GR, Allard JP, et al. Total enteral nutrition support improves body composition of patients with active Crohn's disease. JPEN J Parenter Enteral Nutr 1995;19:95–9.

30. Rombeau JL, Barot LR, Williamson CE, et al. Preoperative total parenteral nutrition and surgical outcome in patients with IBD. Am J Surg 1982;143:139–43.

31. Lashner BA, Evans AA, Hanauer SB. Preoperative total parenteral nutrition for bowel resection in Crohn's disease. Dig Dis Sci 1989;34:741–6.

32. Lin MT, Saito H, Fukushima R, et al. Preoperative total parenteral nutrition influences postoperative systemic cytokine responses after colorectal surgery. Nutrition 1997;13:8–12.

33. Yao GX, Wang XR, Jiang ZM, et al. Role of perioperative parenteral nutrition in severely malnourished patients with Crohn's disease. World J Gastroenterol 2005;11:5732–4.

34. Makhdoom ZA, Komar MJ, Still CD. Nutrition and enterocutaneous fistulas. J Clin Gastroenterol 2000;31:195–204.

35. Teubner A, Morrison K, Ravishankar HR, et al. Fistuloclysis can successfully replace parenteral feeding in the nutritional support of patients with enterocutaneous fistula. Br J Surg 2004;91:625–31.

36. Lloyd DA, Gabe SM, Windsor AC. Nutrition and management of enterocutaneous fistula. Br J Surg 2006;93:1045–55.

37. Coull DB, Tait RC, Anderson JH. Vitamin B-12 deficiency following restorative proctocolectomy. Colorectal Dis 2007;9:562–6.

38. Buckman SA, Heise CP. Nutrition considerations surrounding restorative proctocolectomy. Nutr Clin Pract 2010;25:250–6.

39. Hakala K, Vuoristo M, Luukkonen P, et al. Impaired absorption of cholesterol and bile acids in patients with ileoanal anastomoses. Gut 1997;41:711–77.

40. M'Koma AE, Lindquist K, Liljeqvist I. Biochemical laboratory data in patients before and after restorative proctocolectomy: a study on 83 patients with follow up of 36 months. Ann Chir 1994;48:525–34.

41. ElMuhtaseb MS, Duncan A, Talwar DK, et al. Assessment of dietary intake and trace element status in patients with ileal pouch-anal anastomosis. Dis Colon Rectum 2007;50:1553–7.

42. Pironi L, Miglioli M, Ruggeri E, et al. Nutritional status of patients undergoing ileal pouch-anal anastomosis. Clin Nutr 1991;10:292–7.

43. Steenhagen E, de Roos NM, Bouwman CA, et al. Sources and severity of self-reported food intolerance after ileal pouch-anal anastomosis. J Am Diet Assoc 2006;106:1459–62.

44. Alles MS, Katan MB, Salemans JM, et al. Bacterial fermentation of fructooligosaccharides and resistant starch in patients with an ileal pouch-anal anastomosis. Am J Clin Nutr 1997;66:1286–92.

45. M'Koma AE, Lindquist K, Liljeqvist L. Observations in the blood lipid profile in patients undergoing restorative proctocolectomy. Int J Surg Investig 2000;2: 227–35.

46. Welters CF, Heineman E, Thunnissen FB, et al. Effect of dietary inulin supplementation on inflammation of pouch mucosa in patients with an ileal pouch-anal anastomosis. Dis Colon Rectum 2002;45:621–7.

47. Yan F, Polk DB. Probiotics: progress towards novel therapies for intestinal diseases. Curr Opin Gastroenterol 2010;26:95–101.

48. Laake KO, Bjørneklett A, Aamodt G, et al. Outcome of four weeks' intervention with probiotics on symptoms and endoscopic appearance after surgical reconstruction with a J-configurated ileal-pouch-anal-anastomosis in ulcerative colitis. Scand J Gastroenterol 2005;40:43–51.

49. Cottone M, Orlando A, Modesto I. Postoperative maintenance therapy for inflammatory bowel disease. Curr Opin Gastroenterol 2006;22:377–81.

50. Llopis M, Antolin M, Carol M, et al. *Lactobacillus casei* downregulates commensals' inflammatory signals in Crohn's disease mucosa. Inflamm Bowel Dis 2009; 15:275–83.
51. Gionchetti P, Rizzello F, Morselli C, et al. High-dose probiotics for the treatment of active pouchitis. Dis Colon Rectum 2007;50(12):2075–82.
52. Basse L, Thorbel JE, Lossl, et al. Colonic surgery with accelerated rehabilitation or conventional care. Dis Colon Rectum 2004;47:271–7.
53. Andersen J, Kehlet H. Fast track open ileo-colic resections for Crohn's disease. Colorectal Dis 2005;7:394–7.
54. Fasth S, Hultén L, Magnusson O, et al. The immediate and long-term effects of postoperative total parenteral nutrition on body composition. Int J Colorectal Dis 1987;2:139–45.
55. Fasth S, Hultén L, Magnusson O, et al. Postoperative complications in colorectal surgery in relation to preoperative clinical and nutritional state and postoperative nutritional treatment. Int J Colorectal Dis 1987;2:87–92.
56. Senkal M, Geier B, Hannemann M, et al. Supplementation of omega-3 fatty acids in parenteral nutrition beneficially alters phospholipid fatty acid pattern. JPEN J Parenter Enteral Nutr 2007;31:12–7.
57. Matarese LE, Seidner DL, Steiger E, et al. Practical guide to intestinal rehabilitation for postresection intestinal failure: a case study. Nutr Clin Pract 2005;20: 551–8.
58. Schwartz M, Regueiro M. Prevention and treatment of postoperative Crohn's disease recurrence: an update for a new decade. Curr Gastroenterol Rep 2011;13(1):95–100.
59. Ikeuchi H, Yamamura T, Nakano H, et al. Efficacy of nutritional therapy for perforating and non-perforating Crohn's disease. Hepatogastroenterology 2004;51: 1050–2.
60. Finco C, Magnanini P, Sarzo G, et al. Prospective randomized study on perioperative enteral immunonutrition in laparoscopic colorectal surgery. Surg Endosc 2007;21:1175–9.
61. Lee G, Buchman AL. DNA-driven nutritional therapy of inflammatory bowel disease. Nutrition 2009;25:885–91.
62. Han PD, Burke A, Baldassano RN, et al. Nutrition and inflammatory bowel disease. Gastroenterol Clin North Am 1999;28:423–43.
63. Seidner DL, Lashner BA, Brzezinski A, et al. An oral supplement enriched with fish oil, soluble fiber, and antioxidants for corticosteroid sparing in ulcerative colitis: a randomized, controlled trial. Clin Gastroenterol Hepatol 2005;3:358–69.
64. Trebble TM, Arden NK, Wootton SA. Fish oil and antioxidants after the composition and function of circulating mononuclear cells in Crohn disease. Am J Clin Nutr 2004;80:1137–44.

Nutritional Support in Acute and Chronic Pancreatitis

John P. Grant, MD

KEYWORDS

• Pancreatitis • Nutrition • Nutritional support

ACUTE PANCREATITIS

About 300 per 1 million individuals develop acute pancreatitis each year. The clinical spectrum ranges from a mild, self-limited, edematous form, in which patients often do not seek medical attention; to an acute, necrotizing, or hemorrhagic pancreatitis in which mortality may be as great as 80%. In some patients, the disease develops into a chronic relapsing variant. The clinical diagnosis of acute pancreatitis is based on characteristic nausea and abdominal pain localized to the upper abdomen that typically penetrates through to the back. Patients are often found sitting with their arms folded over in front, bending over at the waist. The diagnosis is confirmed by an increase of the serum concentrations of amylase and lipase, an increased white blood count (WBC), and fever.

Causes of pancreatitis include gallstone disease, abdominal trauma, hyperlipidemia, general anesthesia, viral infections, alcohol, trauma, and some medications (azathioprine, thiazides, and estrogens). Pancreatitis is now recognized as a complex inflammatory condition similar to inflammatory bowel disease. Patients with mutations in genes linked to cationic and anionic trypsinogen, serine protease inhibitor Kazal 1, cystic fibrosis transmembrane conductance regulator, chymotrypsinogen C, and calcium-sensing receptor have been shown to be at increased risk of pancreatitis when exposed to these causes.[1] Obesity seems to increase risks for progression to severe pancreatitis.[2]

DETERMINATION OF SEVERITY

Based on the Atlanta criteria,[3] approximately 75% of patients experience mild disease, with a mortality of less than 1%.[4] Mortality increases up to 20% if the disease progresses to its severe necrotizing form,[5–10] and, in the most severe cases, mortality can increase to 30% to 40%.[9,10] In some patients, the inflammation may lead to

The author has nothing to disclose.
Duke University Medical Center, Durham, NC, USA
E-mail address: grant003@mc.duke.edu

Surg Clin N Am 91 (2011) 805–820
doi:10.1016/j.suc.2011.04.005
0039-6109/11/$ – see front matter © 2011 Published by Elsevier Inc.

complications such as pseudocyst, fistula, and abscess. Several scoring indices have been developed and are used as early predictors of severity and survival.

RANSON SCORE

In 1974, Ranson and colleagues[11] identified 5 criteria related to the severity of pancreatitis (**Box 1**). In their experience, if 3 or more of these criteria were present at the time of admission, more than 60% of patients subsequently expired of the disease during that hospitalization. Six other clinical criteria had a significant impact on outcome if they developed in the first 48 hours after admission.

BEDSIDE INDEX FOR SEVERITY IN ACUTE PANCREATITIS SCORE

The Bedside Index for Severity in Acute Pancreatitis (BISAP) score can be derived on admission based on the following risk factors: blood urea nitrogen (BUN) greater than 25 mg/dL, impaired mental status, presence of the systemic inflammatory response syndrome, age greater than 60 years, and the presence of pleural effusions. The presence of 3 or more factors represents a high risk for morbidity and mortality.[12]

ACUTE PHYSIOLOGY AND CHRONIC HEALTH EVALUATION II SCORE

Studies suggest that the Acute Physiology and Chronic Health Evaluation (APACHE) II score is accurate in predicting prognosis. Although cumbersome to calculate, it can be fully calculated at the time of admission. Internet sites are available to aid in calculations (http://www.sfar.org/scores2/apache22.html). It is recommended that APACHE II scores be generated during the first 3 days of hospitalization and thereafter as needed to help identify and follow high-risk patients.[12] A score greater than or equal to 8 is associated with a poor prognosis.

Box 1
Ranson criteria

- Signs within first 24 hours
  - Age greater than 55 years
  - Blood glucose greater than 200 mg/dL
  - WBC greater than 16,000/mm^3
  - Lactate dehydrogenase greater than 700 IU/L
  - Aspartate aminotransferase greater than 250 U/L
- Signs within first 48 hours
  - Hematocrit decrease greater than 10%
  - Calcium less than 8.0 mg/dL
  - Base deficit greater than 4 mEq/L
  - Blood urea nitrogen increase greater than 5 mg/dL
  - Fluid sequestration greater than 6 L
  - Partial pressure of arterial oxygen (Pao$_2$) less than 60 mm Hg

Data from Ranson JH, Rifkind KM, Roses DF, et al. Prognostic signs and the role of operative management in acute pancreatitis. Surg Gynecol Obstet 1974;139:69–81.

COMPUTED TOMOGRAPHY SEVERITY INDEX

Balthazar and colleagues[13] identified 2 radiographic factors useful in predicting those patients who will develop severe pancreatitis: the amount of edema, or inflammation, and the amount of necrosis of the pancreas on computed tomography (CT). The amount of pancreatic edema is estimated from an unenhanced CT of the pancreas: grade A, normal; grade B, diffuse enlargement of the pancreas without peripancreatic inflammatory changes; grade C, enlarged pancreas with haziness and increased density of peripancreatic fat; grade D, enlarged body and tail of pancreas with fluid collection in peripancreatic spaces; grade E, extensive fluid collections in lesser sac and anterior pararenal space. Each grade is assigned a severity number from grade A = 0 to grade E = 4. The degree of pancreatic necrosis is estimated from enhanced CT of the pancreas, with no necrosis assigned a severity number of 0; up to 30%, 2; from 31% to 50% necrosis, 4; and more than 50%, 6. The severity numbers for edema and necrosis are added together to estimate the severity of the disease (**Table 1**).

Because the full extent of pancreatic necrosis does not usually develop until 72 to 96 hours after the onset of the disease, it might be argued that CT scanning should only be performed in selected patients after 4 to 5 days following admission. However, Vriens and colleagues[14] evaluated application of the Balthazar CT Severity Index within 48 hours of admission and found it to be an excellent prognostic tool for complications and mortality. Patients with a score of 0 to 3 could safely be discharged from the intensive care unit (ICU) and managed in a regular hospital bed, whereas all others were best kept in the ICU.

MECHANISMS LEADING TO SEVERE ACUTE PANCREATITIS

The following scenario for the progression of mild to severe acute pancreatitis, although not proven and likely to change somewhat, is the most favored, based on current research.

Pancreatitis is initiated by release of inappropriately activated zymogen digestive enzymes within the acinar cell, coupled with lysosomal hydrolase cathepsin-B, with conversion of trypsinogen to trypsin and subsequent autodigestion. Any oral intake during the first 24 hours can stimulate the injured pancreas to produce more secretions, producing even more injury. The expanding pancreatic injury results in the release of cytokines (mainly interleukin 1 and tumor necrosis factor) that cause release of nitric oxide, platelet aggregating factor, oxygen free radicals, elastase, and multiple other interleukin products, all leading to development of the systemic inflammatory response syndrome (SIRS). Investigative efforts to suppress or avoid the cytokine response are showing some early promise; however, these efforts have not yet achieved clinical use.

Of recent interest is the role that the intestine likely plays in disease progression. To minimize pancreatic stimulation, it has been standard practice to initiate immediate bowel rest. However, the reduction in luminal nutrients, with possibly glutamine

Table 1 Balthazar CT severity index		
Mild	**Moderate**	**Severe**
0–3	4–6	7–10
Percent Morbidity/Mortality		
3/10	35/6	92/17

depletion or cytokine effect, can lead to loss of gut integrity with increased permeability and release of more cytokines and their products.[15] These products, in turn, lead to vascular leakage, acute respiratory distress syndrome, hypovolemia, and shock.[16,17]

The loss of gut integrity also promotes luminal bacterial interaction with the gut-associated lymphoid tissue and upregulates systemic immunity. Activation of macrophages and stimulation and proliferation of Th1 CD4 helper lymphocytes results in a proinflammatory process. Continued starvation of the patient leads to a reduction in antiinflammatory Th2 lymphocytes and secretory IgA-producing immunocytes, and eventually to a toxin-producing pathogenic bacterial overgrowth of the intestine, further aggravating SIRS.

CLINICAL MANAGEMENT

Clinical management of patients with acute severe pancreatitis must concentrate initially on the restoration of blood volume and electrolyte balance. Replacement of fluid lost or fluid sequestered into third spaces is critical to maintain microcirculation, thereby minimizing pancreatic ischemia and subsequent reperfusion injury. The amount of fluid required is often underestimated, and commonly totals more than 6 L. The adequacy of volume replacement can in part be monitored by normalization of the BUN and serum sodium.

The inciting factor should be addressed, such as removal of a common bile duct gallstone by endoscopic retrograde cholangiopancreatography (ERCP), control of hypertriglyceridemia, and avoidance of any toxins such as alcohol or medications. Subsequent surgical exploration is indicated by the need for continued pressor support, even after adequate volume replacement; development of vital organ failure in spite of adequate support; general deterioration of the medical status; proven or suspected pancreatic abscess; or when the diagnosis is not clear, and some other surgical catastrophe might be present. Whenever possible, a feeding jejunostomy should be placed during any intra-abdominal procedure.

Pulmonary support with oxygen or intubation should be provided as indicated. Broad-spectrum antibiotics are best given to treat specific infections. Prophylactic antibiotic administration remains controversial, with some studies showing reduced need for surgery, decreased incidence of major organ failures, and reduced mortality,[18–20] whereas others do not.[21] Narcotics are required to control pain. Use of H_2 blocker agents remains of unproven value.

NUTRITIONAL SUPPORT

In addition to the clinical interventions mentioned earlier, early initiation of nutritional support seems to have a significant impact on eventual outcome, especially when provided enterally and especially when given to a patient with moderate to severe acute pancreatitis.[22–24] The possible role of nutrition in modulating the cytokine response was first reported by Mochizuki and colleagues[25] in 1984. They reported on the impact of gastric feeding on survival in a guinea pig burn model. They subjected the pigs to a 30% body surface burn and began gastric tube feedings at full support 2 hours or 72 hours later, or at 115% support beginning after 72 hours. Only the animals given full support beginning 2 hours after the burn had a minimal metabolic response, and most survived. All other animals showed a marked hypermetabolic response, and most expired. Although not suspected at that time, the probable explanation for the observed impact of early enteral feeding was that these feedings preserved gut integrity and aborted the early cytokine response, allowing healing and recovery. Subsequently, Wang and colleagues[26] confirmed a similar benefit of early enteral feeding in patients with burns. They found that the resting energy expenditure decreased by an average of 27% in the first 14 postburn days when early enteral feeding was given, compared with delayed enteral feedings (mean resting energy expenditure was 139% of normal in early enterally fed patients and 160% of normal in delayed enterally fed patients). Other studies, reviewed later, confirm that early enteral and parenteral nutrition in pancreatitis, but especially early enteral nutrition, reduce complications and improve survival. Most studies suggest that there is a narrow window of about 72 hours within which this effect can be obtained, consistent again with the known onset of the cytokine response.

OPTIMAL FEEDING FORMULATIONS

Provision of nutrition should minimally stimulate exocrine pancreatic secretions and, perhaps, suppress secretions. Infusion of any hypertonic solution into the jejunum decreases pancreatic exocrine secretion. Intravenous infusions of amino acids and hypertonic glucose have been shown not to stimulate exocrine secretion.[27] However, water and bicarbonate pancreatic exocrine secretion is stimulated by acid and by meat extracts in the duodenum, and by antral distention. Enzyme secretion is stimulated by long-chain fatty acids (LCFA), protein, calcium, and magnesium in the duodenum; and by the process of eating as well as antral distention. Intravenous lipid emulsions and oral medium-chain fatty acids (MCFA) do not seem to stimulate pancreatic secretion. Ideal feeding solutions for patients with acute pancreatitis, which might be expected to decrease exocrine function are discussed later.

Enteral

Enteral feeding includes peptide-based formula, low LCFA (MCFA enriched), hypertonic solutions given into the jejunum. Standard formulas will likely be less well tolerated, but may be satisfactory in some patients. Inadequate data are available to evaluate effectiveness of special formulas such as glutamine-enriched, multifiber, or probiotic supplemented products.

Parenteral

Parenteral feeding includes crystalline amino acids and hypertonic glucose (intravenous fat in sufficient dosage to meet essential fatty acid requirements).

ESTIMATING AND MEETING METABOLIC NEEDS
Caloric

Experience has shown that metabolic expenditure during acute pancreatitis seldom exceeds what might be expected with other stressful events. Four older studies have evaluated the metabolic expenditure of patients with acute pancreatitis (**Table 2**).[28–31]

Although each study was small, it seems that a patient's energy expenditure is somewhere between 1.23 and 1.49 times that predicted from the Harris-Benedict equation. Energy expenditure varies with time and with clinical conditions and that these estimates only represent averages. Owing to patient variability, the best method for determination of energy requirements in acute pancreatitis remains performance of indirect calorimetry whenever it is available.

Table 2 Caloric expenditure in acute pancreatitis			
Author	No. of Patients	RQ	MEE
Van Gossum et al[28]	4	0.81	2080
Bouffard et al[29]	6	0.87	2525
Dickerson et al[30]	5	0.78	26 kcal/kg
Velasco et al[31]	23	0.86	1687
Average ratio MEE/Harris-Benedict EE = 1.24			

Abbreviations: EE, energy expenditure; MEE, measured energy expenditure; RQ, respiratory quotient.

Nitrogen

In general, 1.0 to 1.5 g/kg/d protein are required, depending on the degree of stress. When in doubt, a 24-hour nitrogen balance study can be helpful if renal function is normal. Use of branched-chain enriched amino acid solutions has not been studied specifically in acute pancreatitis but, theoretically, could provide a source of energy for skeletal muscle in the presence of severe glucose intolerance.

Glucose

Providing glucose in excess of maximal glucose use is of no clinical value and may be of some harm. In 1979, Burke, and colleagues[32] showed that the conversion of intravenously administered labeled glucose to labeled carbon dioxide was maximal at a rate of 6 mg/kg/min. They further showed that a maximal benefit of glucose loading during stress with respect to whole body protein synthesis occurred with 4.7 to 6.8 mg/kg/min glucose infusion. Infusions at lower rates resulted in a reduced protein synthesis, and infusions at a higher rate were associated with no further increase in protein synthesis. Black and colleagues[33] studied maximal glucose uptake and use in patients in intensive care compared with nonstressed patients and found a marked decrease in glucose disposal from 9.46 mg/kg/min in normal subjects to only 6.23 mg/kg/min in stressed patients. It is therefore recommended that stressed patients receive a maximum of 5 to 6 mg/kg/min glucose as a caloric substrate.

Attempts at improving glucose use using high-dose insulin have successfully shown depression of blood sugar concentrations,[34] but no study has shown improved glucose oxidation, improved nitrogen balance, or improved whole body protein synthesis. There are some potential adverse side effects of insulin loading that militate against its routine use. Insulin strongly stimulates uptake of amino acids by the skeletal muscle, which, although not clinically confirmed, may alter or deplete the amino acid pool sufficiently to interfere with normal protein synthesis. Another more pertinent side effect of insulin loading is its inhibition of pyruvate dehydrogenase, the critical enzyme for entry of glucose intermediates into the Krebs cycle for oxidative metabolism.[35] As glucose infusion is increased, pyruvate, the anaerobic end product of glucose metabolism, builds up in tissues. A relative block of pyruvate dehydrogenase by increasing concentrations of insulin favors diversion of pyruvate to fat synthesis, an energy consuming process. So instead of benefits from high insulin infusion, energy is consumed in production of an unnecessary substrate: fat. The process of fat synthesis is associated with increased carbon dioxide production, which may stress the respiratory system, especially if significant chronic obstructive pulmonary disease is present. In general, administration of more than 60 units of insulin daily should be avoided, and carbohydrate infusion should be reduced instead.

Fat

At a minimum, essential fatty acids must be given in required doses. Intravenous lipid emulsions seem to be well tolerated, but care must be taken to ensure that the fat is cleared from the blood if it is used as a caloric source. Standard enteral feeding formulas containing fat are often well tolerated, but a product with decreased LCFA and increased MCFA is preferred. The efficiency of fat use as an energy source diminishes as the level of stress increases, rendering fat a poor caloric source in severe pancreatitis.

Other

In addition to provision of adequate nutrients, adequate supplementation of the anabolic electrolytes is critical, because dramatic consumption can occur with onset of anabolism. These electrolytes are potassium, magnesium, and phosphorus. Calcium must also be monitored and supplemented as needed. Ample B-complex vitamins (especially thiamin in an alcoholic patient) and maintenance amounts of fat-soluble vitamins should be given. Consideration should be given to providing oral pancreatic enzymes when an oral diet is resumed.

ENTERAL FEEDING

In many critical care disease states, studies support the concept of an early window of opportunity after admission (36 hours), during which initiation of nutritional support may change the clinical outcome. Similar data are accumulating in the management of acute pancreatitis. Of 6 prospective randomized controlled trials of enteral versus parenteral nutrition, 5 showed significant positive effects on clinical outcome if feedings were started within 48 hours of admission.[36–41] In these 5 studies, although benefits were observed in both feeding groups, enteral nutrition was superior in decreasing infectious morbidity, shortening hospital length of stay, reducing overall complications, and resulting in faster resolution of the SIRS. The sixth study randomized patients after 4 full days of hospitalization, and no significant impact of feeding was observed.[42] In 2000, Schneider, and colleagues[43] evaluated patients with acute severe pancreatitis who were admitted to the ICU and received either nasogastric or jejunostomy enteral nutrition. Patients were only given total parenteral nutrition (TPN) when enteral nutrition was persistently inadequate or when this route was contraindicated (eg, high-volume small bowel fistula). Of 69 patients with acute severe pancreatitis, the median APACHE II score was 18 (range 4–40), and the overall hospital mortality was 39%. Seventeen patients were managed with enteral feedings alone, 10 with TPN alone, and 19 with a combination of both. Twenty-three did not have any nutritional support during their ICU stay. The mortality was higher among patients who received TPN alone compared with those who had at least some enteral nutrition (60% vs 24%).

Other studies have documented that early enteral feeding reduces the incidence of gastric stasis and intestinal ileus.[44–46]

To administer enteral feeding successfully, a clear perception of intolerance must be understood. There are 4 clinical responses to be managed.

Gastric Residuals

Residual volumes have been used by physicians, dietitians, and nurses for many years as objective measures to judge tolerance or intolerance to enteral tube feedings. Recently, studies have raised considerable doubt as to the value of declaring any arbitrary residual volume as unacceptable and have pointed out how rigid rules related to residual volumes have at times rendered enteral nutritional support of limited value. The following are suggestions to improve clinical practice:

- Whenever residual volumes are measured, they should be interpreted along with the appearance of the patient's abdomen and any complaints of fullness or discomfort.
- Abdominal distention can be caused by gas-filled loops of bowel from aerophagia and may not be caused by increased gastric residual volume; this will not improve with interruption of the feedings.
- The amount of residual volume is often greatest during the first several hours after feeding is begun. With continued feeding, the residual volume tends to plateau and then decrease.[47,48]
- The amount of gastric residual volume is dependent on the infusion rate. Computer models have shown that, because of the complex relationship between infusion volume, gastric emptying, and gastric capacity, evaluation of the volume of gastric contents is an unreliable method for monitoring feeding tolerance.[49,50]

Nearly All Patients Show an Increase in Trypsin, Amylase, and Lipase

Although these indicators nearly always increase as enteral feedings are started, these increases are rarely associated with clinical symptoms or any adverse clinical effects. If symptoms are absent, the serologic changes should be ignored, and the feeding solution should be continued.[51]

Exacerbation of Abdominal Pain

Up to 21% of patients may experience an uncomplicated exacerbation of abdominal pain, especially with transition to an oral diet. Returning to enteral feedings usually quickly resolves the symptoms.[52] Only about 4% of patients truly worsen when enteral feedings are begun, and these patients should be transitioned to parenteral feedings.

CLINICAL EXPERIENCE: PARENTERAL NUTRITION DURING ACUTE PANCREATITIS

Parenteral nutrition should only be attempted on failure of enteral feedings. Sax and colleagues[53] randomized 54 patients with mild pancreatitis (1.1 ± 0.2 Ranson criteria) to receive either standard intravenous fluids or TPN. There was no difference between the groups with respect to total hospital days, number of complications of pancreatitis, or days to oral intake. Catheter-related sepsis occurred more frequently in the TPN group than in other patients receiving TPN (10.5% vs 1.5%). Robin and colleagues[54] reported on the administration of TPN to 70 patients with mild to moderate pancreatitis (average Ranson criteria 1.66) and 86 with moderate to severe pancreatitis (average Ranson criteria 2.2). Average age was 39 years, and 79% of the patients developed pancreatitis caused by alcohol intake. Fifty-five percent of patients required insulin (average 69 U/d). Overall mortality was only 4%, and only 3 episodes of catheter-related sepsis occurred. The TPN was well tolerated and nutritional status was improved. Sitzmann and colleagues[55] administered TPN to 73 patients with moderate to severe pancreatitis (average 2.5 Ranson criteria), and 81% had improved nutritional indices following therapy. Sixty percent of patients required insulin for hyperglycemia (average of 35 U/d). Mortality was 10 times greater if a positive nitrogen balance was not achieved. Goodgame and Fisher[56] reported on treatment of 46 patients with severe acute pancreatitis using TPN. They found minimal technical and metabolic complications and reported that nutritional requirements were easily met. In spite of improved nutritional care, little effect was observed on the course of the acute pancreatitis. Of concern was a high incidence of catheter-related sepsis (17% occurring primarily during the first 14 days of therapy).

Perhaps the most interesting report has been that of Kalfarentzos and colleagues[57] in 1991. They administered TPN to 67 patients with severe pancreatitis (>3 Ranson criteria). Average age was 58 years, and 85% of patients developed pancreatitis caused by gallstones. They provided Harris-Benedict recommendation for calories, 1.5 to 2.5 g/kg/d protein, and 300 mL of a 10% lipid emulsion twice a week. The fat emulsion was well tolerated. There was an increased incidence of catheter-related sepsis (8.9% vs 2.9% in other patients receiving TPN). Hyperglycemia occurred in 88% of patients and required an average of 46 U/d insulin. Nutritional status improved in all patients. Twelve patients developed complications of a pseudocyst or pancreatic fistula, all of which resolved while continuing to receive TPN, and none require surgical intervention. However, their most striking finding was a 23.6% complication rate and 13% mortality if TPN were started within 72 hours of onset of symptoms, compared with a 95.6% complication rate and a 38% mortality if started later. Their findings again emphasize the possible role of early nutrition in reduction of the cytokine response.

In 2005, Chandrasegaram and colleagues[58] reported on changes in body composition, plasma proteins, and resting energy expenditure during parenteral nutrition in 15 patients with acute pancreatitis, 13 of whom had severe pancreatitis. Using neutron activation analysis and tritium dilution studies, they found that body composition was preserved during 14 days of parenteral nutrition. In patients without sepsis or recent surgery, body protein stores were significantly increased.

Although enteral nutrition is preferred, there is an apparent beneficial role for parenteral nutrition when enteral feedings are not tolerated.

SUMMARY SUGGESTIONS FOR NUTRITIONAL MANAGEMENT DURING ACUTE PANCREATITIS
Mild Pancreatitis

If admission severity scores are low, observation is indicated. Patients should be placed nil per os until blood chemistries and symptoms nearly resolve, at which time an oral diet can be resumed. If symptoms worsen or persist beyond 5 days, enteral nutrition should be initiated, preferably via a nasojejunal tube, but, if not achievable, via a nasogastric tube, and contrast-enhanced CT should be considered to identify fluid collections, pancreatic necrosis, or other complications that may require intervention.

Moderate Pancreatitis

If symptoms are more significant, or the Balthazar CT Severity Index is 4 to 6, and if intestinal motility is adequate, enteral nutrition via a nasojejunal feeding tube (if not feasible, then a nasogastric tube) should be initiated within 48 hours of admission.

The feeding formula should be peptide based and low in LCFA. If additional fat is necessary, it should be given intravenously or as MCFA. Extra vitamins, trace elements, minerals, and electrolytes may be needed based on the clinical course. Care must be taken to avoid complications of glucose intolerance, giving insulin as required. Jejunal feedings may also be well tolerated by patients who have undergone exploratory laparotomy, at which time a feeding jejunostomy should be placed.

If Balthazar CT Severity Index is 4 to 6, and if intestinal motility is not adequate, patients may initially be followed. If motility recovers, enteral feedings should be started. If no recovery of motility is observed, consideration should be given to initiating intravenous nutrition within 48 hours.

Severe Pancreatitis

When the APACHE II score is greater than or equal to 10 or the Balthazar CT Severity Index is greater than 6, fluid resuscitation should be initiated immediately. Within 48 hours of admission, and after fluid resuscitation, patients should have a nasojejunal tube passed under fluoroscopy, with injection of contrast material to evaluate intestinal motility. If satisfactory antegrade motility is present, jejunal tube feedings should be begun using a peptide-based, low LCFA feeding formula. If retrograde motility is observed, or if an ileus is present, intravenous nutrition should be begun within 48 hours of admission. A balanced amino acid solution should be administered intravenously using hypertonic dextrose and appropriate electrolyte, vitamin, and mineral supplementation. Administration of 3-in-1 solutions seems to be safe, but each patient should be closely monitored to assure that the lipid is cleared from the blood (serum lipid levels should be monitored and ideally kept within normal limits). Close observation for glucose intolerance and catheter-related infections must be maintained to ensure patient safety.

As the severity of acute pancreatitis resolves and gastrointestinal function returns, the patient should be converted to enteral nutrition via nasojejunal feeding. With further improvement, conversion to an oral diet should be attempted.

Resolving Pancreatitis

As the severity of acute pancreatitis resolves, heralded by a decrease in temperature, normalization of the WBC, reduction in serum amylase and lipase, and decrease in abdominal pain, consideration can be given to beginning an oral diet. The risk of beginning an oral diet too soon is stimulation of the pancreas with reactivation of pain and acute pancreatitis. Levy and colleagues[59] studied this problem to determine factors that might predict patients at risk for starting an oral diet. They reported an incidence of recurring pain following refeeding, requiring cessation of feeding in 21% of patients studied. Pain relapse occurred mainly in those patients with a long period of pain, necrotic acute pancreatitis (Balthazar score of ≥3), and with serum lipase concentrations greater than 3 times normal just before refeeding. When refeeding is begun, the diet need not be limited to clear liquids, but can be initiated with a low-fat soft diet and advancement to high-protein, high-calorie, low-fat, solid diet as tolerated.[60] Supplementation with pancreatic enzymes and insulin may be necessary.

SPECIAL CONSIDERATIONS
Pancreatic Necrosis/Abscess

Pancreatic necrosis occurs as diffuse or focal areas of nonviable pancreatic tissue. It usually develops during the first few days of pancreatitis secondary to hypoperfusion. Observation is indicated, because surgery within the first few days of onset of severe acute pancreatitis is associated with rates of death up to 65%. Furthermore, in the early stages, no clear demarcation is evident between viable and nonviable tissue. Delaying pancreatic debridement for at least 2 weeks is recommended. In a recent study, enteral nutrition was considerably more effective in preventing pancreatic necrosis during severe pancreatitis than intravenous nutrition (23% vs 72%).[61]

If infection of the necrotic material is suspected based on leukocytosis and fever, fine-needle aspiration should be performed, guided by either CT or ultrasonography, with Gram staining and culturing of the aspirate. The diagnosis of a pancreatic abscess mandates immediate intervention; antibiotics alone cannot resolve the infection, but are required in the perioperative period. In no event should drainage be delayed for nutritional support. Surgery remains the treatment of choice, with open debridement and wide drainage of the peripancreatic area.[62] Planned reoperations may be required to remove all necrotic material. Recently, various percutaneous drainage approaches have been proposed; however, their results have not been compared prospectively with open surgery. Twenty-four hours after drainage has been accomplished, nutritional support (preferably enteral) should be initiated or resumed.

Pancreatic Pseudocyst

Up to 57% of patients have at least 1 fluid collection evident on CT.[63] Increased serum amylase concentration is the hallmark of a developing pseudocyst and does not necessarily indicate a worsening of the pancreatic inflammation. These collections are usually managed conservatively and resolve spontaneously. If the fluid collections continue to enlarge, cause pain, or compress adjacent organs, then medical, endoscopic, or surgical intervention may be needed. Onset and progression of a fever and an increased WBC suggest development of an infected pseudocyst and mandates immediate evaluation and probable drainage. There seems to be no aggravation of pseudocysts secondary to instillation of enteral feedings into the jejunum, and bowel rest with or without TPN has not been shown to be of any added benefit in their treatment. If the pseudocyst decreases in size in 2 to 3 weeks, surgery should be delayed. If the pseudocyst is unaltered or enlarged, internal surgical drainage should be performed after 6 weeks, when the pseudocyst wall usually matures satisfactorily to hold a suture.

Pancreatic Ascites

Ascites in alcoholic patients with pancreatitis must be differentiated from cirrhotic ascites. A peritoneal aspirate of the ascitic fluid will contain high levels of amylase if the ascites originates from pancreatitis. Although little has been published on the treatment of pancreatic ascites, it seems that some cases resolve spontaneously. In general, it is recommended that TPN, bowel rest, and medical care be provided for at least 2 weeks, anticipating spontaneous resolution. If the ascites persists after 2 weeks, ERCP should be performed to evaluate possible disruption of the pancreatic duct. If leakage is found in the tail or body of the pancreas, a distal pancreatectomy is curative. If a leak is seen from a pseudocyst or from the duct in the head of the pancreas, internal drainage to an intestinal segment should be considered. If no leak is identified on ERCP, either TPN can be continued for another 2 to 4 weeks with a repeat study, or an empirical distal pancreatectomy can be performed.

CHRONIC PANCREATITIS
Malnutrition of Chronic Pancreatitis

Patients with chronic pancreatitis often suffer progressive malnutrition caused by decreased dietary intake, malabsorption, surgical and diagnostic procedures, and recurrent infections. The reduced dietary intake is mostly a consequence of chronic pain, commonly aggravated by oral intake. Unpalatable dietary restrictions for pancreatitis-related diabetes mellitus can also reduce intake. Malabsorption, when present, is caused by pancreatic insufficiency and characterized by steatorrhea.

Suggested Clinical Management

The first effort should consist of manipulation of an oral diet. Carefully designed dietary modifications, with reduced dietary fat, along with provision of pancreatic enzyme supplementation, can be effective in restoring and maintaining nutritional status in up to 80% of patients.[64]

If dietary modulation does not improve nutrient intake and absorption, and especially if nutrient intake is complicated by abdominal pain, consideration should next be given to initiating enteral nutrition. The patient should be hospitalized, and a nasojejunal tube should be placed. A trial of a low-fat, peptide-based, enteral feeding formula should be given, beginning slowly and advancing progressively to full support, and then cycling to nighttime feedings only. If this regimen is successful, consideration can be given to placing a feeding jejunostomy laparoscopically to allow for home enteral nutrition. The first article published using home enteral nutrition in patients with chronic pancreatitis was by Cromer and Grant[65] in 2000. They reported on their experience with home enteral nutrition from 1994 to 1999 in 33 patients referred for intravenous nutrition. These patients underwent placement of a feeding jejunostomy and were discharged on home enteral feedings. Causes for the pancreatitis included 8 alcohol, 10 idiopathic, 6 gallstones, 3 after ERCP, 3 pancreatic cancer, 2 after surgery, and 1 hypertriglyceridemia. All patients were advanced to full enteral support without aggravation of their abdominal pain, and there were no exacerbations of pancreatitis during home care requiring interruption of feedings. Nonetheless, 27 patients required readmission during their home care for complications unrelated to their feedings. Average duration of home enteral feeding was 127 days (range 11–888, with 1 patient still on home therapy after 2067 days). Comparing nutritional status from beginning to end of therapy with respect to blood proteins and body weight, of 26 initially malnourished patients, 16 improved, 4 were unchanged, and 6 became worse (3 had pancreatic cancer, and 3 were poorly compliant with administration of feedings). Of the 33 patients, 26 eventually underwent surgical intervention for debridement (3 deaths), resection, or ductal drainage, following which 19 resumed an oral diet, 4 were still receiving enteral support, and 1 required home intravenous nutrition. They concluded that use of home enteral nutrition was effective in most patients in maintaining or repleting nutritional status, without aggravation of abdominal pain. Surgery could either be delayed until nutritional repletion had been accomplished, or avoided altogether.

In 2002, Yoder and colleagues[66] reported on 33 patients with chronic pancreatitis who were discharged on jejunal feedings using a standard polymeric formula. Seventy-seven percent of patients achieved nutritional goals with minimal complications. In 2005, Stanga and colleagues[67] established home enteral nutrition using jejunal access in 57 patients. They reported a significant reduction in abdominal pain, nausea, vomiting, and diarrhea; decrease in narcotic use from 95% of patients to 27%; and restoration of nutritional status based on weight gain, serum albumin, and subjective global assessment. A standard enteral diet was tolerated by 86% of patients. In addition, they noted a reduction in the need for surgery, compared with that reported in the literature, from a published level between 58% and 67% to only 14%.

NUTRITIONAL NEEDS
Caloric Requirements

Caloric needs are similar to those in other malnourished patients, because there is usually only minimal stress present. Modifications of the Harris-Benedict formula can be used, and the caloric source should be divided between glucose and fat in a balanced standard formula.

Nitrogen Requirements

Nitrogen requirements are also similar to those in other malnourished patients, because there is usually only minimal stress present, and initial nitrogen supplementation should be 0.8 to 1.0 g/kg/d. Once feeding is begun, adjustments can be made in nitrogen support until a neutral or positive balance is achieved.

In addition to standard nutrients, adequate supplementation of the anabolic electrolytes is given (potassium, magnesium, and phosphorus). Calcium is monitored and supplemented as needed. As most patients are vitamin deficient, ample B-complex vitamins must be provided as well as maintenance fat-soluble vitamins orally. Insulin and pancreatic enzymes are administered as indicated.

SUMMARY

Nutrition support can have a significant beneficial impact on the course of moderate to severe acute pancreatitis. Enteral nutrition is preferred, with emphasis on establishment of jejunal access; however, parenteral nutrition can also be of value if intestinal failure is present. Early initiation of nutrition support is critical, with benefits decreasing rapidly if begun after 48 hours from admission. Severe malnutrition in chronic pancreatitis can be avoided or treated with dietary modifications or enteral nutrition.

REFERENCES

1. Whitcomb DC. Genetic aspects of pancreatitis. Annu Rev Med 2010;61:413–24.
2. Martinez J, Sanchez-Paya J, Palazon JM, et al. Is obesity a risk factor in acute pancreatitis? A meta-analysis. Pancreatology 2004;4:42–8.
3. Bradley EL. A clinically based classification system for acute pancreatitis: summary of the International Symposium on Acute Pancreatitis, Atlanta, GA, September 11–13, 1992. Members of the Atlanta International Symposium. Arch Surg 1993;128:586–90.
4. Winslet M, Hall C, London NM, et al. Relationship of diagnostic serum amylase to aetiology and prognosis in acute pancreatitis. Gut 1992;33:982–6.
5. Bradley EL. Indications for surgery in necrotizing pancreatitis: a millennium review. J Pancreas 2000;1:1–3.
6. Ashley SW, Perez A, Pierce EA, et al. Necrotizing pancreatitis: contemporary analysis of 99 consecutive cases. Ann Surg 2001;234:572–80.
7. Buchler MW, Gloor B, Muller CA, et al. Acute necrotizing pancreatitis: treatment strategy according to the status of infection. Ann Surg 2000;232:619–26.
8. Slavin J, Ghaneh P, Sutton R, et al. Management of necrotizing pancreatitis. World J Gastroenterol 2001;7:476–81.
9. Flint R, Windsor J, Bonham M. Trends in the management of severe acute pancreatitis: interventions and outcome. ANZ J Surg 2004;74:335–42.
10. Karsenti D, Bourlier P, Dorval E, et al. Morbidity and mortality of acute pancreatitis. Prospective study in a French university hospital. Presse Med 2002;31: 727–34.
11. Ranson JHC, Rifkind KM, Roses DF, et al. Prognostic signs and the role of operative management in acute pancreatitis. Surg Gynecol Obstet 1974;139:69–81.
12. Papachristou GI, Muddana V, Yadav D, et al. Comparison of BISAP, Ranson's, APACHE-II, and CTSI scores in predicting organ failure, complications, and mortality in acute pancreatitis. Am J Gastroenterol 2010;105:435–41.
13. Balthazar EJ, Robinson DL, Megibow AJ, et al. Acute pancreatitis: value of CT in establishing prognosis. Radiology 1990;174:331–6.
14. Vriens PW, van de Linde P, Slotema ET, et al. Computed tomography severity index is an early prognostic tool for acute pancreatitis. J Am Coll Surg 2005; 201:497–502.

15. Ammori BJ, Leeder PC, Kingm RF, et al. Early increase in intestinal permeability in patients with severe acute pancreatitis: correlation with endotoxemia, organ failure, and mortality. J Gastrointest Surg 1999;3:252–62.
16. Norman J. The role of cytokines in the pathogenesis of acute pancreatitis. Am J Surg 1998;175:76–83.
17. Inagaki T, Hoshino M, Hayakawa T, et al. Interleukin-6 is a useful marker for early prediction of the severity of acute pancreatitis. Pancreas 1997;14:1–8.
18. Nordback I, Sand F, Saaristo R, et al. Early treatment with antibiotics reduces the need for surgery in acute necrotizing pancreatitis-A single-center randomized study. J Gastrointest Surg 2001;5:113–20.
19. Pederzoli P, Bassi C, Vesentini S, et al. A randomized multicenter clinical trial of antibiotic prophylaxis of septic complications in acute necrotizing pancreatitis with imipenem. Surg Gynecol Obstet 1993;176:480–3.
20. Bassi C, Larvin M, Villatoro E. Antibiotic therapy for prophylaxis against infection of pancreatic necrosis in acute pancreatitis. Cochrane Database Syst Rev 2003; 4:CD002941.
21. Nathens AB, Curtis JR, Beale RJ, et al. Executive summary: management of the critically ill patient with severe acute pancreatitis. Proc Am Thorac Soc 2004;1: 289–90.
22. Al Samaraee A, McCallum IJ, Coyne PE, et al. Nutritional strategiew in severe acute pancreatitis: a systematic review of the evidence. Surgeon 2010;8(2):105–10.
23. Dimagno MJ, Wamsteker EJ, Debenedet AT. Advances in managing acute pancreatitis. Med Rep 2009;1:59.
24. Olah A, Romics L Jr. Evidence-based use of enteral nutrition in acute pancreatitis. Langenbecks Arch Surg 2010;395:309–16.
25. Mochizuki H, Trocki O, Dominioni L, et al. Mechanism of prevention of postburn hypermetabolism and catabolism by early enteral feeding. Ann Surg 1984;200: 297–310.
26. Wang S, Wang S, You Z. Clinical study of the effect of early enteral feeding on reducing hypermetabolism after severe burns. Zhonghua Wai Ke Za Zhi 1997; 35:44–7.
27. O'Keefe SJ, Lemmer ER, Ogden JM, et al. The influence of intravenous infusions of glucose and amino acids of pancreatic enzyme and mucosal protein synthesis in human subjects. JPEN J Parenter Enteral Nutr 1998;22:253–8.
28. Van Gossum A, Lemoyne M, Greig PD, et al. Lipid-associated total parenteral nutrition in patients with severe acute pancreatitis. J Parenter Enteral Nutr 1988;12:250–5.
29. Bouffard YH, Delafosse BX, Annat GJ, et al. Energy expenditure during severe acute pancreatitis. J Parenter Enteral Nutr 1989;13:26–9.
30. Dickerson RN, Vehe KL, Mullen JL, et al. Resting energy expenditure in patients with pancreatitis. Crit Care Med 1991;19:484–90.
31. Velasco NF, Papapietro KV, Rapaport JS, et al. Variabilidad del gasto calorico medido en pacientes con pancreatitis aguda: es posible obtener un factor de patologia confiable para estos casos?. Rev Med Chile 1994;122:48–52 [in Spanish].
32. Burke JF, Wolfe RR, Mullany CJ, et al. Glucose requirements following burn injury. Parameters of optimal glucose infusion and possible hepatic and respiratory abnormalities following excessive glucose intake. Ann Surg 1979;190:274–85.
33. Black PR, Brooks DC, Bessey PQ, et al. Mechanisms of insulin resistance following injury. Ann Surg 1982;196:420–35.
34. Taylor BE, Schallom ME, Sona CS, et al. Efficacy and safety of an insulin infusion protocol in a surgical ICU. J Am Coll Surg 2006;202:1–9.

35. Vary TC, Randle PJ. Effects of ischemia on the activity of pyruvate dehydrogenase complex in rat heart. J Mol Cell Cardiol 1984;16:723–33.
36. McClave SA, Greene LM, Snider HL, et al. Comparison of the safety of early enteral versus parenteral nutrition in mild acute pancreatitis. J Parenter Enteral Nutr 1997;21:14–20.
37. Kalfarentzos F, Kehagias J, Mead N, et al. Enteral nutrition is superior to parenteral nutrition in severe acute pancreatitis: results of a randomized prospective trial. Br J Surg 1997;84:1665–9.
38. Windsor AC, Kanwar S, Li AG, et al. Compared with parenteral nutrition, enteral feeding attenuates the acute phase response and improves disease severity in acute pancreatitis. Gut 1998;42:431–5.
39. Olah A, Pardave G, Belogyi T, et al. Early nasojejunal feeding in acute pancreatitis is associated with a lower complication rate. Nutrition 2002;18:259–62.
40. Abou-Assi S, Craig K, O'Keefe SJ. Hypocaloric jejunal feeding is better than total parenteral nutrition in acute pancreatitis: results of a randomized comparative study. Am J Gastroenterol 2002;97:2255–62.
41. Gupta R, Patel K, Calder PC, et al. A randomized clinical trial to assess the effect of total enteral and total parenteral nutritional support on metabolic, inflammatory, and oxidative markers in patients with predicted severe acute pancreatitis (APACHI II > or = 6). Pancreatoloty 2003;3:406–13.
42. Louie BE, Noseworthy T, Hailey D, et al. Enteral or parenteral nutrition for severe pancreatitis: a randomized controlled trial and health technology assessment. Can J Surg 2005;48:298–306.
43. Schneider H, Boyle N, McCluckie A, et al. Acute severe pancreatitis and multiple organ failure: total parenteral nutrition is still required in a proportion of patients. Br J Surg 2000;87:362–73.
44. Cravo M, Camilo ME, Marques A, et al. Early tube feeding in acute pancreatitis: a prospective study. Clin Nutrit 1989;8(Suppl):14.
45. Eatock FC, Brombacher GD, Steven A, et al. Nasogastric feeding in severe acute pancreatitis may be practical and safe. Int J pancreatol 2000;28(1):23–9.
46. Eatock FC, Chong P, Menezes N, et al. A randomized study of early nasogastric versus nasojejunal feeding in severe acute pancreatitis. Am J Gastroenterol 2005;100(2):432–9.
47. McClave SA, Snider HL, Lowen CC, et al. Use of residual volume as a marker for enteral feeding intolerance: prospective blinded comparison with physical examination and radiographic findings. JPEN J Parenter Enteral Nutr 1992;16:99–105.
48. McClave SA, Snider HL. Clinical use of gastric residual volumes as a monitor for patients on enteral tube feeding. J Parenter Enteral Nutr 2002;26(6 Suppl):S43–8.
49. Lin HC, Van Citters GW. Stopping enteral feeding for arbitrary gastric residual volume may not be physiologically sound: results of a computer simulation model. J Parenter Enteral Nutr 1997;21:286–9.
50. Burd RS, Lentz CW. The limitations of using gastric residual volumes to monitor enteral feedings: A mathematical model. Nutr Clin Pract 2001;16:349–54.
51. O'Keefe SJ, Broderick T, Turner, et al. Nutrition in the management of necrotizing pancreatitis. Clin Gastroenteral Hepatol 2003;1(4):315–21.
52. Levy P, Heresbach D, Pariente EA, et al. Frequency and risk factors of recurrent pain during refeeding in patients with acute pancreatitis: a multivariate multicenter prospective study of 116 patients. Gut 1997;40(2):262–6.
53. Sax HC, Warner BW, Talamini MA, et al. Early total parenteral nutrition in acute pancreatitis: lack of beneficial effects. Am J Surg 1987;153:117–24.

54. Robin AP, Campbell R, Palani CK, et al. Total parenteral nutrition during acute pancreatitis: clinical experience with 156 patients. World J Surg 1990;14:572–9.

55. Sitzmann JV, Steinborn PA, Zinner MJ, et al. Total parenteral nutrition and alternate energy substrates in treatment of severe acute pancreatitis. Surg Gynecol Obstet 1989;168:311–7.

56. Goodgame JT, Fischer JE. Parenteral nutrition in the treatment of acute pancreatitis. Ann Surg 1997;186:651–8.

57. Kalfarentzos FE, Karavias DD, Karatzas TM, et al. Total parenteral nutrition in severe acute pancreatitis. J Am Coll Nutr 1991;10:156–62.

58. Chandrasegaram MD, Plank LD, Windsor JA. The impact of parenteral nutrition on the body composition of patients with acute pancreatitis. JPEN J Parenter Enteral Nutr 2005;29:65–73.

59. Levy P, Heresbach D, Pariente EA, et al. Frequency and risk factors of recurrent pain during refeeding in patients with acute pancreatitis: a multivariate multicentre prospective study of 116 patients. Gut 1997;40:262–6.

60. Sathiaraj E, Murphy S, Mansard MJ, et al. Clinical trial: oral feeding with a soft diet compared with clear liquid diet as initial meal in mild acute pancreatitis. Aliment Pharmacol Ther 2008;28:777–81.

61. Wu XM, Ji KQ, Li GF, et al. Total enteral nutrition in prevention of pancreatic necrotic infection in severe acute pancreatitis. Pancreas 2010;39:248–51.

62. Sakorafas GH, Lappas C, Mastoraki A, et al. Current trends in the management of infected necrotizing pancreatitis. Infect Disord Drug Targets 2010;10:9–14.

63. Robert JH, Frossard JL, Mermillod B, et al. Early prediction of acute pancreatitis: prospective study comparing computed tomography scans, Ranson, Glascow, Acute Physiology and Chronic Health Evaluation II scores, and various serum markers. World J Surg 2002;26:612–9.

64. Meier R. Nutrition in chronic pancreatitis. In: Buechler M, Friess H, Uhl W, et al, editors. Chronic Pancreatitis. Berlin: Blackwell Science; 2002. p. 421–7.

65. Cromer M, Grant JP. Outcome study of home enteral nutrition patients with chronic pancreatitis. ASPEN 24th Clinical Congress Poster Session. Nashville (TN), January 25, 2000.

66. Yoder AJ, Parrish CR, Yeaton P. A retrospective review of the course of patients with pancreatitis discharged on jejunal feedings. Nutr Clin Pract 2002;17:314–20.

67. Stanga Z, Giger U, Marx A, et al. Effect of jejunal long-term feeding in chronic pancreatitis. J Parenter Enteral Nutr 2005;29:12–20.

The Surgical Treatment of Type Two Diabetes Mellitus

Walter J. Pories, MD[a,b,]*, James H. Mehaffey, BS[c],
Kyle M. Staton, BS[d]

KEYWORDS

• Diabetes mellitus • Bariatric surgery • RYGB • Gastric bypass

The concept that surgery can produce full and durable remission of type 2 diabetes mellitus (T2DM) seems to not make sense. How could a simple operation such as the gastric bypass (**Fig. 1**), a procedure that merely bypasses a segment of the intestine, reverse the most expensive, chronic, and deadly illness of the developed world?

It is a difficult question to answer because T2DM is still not well understood. According to the American Diabetes Association in 2009, the disease "is a metabolic disorder characterized by consistently elevated blood glucose" caused by secretion of insufficient amounts of insulin or by "insulin resistant" target cells, especially in muscle, which have an inadequate response to the insulin released. However, that classification of hyperglycemia allows the inclusion of two sharply different forms of diabetes: type 1 and type 2, as well as elevations of blood glucose due to other causes such as Cushing disease or the administration of steroids.

The authors have nothing to disclose.
[a] Division of Bariatric Surgery, Department of Surgery, The Brody School of Medicine, East Carolina University, 600 Moye Boulevard, Brody Medical Science 4W-48, Mail Stop 639, Greenville, NC 27834, USA
[b] Uniformed Services, University of the Health Sciences, 4301 Jones Bridge Road, Bethesda, MD 20814, USA
[c] The Brody School of Medicine at East Carolina University, 904 Spring Forest, Apartment E2, Greenville, NC 27858, USA
[d] The Brody School of Medicine at East Carolina University, 402-31 Treybrooke Circle, Greenville, NC 27834, USA
* Corresponding author. Department of Surgery, The Brody School of Medicine at East Carolina University, East Carolina University, 600 Moye Boulevard, Brody Medical Science 4W-48, Mail Stop 639, Greenville, NC 27858.
E-mail address: pories@aol.com

Surg Clin N Am 91 (2011) 821–836
doi:10.1016/j.suc.2011.04.008
0039-6109/11/$ – see front matter © 2011 Published by Elsevier Inc.

surgical.theclinics.com

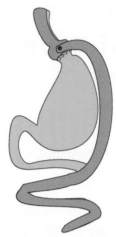

Fig. 1. Roux-en-Y Gastric Bypass, also known as the Greenville Gastric Bypass first described in 1980. This procedure is a prototypical gastric bypass. (*Courtesy of* Walter J. Pories, MD, Greenville, NC.)

TYPE 1 AND TYPE 2 DIABETES: TWO DIFFERENT DISEASES WITH THE SAME NAME

If the discussion is limited to the two variations of diabetes, there are two "types." Type 1 diabetes mellitus (T1DM), also known as juvenile onset or insulin-dependent diabetes, is the result of the patient's immune system, apparently stimulated by a viral infection, attacking and destroying pancreatic β-cells, the only cells in the body that synthesize and secrete insulin. Often, in a matter of just a few weeks, the destruction of the β-cells results in insulin levels that are too low to sustain life. Autoimmune, genetic, and environmental factors are among the major predisposing and contributing causes leading to the development of T1DM, which currently accounts for 5% to 10% of all cases of diabetes. Currently, there is no way to prevent T1DM, although promising research into preventative vaccinations is under way.[1] The progress in the prevention and control of T1DM is remarkable. A universally fatal disease only 100 years ago now responds well to treatment with insulin, insulin pumps, diet, and exercise, allowing patients with T1DM to live into their sixties. Transplantation of islets or intact pancreas from organ donors is now proving to be modestly successful.

The efforts to control T2DM offer a much less encouraging story. This disease differs sharply from T1DM and it accounts for more than 90% of cases. The onset of T2DM is gradual and occurs primarily in the later years of life. The cause or causes are unknown, although it has a genetic predisposition.

Obesity is often considered a cause of the disease because the prevalence of T2DM has risen parallel to the increases in the body mass index (BMI), which is measured in kilograms per meters squared. However, even this association is clouded. Although the increasing prevalence of obesity is accompanied by a similar rise in T2DM, 10% of patients with T2DM are lean, and two-thirds of the severely obese are not diabetic.

On the other hand, these two apparently distinct diseases show considerable overlap. The complications of the two types are the same: blindness, peripheral vascular disease leading to amputations, renal failure, and a four times higher prevalence of stroke and heart disease. Whether these complications are due to the hyperglycemia, high insulin levels, insulin resistance, or other factors is still not clear.

THE SILENT EPIDEMIC

The United States public responds rapidly to the spread of infectious disease, whether it is a localized outbreak of food-borne salmonella or an increased reporting of the flu. However, there has been remarkably little concern about the rapid increase of T2DM, a far more deadly disease. In spite of the development of new drugs, investigations into molecular pathways, and public education efforts, the number of Americans diagnosed with T2DM tripled from 1980 to 2007, rising from 5.6 million to 17.4 million cases. Estimates of undiagnosed cases of T2DM in the United States continue to rise steadily. The World Health Organization estimates that by 2030 the United States will have 30.3 million cases. Within the United States, 1 in 10 people over the age of 20 and 1 in 4 people over the age of 60 currently suffer from T2DM.

The epidemic of diabetes appears to be worsening. A recent study estimated that one in three Americans born in the year 2000 will develop diabetes during the course of their lifetime. African Americans, Hispanic or Latino Americans, American Indians, and native Hawaiians or other Pacific Islanders are at particularly high risk for T2DM and its complications. African Americans have a 70% higher probability of developing diabetes over their lifetime in comparison with white Americans. The Southeastern regions of the United States currently have higher rates of diabetes than other regions.

T2DM: A SYSTEM-WIDE DISEASE

T2DM is associated with other metabolic abnormalities in a complex known as the "metabolic syndrome," a term that includes a broad spectrum of disease, including obesity, hypertension, nonalcoholic steatohepatitis (NASH), gastroesophageal reflux disease (GERD), sleep apnea, cardiopulmonary failure, asthma, polycystic ovary disease, infertility, cancer, atherosclerosis, depression, deep venous disease, pulmonary emboli, arthritis of weight-bearing joints, epigenetic changes in offspring, neuropathy, increased risk of infection, and renal failure.[2]

T2DM has serious social implications for patients and their families because it is a chronic, lifelong disease. Because the disease is systemic in nature, the treatment generally requires lifelong medication and daily blood glucose checks, as well as major changes in lifestyle. Successful management of diabetic patients necessitates strict adherence to diet regimens and adoption of healthier daily habits pertaining to exercise and physical activity in addition to pharmacologic intervention. As with most chronic diseases, living with T2DM results in a lower quality of life that must be taken into account when considering the nominal success of medical management compared with surgical intervention, which is the only known "cure" for the disease.

THE FAILURE OF CURRENT THERAPIES

A medical cure for patients suffering from T2DM does not exist.[3] At best, current medical therapies are targeted to lower blood glucose and decrease peripheral insulin resistance associated with T2DM. Medical treatment has had limited success maintaining safe blood glucose levels in patients as evidenced in part by the high number of diabetic amputations and blindness. In the United States, over 60% of all nontraumatic amputations of the lower extremity are in patients with diabetes, with more than 85% being precipitated by a foot ulcer deteriorating to deep infection or gangrene.[4] With a 3% to 8% prevalence of foot ulcers in the diabetic population due to uncontrolled high blood glucose, this serious health problem requires immediate attention. Over 90% of patients who have diabetes for over 10 years will suffer from diabetic retinopathy and it is the leading cause of blindness in diabetic patients.[5] Diabetes is the number one cause of new onset blindness in all persons age 20 to 74, and approximately 24,000 new cases of blindness due to diabetic retinopathy are reported each year.[1] With the minimal success of medical treatment, attention must be given to a more permanent cure for this disease that has debilitated so many patients.

The chronic progressive nature of T2DM results in a costly medical management with significant financial consequences. In 2007, the total estimated cost of diabetes was $174 billion, including $116 billion in excess medical expenditures and $58 billion in reduced national productivity. Of the latter, $26.9 billion is from loss of productivity due to early mortality, $20 billion is from reduced productivity at work, and $0.8 billion is from unemployment caused by disease-related disability. Medical expenditures, on average, are 2.3 times higher for diabetic patients than for patients without the disease. Within the United States, one in five health care dollars is used for the treatment of a diabetic patient. These statistics illustrate both the weakness of medical treatment and the need for a better treatment to combat diabetes.[1,6]

Numbers alone fail to represent the full spectrum of negative effects associated with T2DM; the costly and frustratingly ineffective medical management of the disease further exacerbates the associated consequences.[7] Current medical management of diabetes leaves much to be desired, requiring constant vigilance from both the patient and the physician. The problem is that family physicians lack the tools to control obesity (perhaps not a cause but certainly a factor in T2DM), and to regulate diets, exercise, behavior, and appropriate control of glucose levels, especially since tight control has proved to be dangerous.[8] Further, medical treatment provides little to no amelioration of symptoms and lacks the capacity to cure the underlying disease.[6,9]

The statistics are disturbing, but abstract. They come into sharp focus, however, with the recognition that T2DM is the primary cause of blindness, kidney failure, and amputation in the United States, as well as a leading cause of stroke and heart attacks.

BARIATRIC SURGERY: A SURPRISING ANSWER

In 1980, during a prospective clinical trial of the Greenville gastric bypass, the authors were the first to note the remission of T2DM. We were puzzled by the postoperative euglycemia in five consecutive patients and, initially, ascribed the normal glucose levels to a misdiagnosis of diabetes and laboratory errors. However, we were convinced by the sixth patient (**Table 1**) who was admitted on November 16, 1980 with a plasma glucose of 495 mg/dL in spite of the preoperative administration of 90 units of insulin. The operation was conducted with intravenous insulin control, and we were prepared for difficulties in controlling her glucose in the postoperative period. However, on the first postoperative day, her insulin requirement was only 8 units and November 22 (postoperative day 6), was the last day that she required insulin. The remission has lasted through 10 years of follow-up.

When our series of the Greenville Roux-en-Y gastric bypass (RYGB) reached 608 patients, 165 patients had T2DM and another 165 had impaired glucose tolerance (IGT). Omitting those that had their operation within the previous 6 months, we found that 121 out of 146 (83%) of the T2DM patients and 150 or the 152 (99%) of the IGT patients had returned to euglycemia.[10] These results were later corroborated by Schauer and colleagues,[11] who also found a full rate of remission of T2DM in 83% of a total of 1160 patients. Nor were these changes merely in blood chemistry. A comparison was made of 154 patients who underwent RYGB with another 78 patients who were scheduled for, but did not undergo the surgery because of a lack of insurance coverage, or for personal reasons. Those patients who underwent RYGB surgery had a mortality rate of 14 out of 154 (9%) in 9 years, or 1% per year, versus those who

Table 1
Remission of T2DM following the Greenville gastric bypass operation[a]

Date	Glucose	Insulin Given
16 November 1980 Preoperative/Operative	495	90
17 November	281	8
18 November	308	16
19 November	240	8
20 November	210	4
21 November	230	8
22 November	216	4
28 November	193	0
30 November	153	0
14 December	155	0

[a] The sixth diabetic patient undergoing Roux-en-Y Gastric Bypass by Pories et al. She was admitted on November 16, 1980, with a plasma glucose of 495 mg/dL in spite of the preoperative administration of 90 units of insulin. The operation was conducted with intravenous insulin and preparations were made for difficulties in controlling her glucose in the postoperative period. However, on the first postoperative day, her insulin requirement was only 8 units and November 22, the 6th postoperative day, was the last time she required insulin. The remission lasted at least through 10 years of follow-up.

Data from Pories W. "Understanding Diabetes: what can we learn from bariatric surgery?" Presented at Surgical Grand Rounds. Boston (MA): Cleveland Tufts Medical Center; 2010.

did not, who had a mortality rate of 22 out of 78 (28%), or 4.5% per year, a reduction of mortality by 78% ($P<.003$).[12] Similar reductions of mortality were reported by Sjostrom.[13] Meta-analysis, led by Buchwald and colleagues,[14] showed similar reductions. In a review of 621 studies published in the English language from 1990 to 2006, including 135,000 patients and 888 treatment arms, there was 83.7% resolution of T2DM after RYGB. Of interest was the finding that a more extensive exclusion of food from the foregut by the biliopancreatic diversion produced a 98.9% resolution rate. T2DM was resolved in 98.9% of patients undergoing biliopancreatic diversion; whereas adjustable gastric banding, an operation that only reduces intake, produced a rate of remission of only 47.9% and did so only after 2 to 3 years. Scopinaro and colleagues[15] reported a 97% diabetes remission rate in 312 patients, which was maintained at 10 years postoperative follow-up in patients undergoing biliopancreatic diversion. In short, the rate of remission is "dose related" to the degree of exclusion of food from the gut.[16]

Although the mechanism behind the resolution of T2DM following gastric bypass remains elusive, recent evidence demonstrates that the results are not caused solely by weight loss. In most cases, remission is observed directly after surgery (**Fig. 2**), whereas it is usually weeks to months following the operation before any substantial weight loss has occurred. Recently researchers have provided evidence that these results may be achievable in the nonobese population as well. Several human studies have shown dramatic diabetes control in patients with BMI less than 35 kg/m^2. Lee and colleagues[17] showed that 89.5% of diabetic patients with BMI less than 35 kg/m^2 had returned to euglycemia 1 year after gastric bypass. Lee and colleagues[17] also found the mean hemoglobin A1C level reduced from 7.3% preoperatively to 5.6% at 1 year postoperatively. The benefits of diabetes resolution accomplished by surgery are significant and clear. Diabetes-related mortality rates were followed for a period of 7 years after RYBG and were found to be decreased 92% in comparison with control patients. Christou and colleagues[18] used a retrospective review of 23,803 morbidly obese

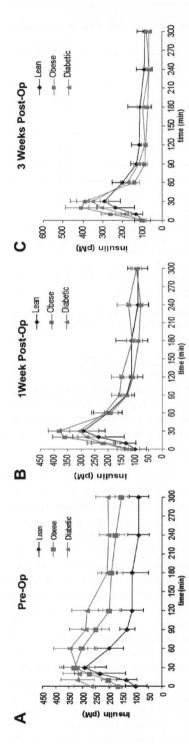

Fig. 2. Gastric bypass patient response to Oral Glucose Tolerance Test (OGTT) at different stages of treatment. (*A*) Before operation: reveals abnormal OGTT in diabetic and obese patients. (*B, C*) Demonstrates normalization of OGTT at 1 week and 3 weeks post-operation in diabetic and obese patients, respectively. (*Data from* Pories WJ, et al. Diabetes the evolution of a new paradigm. Ann Surg 2004;239(1):12–3.)

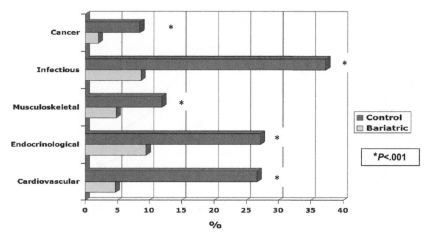

Fig. 3. Comparison of 5-year comorbidities between bariatric surgery patients and a matched group who did not have bariatric surgery. All comorbidities (cancer, infections, musculoskeletal, endocrinological, and cardiovascular) were found to have significant reductions (P<.001). (*Data from* Christou NV, Sampalis JS, Liberman M, et al. Surgery decreases long-term mortality, morbidity, and health care use in morbidly obese patients. Ann Surg 2004;240(3):416–23.)

patients, 5347 of whom had diabetes, to show that survival rates were increased, and comorbidities were decreased in surgical patients compared with the nonsurgical group (P<.001) (**Fig. 3**). Survival benefits occur as early as 6 months postoperatively for patients aged less than 65 years and as early as 11 months in patients aged more than 65 years.[6,19] Despite these compelling data, the decision to operate should be made based on a risk factor assessment for each patient.

MECHANISM OF REMISSION

One theory explaining resolution of T2DM in patients undergoing gastric bypass implicates foregut factors as contributors to diabetes. When foregut diversion occurs, as it does with RYGB, absence of such factors improves glycemic control. Because glycemic response to surgery seems to correlate with the extent of the foregut diversion (RYGB>Billroth II>Billroth I>lap band), it is hypothesized that the distal stomach and duodenum play an integral role.[20,21] In fact, follow-up studies done at our group examining nonobese patients undergoing gastric bypass or resection for cancer or ulcer disease, supports this hypothesis.[22] Zervos and colleagues[22] demonstrated that the same significant cure rates of T2DM seen in morbidly obese (BMI>35 kg/m^2) patients, 83%, can be reproduced in less obese (BMI 30–35 kg/m^2), overweight, or nonobese (BMI<30 kg/m^2) patients undergoing RYGB surgical anatomic derangements.

The rapid resolution of T2DM following the RYGB indicates that resolution of T2DM cannot be explained solely by decreased caloric intake and weight loss. This concept has been validated in a lean-animal model of diabetes in which nonobese Goto-Kakizaki rats rapidly resolve their spontaneous diabetes after gastric bypass, independent of weight loss or caloric intake, and quickly relapse after normal anatomy is restored.[23] Rubino and colleagues[23] performed oral glucose tolerance test (OGTT) in three groups of diabetic rats. Group 1 was managed by diet only, Group 2 had a sham procedure with no change in anatomy, and Group 3 underwent a gastrointestinal bypass. Only Group 3 showed an improvement in glucose tolerance (**Fig. 4**).

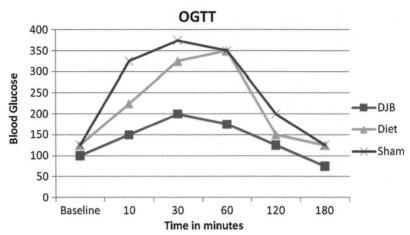

Fig. 4. The glycemic response curve after an OGTT in nonobese Goto-Kakizaki rats. There are three test groups: (1) those that underwent a duodenal-jejunal bypass (DJB), (2) those that underwent a sham procedure where there was no change in anatomy, and (3) those that had no procedure except a low-fat diet. There is normalization of the DJB group but no significant change in the sham and diet group. (*Data from* Rubino F, et al. Effect of duodenal-jejunal exclusion in a non-obese animal model of type 2 diabetes: a new perspective for an old disease. Ann Surg 2004;239:1–11.)

These animal models have provided the ability to reach beyond speculation in explaining the effects of gastric or proximal intestinal diversion on T2DM, leading to a few human studies describing small numbers of nonobese patients who underwent ileal interposition or minilaparoscopic gastric bypass with the sole intent of resolving diabetes or the metabolic syndrome. Each study has shown improvement in glycemic control in diabetic patients, albeit less pronounced than that observed in patients undergoing gastric bypass or restrictive procedures for obesity.[24–26]

Since the discovery that gastric bypass surgery leads to the rapid reversal of T2DM in morbidly obese patients, researchers have been searching for possible mechanisms to explain the result. One experiment compared the results of oral versus intravenous glucose tolerance tests in patients with T2DM with those of healthy individuals to determine the importance of gut signaling in the insulin response. The results suggest that signaling from the gut inhibits glucagon suppression in response to an oral glucose bolus compared with an equivalent intravenous load. The leading theory aimed at explaining this observation implicates the so-called enteroinsular axis, a group of hormones secreted by the gut that have a significant effect on beta cell secretion of insulin, insulin resistance in the periphery, glycogenolysis, and gluconeogenesis.[27] The two most established members of the incretin family of hormones are glucagon-like peptide (GLP-1), which increases in concentration from the proximal to the distal gut, and pro-glucose-dependent insulinotropic polypeptide (GIP), which decreases distally. They are known to have favorable effects on glycemic control, although their exact mechanisms are uncertain. Incretins are secreted in response to nutrient ingestion and are known to increase beta cell mass and to decrease insulin resistance. One theory, proposed for the pathogenesis of diabetes infers that anti-incretin hormones are released by the stimulated foregut, exacerbating diabetes in the presence of normal anatomy, but improving diabetes when the unstimulated (bypassed) foregut fails to secrete these anti-incretin factors. In addition to the effects of increased levels of such hormones on the bypassed and unstimulated foregut, it has been further theorized that relatively undigested foodstuffs exposed to the distal intestinal mucosa (as occurs with gastric bypass or biliopancreatic diversion) may also cause rapid and significant increase in incretins.[28]

There is some dispute in the literature regarding the exact mechanism that leads to the defect in incretin signaling from the gut. Currently, there are two theories, the "foregut hypothesis" and the "hindgut hypothesis," each of which argue that the signaling from its respective portion is critical in its effects on the diabetic state. Several studies have been done to determine which is most important, but there is no clear answer yet. The foregut hypothesis states that the surgical bypass of the duodenum either gives rise to an antidiabetic signal or prevents the diabetic signal. It is not clear what the signal may be, but GIP is a favored molecule for this mechanism because it is produced by K cells in the duodenum, and decreased GIP secretion has been shown to protect against obesity and metabolic malfunctions associated with T2DM. The hindgut hypothesis states that the surgical rerouting of nutrients to the ileum allows for increased secretion of GLP-1, leading to increased glucagon suppression and insulin sensitivity. One issue with the hindgut hypothesis are the data from the old bariatric vertical banded gastroplasty (VBG) procedure, which indicated an improvement in T2DM in some patients despite the lack of nutrient rerouting to the ileum. The VBG procedure is no longer performed, due to safety concerns. Therefore, more research needs to be done with nutrient-limiting procedures without gastric rerouting before there is sufficient data to be certain which portion of the gut plays the most significant role in hormonal signaling in the diabetic state. Investigation into the pathophysiological basis of diabetes continues with the hope of discovering optimal therapeutic targets. However, currently, RYGP is the only option that has been shown to cure T2DM.[12,21]

OPERATIVE PROCEDURES

The four operations shown in **Fig. 5** are the most commonly performed bariatric surgical operations. They are described below in detail but, in essence, all represent approaches to reducing contact between food and the gut. The band does so by

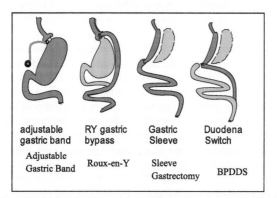

Fig. 5. The four bariatric procedures currently accepted for weight loss in obese patients and treatment of metabolic syndrome: (1) adjustable gastric banding, a strictly restrictive procedure; (2) RYGB, which has both restrictive and malabsorptive components and has been successful in the treatment of metabolic syndrome with a cure rate of 83%; (3) sleeve gastrectomy, another strictly restrictive procedure used for treatment of morbid obesity; and (4) biliopancreatic diversion with duodenal switch, a more radical restrictive and malabsorptive procedure with high efficacy as a treatment of metabolic syndrome eliciting a 95% cure rate. (*Courtesy of* Walter J. Pories, MD, Greenville, NC.)

decreasing intake, the others add to this effect by altering the intestinal signaling systems.

Laparoscopic Adjustable Gastric Band

Laparoscopic adjustable gastric banding is solely a restrictive procedure. A band is wrapped around the proximal stomach, just below the gastroesophageal junction. Weight loss is achieved through the reduction of the gastric reservoir to about 30 cc and delayed emptying due to the restriction of the gastric outlet to about 1 cm. After only a few bites of food, the stomach becomes distended, limiting the patient's intake. The amount of gastric restriction is adjusted through injection or withdrawal of saline from the inflatable plastic core of the band.[29] The idea of gastric banding began in 1976 with Wilkonson, who originally used Marlex mesh to form the stomach into a smaller hourglass shape. Wilkonson later revised his procedure to include wrapping the entire stomach with Marlex mesh. Molina next explored the use of nylon and other materials for the band itself. The adjustable silicone gastric banding (ASGB) was introduced by Kuzmak in 1989. ASGB uses a Dacron-reinforced silicone band with an inflatable inner section. A nonkinking tube leading to a self-sealing subcutaneous reservoir containing saline connects to the inflatable inner section. With the use of an electronic sensor, safe and effective adjustment of the band is possible. During the 1990s, a shift was made toward the laparoscopic placement of the band instead of an open procedure in an attempt to reduce the morbidity and injury related to the procedure. The benefits of laparoscopic adjustable gastric banding include two favorable features: (1) no actual cutting or stapling of the stomach and (2) a calibrated pouch and stoma size which are adjustable to meet specific patient needs. Laparoscopic removal of the band is possible allowing this procedure to be fully reversible procedure and, typically, only a short hospital stay is required rarely exceeds 48 hours.[29]

RYGB

Gastric bypass is considered a malabsorptive and restrictive procedure because it both decreases the absorptive surface area and reduces the size of the stomach. The gastric bypass procedure was first described by Mason and Ito[30] in 1967. It has undergone many modifications and improvements over the past 45 years. The first procedure had three major components: a small gastric pouch to limit intake, a gastrojejunostomy to limit gastric emptying, and a bypass of the stomach and duodenum to interfere with absorption and digestion.[31] As time progressed, several changes were made to overcome the common problems associated with the procedure. A major obstacle in the development of a superior gastric bypass procedure was the problem of biliary reflux common in the original procedure. In 1977, Griffin and colleagues[32] published the first report describing the Roux-en-Y modification to prevent the biliary reflux common with the original jejunal loop reconstruction. Buchwald[31] showed endoscopic, chemical, and histologic evidence that the Roux-en-Y modification was superior to the jejunal loop in preventing bile reflux. In 1987, Torres and Oca[33] described the long limb gastric bypass (LLGB) in a failed Roux-en-Y bypass patient, by moving to a 150 cm Roux-en-Y limb in the jejunum as opposed to the 75 cm limb previously used. The LLGB demonstrated superior weight loss with no significant rise in malnutrition or other complications.

The Greenville gastric bypass limited the gastric pouch size to 20 to 30 mL, which resulted in an early feeling of satiety due to decreased release of ghrelin from the P/D1 cells lining the fundus of the stomach.[6] Ghrelin is the counterpart of the satiety hormone leptin that is secreted from adipose tissue. A small gastric pouch also induces dumping syndrome, a desired side effect of the surgery. Dumping syndrome occurs when food is moved too quickly from the stomach to the intestine, resulting in abdominal pains, sweating, palpitations, light headedness, and diarrhea.[31] The symptoms are generally associated with a spike in enteroglucogon, a peptide hormone secreted by mucosal cells of the intestine to delay gastric emptying. Dumping encourages patients to not try to overcome their bypass by eating many small snacks throughout the day that are high in carbohydrates, especially sugar, which increases the symptoms. Another modification added by the Greenville gastric bypass was the reduction of the gastrojejunal anastomosis to 8 to 10 mm from the 2 to 5 cm used in the original operation. The wider anastomosis led to severe dumping syndrome and provided for a less pronounced reduction in ghrelin secretion, which prolonged the onset of the satiety signal during eating. The original procedure described by Mason provided for a single staple line in which the stomach was divided to create the gastric pouch, but which resulted in gastric rupture in a majority of patients. After adding the modification of a double staple line, the 10-year complication rate due to gastric rupture decreased to 20%. The Greenville gastric bypass adds a third suture line, which reduced the gastric rupture rate to less than 2%. Later, it was determined that the stomach did not need to be physically separated from the pouch because this added technical challenges to the procedure and had a 6% failure rate due to formation of a gastrogastric fistula.[34]

Today the procedure is usually performed as a laparoscopic operation, resulting in a less invasive method and a shorter recovery. As with all operations, the laparoscopic procedure is similar to the open technique but has some variations due to the nature of the approach. In 1994, Wittgrove and colleagues[35] described an endoscopic procedure to introduce the anvil of an end-to-end stapler into the gastric pouch, allowing a good line for gastric division. Torre and Scott[36] improved the technique in 1999 by introducing the anvil intra-abdominally to achieve control that is more precise. The same year, Higa and colleagues[37] described a hand-sewn procedure to reduce the incidence of gastrojejunal leakage.[34] When performing any gastric bypass procedure, it is critical to ensure that all anastomoses are secure without leakage. The gastric staple lines should also be double checked to confirm that there is no leakage. After checking all anastomoses, the bowel should be checked for viability and blood supply by observing the color. If the blood supply to the bowel is insufficient, the procedure needs to be redone. In the instance of a failed bariatric procedure, an operation can be done in which the gastric pouch is separated from the stomach vertically and anastomosed, end to end, to the Roux-en-Y loop.[38]

Sleeve Gastrectomy

The sleeve gastrectomy was first performed as an open procedure but now is done almost exclusively laparoscopically. It is a restrictive procedure that reduces the size of the stomach 85% by excising the greater curvature and reconstructing a tubularized stomach conduit. The resultant smaller stomach inhibits patients from overeating and provides for an earlier decrease in release of ghrelin, leading to satiety earlier during the meal.[39] Since there is no malabsorptive component to the procedure, maximal weight loss is generally not accomplished with the sleeve gastrectomy alone. In many severely obese patients who are high-risk surgery candidates, the procedure is used as stage one of a two-stage approach to weight loss. After the laparoscopic sleeve gastrectomy the patient will be reassessed and usually will undergo a Roux-en-Y gastric bypass 6 to 18 months later, after showing a reduction in operative risk and stabilization in weight.[40]

Biliopancreatic Diversion with Duodenal Switch

The biliopancreatic diversion with duodenal switch (BPDDS) bypass represents a combination of the gastric bypass and the intestinal bypass. It was found to produce a greater weight loss than is achievable with Roux-en-Y gastric bypass alone, but is associated with more complications. The BPDDS procedure includes a distal gastrectomy in addition to intestinal bypass. The safety of the BPDDS primarily depends on the strength and security of the anastomoses, whether hand sewn or stapled, and the maintenance of viable intestine. The integrity of the anastomoses is commonly tested using air or methylene blue. If the color of the gut is in question, blood flow must be assured, or the operation must be redone. Due to the increased risks associated with the BPDDS, most facilities prefer the Roux-en-Y procedure for surgical treatment of bariatric patients. However, the BPDDS is commonly used for surgical repair of previous unsuccessful bariatric surgical procedures.[41]

SAFETY

An increasing number of clinicians believe that, given the success of bariatric operations in treating diabetes, the profession should now advance toward the establishment of specific surgical treatments for diabetes. Before this move can be made, the benefits of the procedures must be weighed against the risks, and all possible complications and mortality of all procedures must be considered. Contrary to commonly held misperceptions, bariatric surgery is strikingly safe, both during the procedure and postoperatively. Buchwald and colleagues'[42] meta-analysis of 361 studies encompassing greater than 85,000 patients, early ($\leq$30 days) or late (30 days–2 years) mortality was 0.28% (95% CI 0.22–0.34) and 0.35% (0.12–0.58), respectively. This is consistent with more recent studies that report bariatric surgery mortality rates ranging from 0.25% to 0.5%. Most gastric bypasses are now conducted laparoscopically, which has led to a decrease in the invasiveness of the procedure. Rubino and colleagues[6] state "these mortality rates are comparable to those of patients undergoing laparoscopic cholecystectomy (0.26–0.6%), a commonly performed elective procedure." The recently accepted classification of obesity as a genuine disease has yet to change the perception of bariatric surgery. Many within the medical community consider bariatric surgery too drastic a procedure to be considered an elective procedure. Yet these same physicians consider coronary artery bypass graft, with mortality rates of 3.5%, a safe and effective treatment of coronary artery disease. Given the 0.5% mortality rates associated with bariatric surgery, there should be no reservations about further exploring the surgical treatment of obesity as well as T2DM.[6] Both the potential long-term benefits conferred by surgery and the low complication rates must be examined. Upon close examination, it will be found that surgery is a safe and effective treatment option.

INDICATIONS FOR BARIATRIC SURGERY

The basic indications suggested by the 1991 National Institutes for Health conference[43] still serve as the guidelines for most insurance carriers, with a few modifications:

1. Diets, exercise, behavioral modification, and drugs are not effective for the long-term management of the severely obese.
2. Patients should be considered as candidates for bariatric surgery if they
   a. are between the ages of 18 and 65 years
   b. have a BMI greater than or equal to 40 or a BMI greater than or equal to 35 with significant comorbidities
   c. understand the consequences of the surgery
   d. have no evidence of uncontrolled substance or alcohol abuse
   e. agree to long-term follow-up.

3. The surgery should be performed in a Bariatric Surgery Center of Excellence, certified by the American Society for Metabolic and Bariatric Surgery or the American College of Surgeons.

SURGICAL RECOMMENDATIONS

With four legitimate options available for the surgical treatment of obesity and T2DM, alternatives providing the best long-term solution with the least likelihood of a negative result must be examined. With over 20 years of data from thousands of patients, it is evident that each of the four operations has a place in the surgical armamentarium. The band may well be a good choice for a severely obese child or adolescent because it is fully reversible. In contrast, the duodenal switch may be the best operation for an older patient with a long history of T2DM. As with any abdominal surgery, there are risks, including bleeding, infection, and leak, in addition to those postoperative complications that accompany restrictive and malabsorptive surgeries such as malnutrition, emotional problems, internal hernias, and severe dumping syndrome. With the founding of Bariatric Surgery Centers of Excellence there is greater accountability, including quality control and site inspections, resulting in a risk comparable to childbirth (.11%).[44] In fact, the gastric bypass reduces the mortality from the metabolic syndrome; therefore, the surgical treatment is safer than medical therapy. Despite the higher weight loss and T2DM remission (95%) rates achieved with the BPDDS operation, there are significant risks with a procedure of this radical extent due to the large intestinal bypass. The other strictly restrictive procedures do not provide the high rate of T2DM remission achieved with the malabsorptive procedure; however, weight loss is significant and durable.[45] Pories[46] are confident with the recommendation of the Roux-en-Y procedure for the treatment of T2DM in both morbidly obese and overweight individuals.

COST

The metabolic syndrome is our worst and costliest epidemic, far exceeding breast cancer and HIV or AIDS. Countless comorbidities are associated with metabolic syndrome, including hypertension, NASH, GERD, sleep apnea, cardio-pulmonary failure, asthma, polycystic ovary disease, infertility, cancer, atherosclerosis, depression, deep venous disease, pulmonary emboli, arthritis of weight-bearing joints, epigenetic changes in offspring, and renal failure. Data from Pories[46] demonstrate that, before surgery, patients suffering from metabolic syndrome spend $10,592 per year on diabetic medications alone. After undergoing the Roux-en-Y procedure, the average expenditure falls to $1,875, a savings of over $8,700 a year. In analyses that used a lifetime timeline, projected future costs based on age and obesity, and discounted costs and health utilities at 3% per year, the cost to utility ratio for bariatric surgery versus no surgery was approximately $1,400 per quality-adjusted life-year gained.[47] T2DM is one of the fastest growing chronic debilitating diseases that will affect over 30 million Americans in our lifetime. Surgical intervention is the most cost-efficient treatment and is the only known cure to date.

SUMMARY

The significance of bariatric surgery is twofold. It offers hope and successful therapy to the severely obese; those with T2DM, sleep apnea, or polycystic ovary disease; and others plagued by the comorbidities of the metabolic syndrome. Even more important, however, is the provision of a model for the study of these chronic diseases, a model that allows the study of the abnormal molecular signals in man and, it is hoped, the future development of pharmaceutical approaches that will render surgery unnecessary.

REFERENCES

1. American Diabetes Association. Diabetes statistics 2009. Retrieved November 12, 2010, from American Diabetes Association. Available at: http://www.diabetes.org/diabetes-basics/diabetes-statistics/. Accessed April 15, 2011.
2. Ali MR, Marquire MB, Wolfe BM. Assessment of obesity-related comorbidities: a novel scheme for evaluating bariatric surgical patients. J Am Coll Surg 2006; 202:70–7.
3. American Diabetes Association. American Diabetes Association's clinical practice guidelines. Diabetes Care 2009;32:S1–97.
4. Jan Apelqvist JL. What is the most effective way to reduce incidence of amputation in the diabetic foot? Diabetes Metab Res Rev 2000;16(Suppl 1):S75–83.
5. Wiener RS, Wiener DC. Benefits and risks of tight glucose control in critically ill adults: a meta-analysis. JAMA 2008;300:933–44.
6. Rubino F, Schauer PR, Kaplan LM, et al. Metabolic surgery to treat type 2 diabetes: clinical outcomes and mechanisms of action. Annu Rev Med 2010;61:393–411.
7. World Health Organization. Diabetes fact sheet 2009. Retrieved October 11, 2010, from World Health Organization. Available at: http://www.who.int/mediacentre/factsheets/fs312/en/. Accessed April 15, 2011.
8. Action to Control Cardiovascular Risk in Diabetes Study Group, Gerstein HC, Miller ME, et al. Effects of intensive glucose lowering in type 2 diabetes. N Engl J Med 2008;358:2545–59.
9. Nathan DM, Buse JB, Davidson MB, et al. Medical management of hyperglycemia in type 2 diabetes: a consensus algorithm for the initiation and adjustment of therapy. Diabetes Care 2008;31:173–5.
10. Pories WJ, Caro JF, Flickinger EG, et al. The control of diabetes mellitus (NIDDM) in the morbidly obese with the Greenville gastric bypass. Ann Surg 1987;206:316–23.
11. Schauer PR, Burguera B, Ikramuddin S, et al. Effect of laparoscopic Roux-en-Y gastric bypass on type 2 diabetes mellitus. Ann Surg 2003;238:467–85.
12. Pories WJ. Diabetes the evolution of a new paradigm. Ann Surg 2004;239:12–3.
13. Sjostrom L. Bariatric surgery and reduction in morbidity and mortality: experiences from the SOS study. Int J Obes (Lond) 2008;32(Suppl 7):S93–7.
14. Buchwald H, Estok R, Fahrbach K, et al. Weight and type 2 diabetes after bariatric surgery: systematic review and meta-analysis. Am J Med 2009;122(3): 248–56.e5.
15. Scopinaro N, Papadia F, Marinari G, et al. Long-term control of type 2 diabetes mellitus and the other major components of the metabolic syndrome after biliopancreatic diversion in patients with BMI <35 kg/m2. Obes Surg 2007;17:185–92.
16. Dixon JB, O'Brien PE, Playfair J, et al. Adjustable gastric banding and conventional therapy for type 2 diabetes: a randomized controlled trial. JAMA 2008; 299:316–23.
17. Lee WJ, Wang W, Lee YC, et al. Effect of laparoscopic mini-gastric bypass for type 2 diabetes mellitus: comparison of BMI>35 and <35 kg/m2. J Gastrointest Surg 2008;12:945–52.
18. Christou NV, Sampalis JS, Liberman M, et al. Surgery decreases long-term mortality, morbidity, and health care use in morbidly obese patients. Ann Surg 2004;240(3):416–23.

19. Rubino F, Kaplan LM, Schauer PR, et al. The Diabetes Surgery Summit consensus conference: recommendations for the evaluation and use of gastrointestinal surgery to treat type 2 diabetes mellitus. Ann Surg 2010;251:399–405.
20. Hickey MS, Pories WJ, MacDonald KG Jr, et al. A new paradigm for type 2 diabetes mellitus: could it be a disease of the foregut? Ann Surg 1998;227:637–44.
21. Rubino F, Forgione A, Cummings DE, et al. The mechanism of diabetes control after gastrointestinal bypass surgery reveals a role of the proximal small intestine in the pathophysiology of type 2 diabetes. Ann Surg 2006;244:741–9.
22. Zervos EE, Agle SC, Warren AJ, et al. Amelioration of insulin requirement in patients undergoing duodenal bypass for reasons other than obesity implicates foregut factors in the pathophysiology of type II diabetes. J Am Coll Surg 2010;210(5): 564–72, 572–4.
23. Rubino F, Marescaux J. Effect of duodenal-jejunal exclusion in a non-obese animal model of type 2 diabetes: a new perspective for an old disease. Ann Surg 2004; 239:1–11.
24. Ferzli GS, Dominique E, Ciaglia M, et al. Clinical improvement after duodenojejunal bypass for nonobese type 2 diabetes despite minimum improvement in glycemic homeostasis. World J Surg 2009;33:972–9.
25. DePaula AL, Macedo AL, Mota BR, et al. Laparoscopic ileal interposition associated to a diverted sleeve gastrectomy is an effective operation for the treatment of type 2 diabetes mellitus patients with BMI 21–29. Surg Endosc 2009;23:1313–20.
26. Fried M, Ribaric G, Buchwald JN, et al. Metabolic surgery for the treatment of type 2 diabetes in patients with BMI <35 kg/m2: an integrative review of early studies. Obes Surg 2010;20:776–90.
27. Salameh BS, Khoukaz MT, Bell RL. Metabolic and nutritional changes after bariatric surgery. Expert Rev Gastroenterol Hepatol 2010;4:217–23.
28. Laferrère B. Does surgically induced weight loss decrease mortality? Nat Clin Pract Endocrinol Metab 2008;4(3):136–7.
29. Sultan S, Parikh M, Youn H, et al. Early US outcomes after laparoscopic adjustable gastric banding in patients with a body mass index less than 35 kg/m2. Surg Endosc 2009;23:1569–73.
30. Mason EE, Ito C. Gastric bypass in obesity. Surg Clin N Am 1967;47:1345–51.
31. Buchwald H. Surgery, overview of bariatric surgery. Presented at the American College of Surgeons Committee on Emerging Surgical Technology and Education Symposium. New Orleans (LA), 87th Annual Clinical Congress. October, 2011.
32. Griffen WO, Young VL, Stevenson CC. A prospective comparison of gastric and jejunoileal bypass procedures for morbid obesity. Ann Surg 1977;186:500–9.
33. Torres J, Oca C. Gastric bypass lesser curvature with distal Roux-en-Y. Bariatric Surg 1987;5:10–5.
34. Albrecht RJ, Pories WJ. Surgical intervention for the severely obese. Clin Endocrinol Metab 1999;13(1):149–72.
35. Wittgrove AC, Clark GW, Tremblay LJ. Laparoscopic Gastric Bypass Roux-en-Y: Preliminary Report of Five Cases. Obes Surg 1994;4(4):353–7.
36. de la Torre RA, Scott JS. Laparoscopic Roux-en-Y gastric bypass: a totally intra-abdominal approach–technique and preliminary report. Obes Surg 1999;9(5):492–8.
37. Higa KD, Boone KB, Ho T, et al. Laparoscopic Roux-en-Y gastric bypass for morbid obesity: technique and preliminary results of our first 400 patients. Arch Surg 2000;135(9):1029–33 [discussion: 1033–4].
38. Howard L, Carter J, Alger S, et al. Gastric bypass and vertical banded gastroplasty—a prospective randomized comparison and 5year follow-up. Obes Surg 1995;5(1):55–60.

39. Langer FB, Hoda MA, Wenzl E, et al. Sleeve gastrectomy and gastric banding: effects on plasma ghrelin levels. Obes Surg 2005;15:1024–9.
40. Cottam D, Qureshi FG, Mattar SG, et al. Laparoscopic sleeve gastrectomy as an initial weight-loss procedure for high-risk patients with morbid obesity. Surg Endosc 2006;20:859–63.
41. Hess DS, Hess DW. Biliopancreatic diversion with a duodenal switch. Obes Surg 1998;8:267–82.
42. Buchwald H, Avidor Y, Braunwald E, et al. Bariatric surgery: a systematic review and meta-analysis. JAMA 2004;292:1724–37.
43. Anonymous. NIH conference, Gastrointestinal surgery for severe obesity. Consensus Development Conference Panel. Ann Intern Med 1991;115(12):956–61.
44. Pratt GM, McLees B, Pories WJ, et al. The ASBS Bariatric Surgery Centers of Excellence program: a blueprint for quality improvement. Surg Obes Relat Dis 2006;2:497–503.
45. Adams TD, Gress RE, Smith SC, et al. Long-term mortality after gastric bypass surgery. N Engl J Med 2007;357:753–61.
46. Pories W. "Understanding Diabetes: what can we learn from bariatric surgery?" Presented at Surgical Grand Rounds. Boston (MA): Cleveland Tufts Medical Center; 2010.
47. McEwen LN, Coelho RB, Baumann LM, et al. The cost, quality of life impact, and cost-utility of bariatric surgery in a managed care population. Obes Surg 2010; 20:919–28.

Nutritional Support of the Obese and Critically Ill Obese Patient

Haytham M.A. Kaafarani, MD, MPH, Scott A. Shikora, MD*

KEYWORDS

• Nutrition • Obese • Critically ill • Bariatric

The World Health Organization (WHO) defines overweight as a body mass index (BMI) greater than or equal to 25 kg/m^2 and obesity as a BMI greater than or equal to 30 kg/m^2.[1] Worldwide, it is estimated that 1.6 billion adults are currently overweight, and at least 400 million are obese. In the United States, The Centers for Disease Control and Prevention (CDC) report that the prevalence of obesity has been steadily increasing in the last 2 decades. Currently, the overall rate of obesity is estimated at 33%; only 2 states (Colorado and the District of Columbia) have obesity rates less than 20%.[2,3] More than 16 million Americans are morbidly (or extremely) obese,[4] defined as a BMI greater than or equal to 40 kg/m^2. Obesity is classified in **Table 1**.

From a public health perspective, it is estimated that obesity is currently a leading cause of preventable death, second only to tobacco.[5] Several serious health morbidities are associated with obesity, including type 2 diabetes mellitus, hypertension, coronary artery disease, obstructive sleep apnea, cerebrovascular disease, osteoarthritis, and depression. Recent research has determined that obesity-related medical costs in the United States have now reached $168 billion yearly or about 17% of the total US medical costs.[6] This figure is expected only to increase in the future.

Presently, bariatric surgery (commonly referred to as weight-loss surgery) has been shown to be the only therapeutic option that provides meaningful and sustainable weight loss. The current operations have favorable safety and efficacy profiles that have resulted in a large increase in popularity.[7] Results are achieved in all of the currently performed bariatric procedures by manipulating the anatomy and/or physiology of the gastrointestinal tract. As a consequence, there is the potential for nutritional deficiencies and derangements must be considered and prevented or treated. Therefore, for all bariatric procedures, patients are required to modify their usual diet and to take vitamin supplements.

Department of Surgery, Tufts Medical Center and Tufts University School of Medicine, 800 Washington Street, Box 437, Boston, MA 02111, USA
* Corresponding author.
E-mail address: sshikora@tuftsmedicalcenter.org

Surg Clin N Am 91 (2011) 837–855
doi:10.1016/j.suc.2011.04.009
0039-6109/11/$ – see front matter © 2011 Elsevier Inc. All rights reserved.

Table 1
Classification of obesity per BMI

BMI Range (kg/m^2)	Classification	Common Nomenclature
25–29.9	Not applicable	Overweight
30–34.9	Class I	Obese
35–39.9	Class II	Moderately obese
40–49.9	Class III	Severely, extremely, or morbidly obese
≥50	Class IV	Super obese

With the increased prevalence of obesity worldwide and in the United States, and the dramatic increase in the number of bariatric surgery procedures, it is likely that all clinicians, including the general surgeon, the primary care physician, and the intensivist, will have opportunities to treat obese bariatric and nonbariatric obese patients with increasing frequency, and that some of these patients will be, or will become, critically ill. In addition to treating disease, this care will likely include the institution of nutritional support, both oral as well as interventional. Similar to most other care issues of the obese patient, the provision of nutrition can be challenging, especially as it relates to intensive care patients.

This article reviews the nutritional assessment and management of the bariatric and critically ill obese patient.

NUTRITION OF THE BARIATRIC PATIENT

It is not appropriate to discuss the nutritional assessment and management of bariatric patients without a basic understanding of the currently available bariatric procedures.

Overview of Bariatric Surgery

Bariatric surgery is currently the only treatment modality of obesity that has been able to produce sustainable weight loss and reversal of the related adverse health effects of obesity. Several studies have clearly shown that bariatric surgery is effective in mitigating the ill effects of obesity, treating its comorbidities, improving quality of life, and reducing mortality.[8–20]

Accordingly, bariatric surgical procedures are rapidly increasing in frequency and are becoming some of the most commonly performed procedures in general surgery. In a study by Pierce and colleagues[21] presented at the 2010 annual meeting of the American Society for Metabolic and Bariatric Surgery, laparoscopic gastric bypass was the second most frequently performed general surgery procedure after laparoscopic cholecystectomy. The sharp increase in the number of bariatric procedures performed in the United States and globally is not only related to the increased rates of obesity but also to the introduction of minimally invasive laparoscopic techniques that dramatically improved the surgical safety profile of these procedures. As stated previously, all of these procedures result in acute changes in the gastrointestinal anatomy and physiology and, as a result, increase the risk for nutritional deficiencies. They induce weight loss by 3 mechanisms: (1) restriction of the amount of food intake, (2) malabsorption of nutrients, and (3) alteration of gut and hormonal metabolism (eg, ghrelin, peptide YY [PYY]).[22–24] Pure malabsorptive (nonrestrictive) procedures such as the jejunoileal bypass or the biliopancreatic diversion, with or without duodenal switch, are uncommonly performed nowadays because of their high incidence of postoperative metabolic complications, specifically protein, calorie, and vitamin deficiencies. The 3 most commonly performed bariatric procedures today are: (1) gastric bypass, (2) adjustable gastric banding, and (3) sleeve gastrectomy.

Gastric bypass

Developed initially in the 1960s after the unintended sustainable weight loss of patients undergoing partial gastrectomy was noted,[25] gastric bypass has undergone many alterations and modifications in the last 4 decades. The laparoscopic Roux-en-Y gastric bypass (LRYGB) is currently considered the de facto gold standard and is thus the most commonly performed bariatric procedure. Surgery consists of creating a small gastric pouch of 15 to 30 cm^3 that drains directly into a limb of jejunum described as either the roux limb or the alimentary limb. The limb of proximal jejunum that is in continuity with the gastric fundus and duodenum, referred to as the biliopancreatic limb, drains through a jejunojejunostomy created typically 100 to 150 cm distally to the gastrojejunostomy (**Fig. 1**). LRYGB has many hypothetical mechanisms of action for weight loss and improvement of obesity-related conditions such as type 2 diabetes mellitus. It is restrictive in that the gastric capacity is only 15 to 30 cm^3. It has also been shown to inhibit the appetite hormone ghrelin while stimulating the release

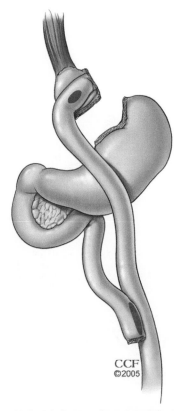

CCF
©2005

Fig. 1. Laparoscopic Roux-en-Y Gastric bypass. (*Reprinted from* Cleveland Clinic Center for Medical Art & Photography; with permission © 2005–2011. All rights reserved.)

of incretins such as PYY and GLP-1, and it is also malabsorptive for dietary fat.[23,24,26,27]

Adjustable gastric banding

Laparoscopic adjustable gastric banding (LAGB) is a purely restrictive procedure in which an inflatable silicone rubber band is wrapped around the upper stomach to create a small gastric pouch of 15 to 30 cm^3. The silicone band is connected via a hollow tube to a subcutaneous port, through which intermittent syringe injections of saline help tailor the amount of stomach restriction desired for appropriate weight loss. There are no apparent effects on gut hormones or malabsorption associated with this procedure (**Fig. 2**).

Gastric sleeve

Recent evidence is accumulating to suggest that laparoscopic sleeve gastrectomy (LSG), initially conceived as a staged step of a duodenal switch procedure or a gastric bypass, can be used as a definitive stand-alone procedure for weight loss.[28] A partial gastrectomy is performed in which most of the greater curvature of the stomach is removed, thus creating a gastric tube (or sleeve) of smaller capacity (120–150 cm^3). Food travels through the tube and pylorus, because no gastrointestinal anastomosis is required. The mechanism of action of LSG is not yet known. It likely is a restrictive procedure, but its potential effects on gut hormones or gastrointestinal physiology have not yet been determined (**Fig. 3**).

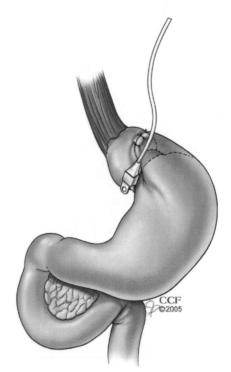

Fig. 2. Laparoscopic adjustable gastric banding. (*Reprinted from* Cleveland Clinic Center for Medical Art & Photography; with permission © 2005–2011. All rights reserved.)

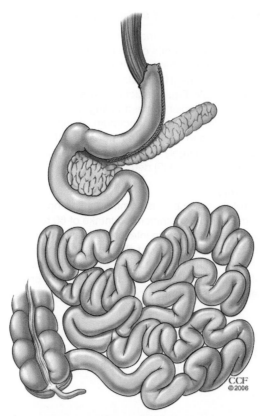

Fig. 3. Laparoscopic sleeve gastrectomy. (*Reprinted from* Cleveland Clinic Center for Medical Art & Photography; with permission © 2005–2011. All rights reserved.)

Perioperative Nutritional Management of Bariatric Patients

Before surgery

A routine and comprehensive preoperative nutritional assessment of patients undergoing bariatric surgery is warranted.[29,30] This evaluation is usually performed by a registered dietitian with a background in bariatric surgery. Information is gathered regarding usual eating patterns, weight history, and prior weight-loss attempts. Many patients have maladaptive dietary habits and even preoperative nutritional deficiencies that might persist after surgery. For example, many obese people are already vitamin D deficient before surgery.

After surgery

Patients undergoing LRYGB, LAGB, or LSG are usually placed on a dietary regimen that is sequentially advanced from clear liquids to solids in the subsequent days and weeks.[31] It is highly encouraged, and arguably necessary, that nutritional and dietary guidance is provided to the patient during the short postoperative stay by consultation with a dedicated bariatric dietitian.[31] In addition, vitamin supplementation is instituted shortly after hospital discharge to minimize the risk for the development of vitamin deficiencies.

Long-term Nutritional Management of Bariatric Patients

The nutritional consequences of bariatric surgery depend on the specific procedure performed as well as the dietary habits of the patient. Each procedure can affect the postoperative nutritional status differently. It is therefore essential to have a basic understanding of the locations along the gastrointestinal tract at which the various nutrients are absorbed. For example, **Fig. 4** depicts the absorption sites for the various nutrients. Reviewing it allows a simpler understanding of how a gastric bypass diverts nutrients away from the stomach and duodenum, resulting in a higher risk of deficiencies of iron, vitamin B_{12}, and folate. The nutritional deficiencies following bariatric procedures can be divided largely into 3 types: (1) protein-calorie malnutrition, (2) vitamin/mineral deficiencies, and (3) dehydration.

Protein-calorie malnutrition

Mild intolerance of protein-rich meals is common following weight-loss surgery, and patients often fail to meet their recommended intake of 60 to 120 g of protein daily.[31] Once a common complication following intestinal bypasses, protein malnutrition rarely complicates the postoperative course of the current popular bariatric procedures, such as LRYGB, mainly because gastric bypass results in loss of fat stores with relative preservation of lean body tissue,[32] because ingested protein is generally well absorbed. Nonetheless, postoperative protein malnutrition is still being reported,

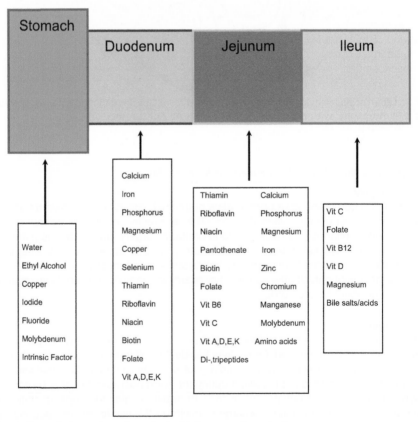

Fig. 4. Sites of absorption of nutrients in the gastrointestinal tract.

mainly in the setting of dysfunctional eating habits or protracted postoperative vomiting. Protein malnutrition following bariatric surgery is difficult to diagnose, primarily because patients may rapidly lose lean body mass while their serum protein levels remain at normal levels until late in the course when the malnutrition is profound.[18,33,34] Therefore, we strongly recommend that all bariatric patients be monitored for the potential development of protein malnutrition during the weight-loss, weight-regain, and weight-plateau phases following bariatric surgery. Protein intake should be monitored not only by serum protein levels but also by dietary habits and bowel activity. Protein supplementation (eg, protein shakes) should be prescribed promptly when the intake is persistently less than 60 g per day.[31] Suboptimal protein intake is often accompanied by decreased caloric intake, leading to a state of protein-calorie malnutrition. In severe malnutrition, enteral or parenteral nutrition should be considered, especially when oral supplementation has proved insufficient or unsuccessful. In the case of refractory protein-calorie malnutrition, common channel lengthening, or even reversal of the gastric bypass, might be necessary. In comparison, protein deficiency after LGB is rare and, when it occurs, is solely related to poor intake. Patients having biliopancreatic diversion are clearly more prone to protein-calorie malnutrition than patients having LRYGB. Patients undergoing biliopancreatic diversion, with or without duodenal switch, must be closely monitored. Reliable data on the incidence of protein-calorie malnutrition with LSG are still lacking.

Vitamin/mineral deficiencies

Vitamin and mineral deficiencies are more common than protein-calorie malnutrition following LRYGB, thus justifying lifelong supplementation of many of these nutrients. Because these deficiencies can develop gradually during many postoperative years, and because their clinical manifestations are often subtle, a policy of lifelong surveillance can be supported. In general, the pure restrictive procedures such as LGB result in a lower incidence of vitamin and mineral deficiency. With LRYGB, iron, folate, calcium, and vitamin B_{12} deficiencies can occur as nutrients are diverted away from the duodenum and proximal jejunum. With malabsorptive procedures such as the biliopancreatic diversion, patients risk additional deficiencies of fat-soluble vitamins (A, D, E, and K), zinc, sodium, chloride, and magnesium. **Box 1** delineates the current protocols for vitamin/mineral deficiencies surveillance and supplementation that are followed at the Weight and Wellness Center at Tufts Medical Center.

Iron Patients undergoing LRYGB, especially menstruating women, are susceptible to microcytic anemia for 2 main reasons: (1) bypass of the duodenum and proximal jejunum where most of the gastrointestinal absorption of iron normally occurs, and (2) the lack of gastric acid that is necessary for iron absorption. It has been shown that LRYGB decreases the production of gastric acid by the gastric pouch at baseline and on stimulation.[35] Furthermore, patients occasionally cannot tolerate eating meat following weight-loss surgery; Avinoah and colleagues[33] showed that patients who do not, or cannot, eat meat are particularly prone to iron deficiency. Therefore, iron levels must be monitored in all patients having bariatric surgery, and deficiencies require treatment as appropriate.[31] For patients at risk (and, arguably, for all patients), routine supplementation with 325 mg of oral ferrous sulfate daily is recommended. For patients in whom iron deficiency had already been documented, supplementation with 325 mg of oral ferrous sulfate 1 to 3 times a day is warranted. Ferrous fumarate or gluconate may be used as an alternative source of iron. Vitamin C should be prescribed simultaneously, because vitamin C improves the absorption of iron and increases the levels of ferritin.[31] Because iron interferes with the absorption of some

---

Box 1
Vitamin/mineral supplementation protocols for treating deficiencies (Weight and Wellness Center, Tufts Medical Center, Boston, MA)

All Patients After Surgery

- Complete multivitamin infusion with iron by mouth every day.
- Calcium with vitamin D 1200 to 1500 mg by mouth every day.
- Patients should be advised against taking a calcium supplement that does not include vitamin D (400 IU/d).

Specific Vitamin/Mineral

- Iron
  - Fe saturation <10% and ferritin <10 ng/mL or Fe saturation <7% (regardless of ferritin).
    - Supplement with $FeSO_4$ 325 mg plus 250 mg vitamin C by mouth every day.
    - Increase to 3 times a day as tolerated. Patient is instructed to take with orange juice.
- Folate
  - If red blood cell folate level is low:
    - First replete vitamin B_{12} if it is low.
    - 1 mg of folate by mouth every day for 3 months
- Vitamin B_{12}
  - If neurologic symptoms (regardless of level) or if level is <100 μg/dL:
    - Vitamin B_{12} 1000 μg intramuscularly every week for 4 weeks, then 1000 μg intramuscularly every month for 4 months and recheck.
    - If level is 100 to 150 pg/dL:
      - Vitamin B_{12} 1000 μg intramuscularly every month, and recheck in 3 to 4 months.
    - If level is 150 to 250 pg/dL:
      - Vitamin B_{12} 1000 μg by mouth every day, and recheck in 3 to 4 months.
      - Vitamin B_{12} can also be administered sublingual or by nasal spray.
- Vitamin D
  - If low serum vitamin D level:
    - Vitamin D 50,000 IU by mouth every week for 6 to 8 weeks; recheck level in 3 to 6 months.
    - If vitamin D level in 3 to 6 months is normal, go back to baseline postoperative supplements, and recheck in 3 months.
    - Ensure that the patient is taking 1200 to 1500 mg elemental calcium per day.

---

nutritional elements (eg, calcium, zinc, magnesium), supplemental iron should not be ingested at the same time as these nutrients.[36] Intravenous iron infusions should be reserved for refractory cases of iron deficiency.

Folate (vitamin B9) Folic acid absorption occurs mainly in the proximal small bowel; however, following LRYGB, folic acid can be absorbed in the mid and distal small bowel. Therefore, folate deficiency is believed to occur because of inadequate intake rather than malabsorption, and can easily be prevented with routine multivitamin intake (including 400 μg/d of folate).[31] The risk of macrocytic anemia or, in more severe cases, leucopenia, thrombocytopenia, or glossitis resulting from folate deficiency has also been suggested to be higher in bariatric patients who do not tolerate meat well.[33] Diagnosing folate insufficiency is challenging, because serum folate levels reflect acute dietary intake rather than chronic or subacute deficiency.[34] Red blood cell folate levels are more reflective of tissue levels than simple serum levels, but the clinical significance of decreased red cell folate levels is still not clear. If deficiency is suspected, prompt supplementation with 1 mg of folate daily is usually adequate.[37]

Vitamin B$_{12}$ The absorption of B$_{12}$ is a complex process that starts in the stomach with the release of B$_{12}$ from the ingested nutrients, and its subsequent binding to a protein called R-protein. This process requires gastric acid. In the duodenum, R-protein is cleaved off the B$_{12}$, and a B$_{12}$-intrinsic factor (B$_{12}$-IF) complex is formed. The B$_{12}$-IF complex then travels through the small intestine, and B$_{12}$ is absorbed in the distal ileum. With less gastric acid production by the gastric pouch and complete bypassing of the duodenum, vitamin B$_{12}$ deficiency following LRYGB is common, especially in patients with suboptimal intake of meat. Some studies have even suggested that the incidence of vitamin B$_{12}$ deficiency following LRYGB is between 26% and 70%.[38–41] Such deficiency does not usually develop until 1 or 2 years after surgery because of the large body stores of B$_{12}$. However, when vitamin B$_{12}$ deficiency occurs, it can result in macrocytic anemia, bone marrow megaloblastosis, and, rarely, irreversible neuropathy. It is generally recommended that all patients undergoing bariatric surgery receive 500 to 600 µg of oral vitamin B$_{12}$ daily. If a deficiency is detected, the daily dose should be increased to 1000 µg. Parenteral, usually intramuscular, supplementation with 1000 µg of vitamin B$_{12}$ monthly, or 1000 to 3000 µg every 6 to 12 months, should be given when oral supplementation fails to correct the deficiency.[31] B$_{12}$ supplementation can also be administered transnasally or sublingually. Like the other micronutrients, B$_{12}$ malabsorption does not occur after LGB, thus, deficiencies would be less common than with LRYGB or biliopancreatic diversion and would be solely the result of poor dietary intake. There are currently few data on B$_{12}$ deficiency after LSG, but it might be predicted that B$_{12}$ deficiency could develop following the procedure because the resected stomach contains most of the acid and intrinsic factor–producing parietal cells.

Vitamin D and calcium Calcium absorption is suboptimal following LRYGB, mainly because most intestinal calcium absorption occurs normally in the duodenum and proximal jejunum with the help of gastric acid. The data regarding the effect of bariatric surgery on vitamin D levels are less conclusive.[31] However, patients having gastric bypass are at a higher risk than the general population for bone abnormalities and disruption of the normal calcium homeostasis, with resultant bone abnormalities including osteoporosis.[42–48] Increasing levels of alkaline phosphatase and osteocalcin, as well as parathyroid hormone levels, can be early indications of vitamin D or calcium deficiency, although measurement of bone density may be the only accurate indicator of calcium deficiency. Daily recommendations for calcium supplementation are 1200 to 2000 mg of calcium citrate with vitamin D (400–800 units/d).[49]

Thiamine (vitamin B$_1$) Thiamine deficiency following bariatric surgery is rare, but may occasionally be seen, especially in patients with persistent postoperative vomiting. Rehydration of these dehydrated patients with a glucose-containing intravenous solution without thiamine can result in the serious Wernicke-Korsakoff syndrome, characterized by confusion, nystagmus, ataxia, ophthalmoplegia, and psychosis. These patients should initially be given glucose-free intravenous fluid and 100 mg thiamine before administering fluid with glucose. The appropriate dose and duration for prophylaxis or treatment of Wernicke-Korsakoff encephalopathy is controversial,[49] but, in patients with persistent postoperative vomiting, parenteral thiamine treatment for 6 months should prevent deficiency.[43] It is the protocol in our program to administer 100 mg of thiamine to all bariatric patients presenting to the Emergency Department regardless of the reason for presentation. In addition, all patients are given a 100-mg dose of thiamine after surgery.

Selenium There are insufficient data to support empiric selenium supplementation of patients undergoing bariatric surgery, although the incidence of asymptomatic selenium deficiency can be as high as 25%.[31]

Zinc Zinc deficiency can occur following bariatric surgery, and may be reversed with zinc supplementation. Hair loss in bariatric patients has been hypothesized to result from zinc deficiency, although the causal relationship between the 2 is unclear at best.[36,50]

Vitamins A, E, and K Deficiencies in the fat-soluble vitamins A, E, and K are rare following bariatric surgery, but occur more commonly with the biliopancreatic diversion. Even when these deficiencies do occur, they usually have no obvious clinical significance.

Potassium and magnesium Hypokalemia and hypomagnesemia are common in the short-term and long-term phases following bariatric surgery, especially with the existence of persistent vomiting. Both are easily correctable in both settings, usually with oral supplementation.

Dehydration

Dehydration is common following bariatric surgery, especially in warmer climates, during hot weather, or after vigorous activity. However, decreased fluid intake in the setting of high fluid requirements is usually the cause. In the case of LRYGB and LGB, the patient's ability to drink large amounts of water is restricted. Patients must learn how to drink small sips of water frequently rather than attempt to take large amounts at one time.[50] In addition, vomiting and/or diarrhea could exacerbate a bariatric patient's dehydration. Patients should be instructed to keep a fluid container available to them at all times. Although the amount of fluid intake varies per patient depending on their specific body physiology and their daily activity, an intake of 1.9 L of fluid a day is usually recommended.

NUTRITION OF THE CRITICALLY ILL OBESE PATIENT

As the prevalence of obesity continues to increase, the number of obese and morbidly obese patients admitted to intensive care units continues to increase as well. Hospitalized obese patients, particularly those with critical illness, are at an independently higher risk of morbidity and mortality than is the nonobese patient population.[51] Managing the critically ill obese patient is especially challenging because several unique problems can arise; obese patients often present the need for special equipment (eg, oversized beds, oversized computed tomography machines), more challenging fluid status management, more aggressive deep vein thrombosis prophylaxis, and more careful sedation and drug dosing.[52] Nutritional support of the obese patient is particularly complex because of the balance needed between avoiding overfeeding (weight loss is not the goal in critical illness), and the need to minimize the catabolic state in order to optimize the body's response to injury and allow tissue healing. Despite the excessive stores of adipose tissue, critically ill obese patients should receive early and timely nutrition (as should all critically ill patients), because protein-calorie malnutrition can and does occur in obese patients. However, unique feeding strategies are required, because the routine or standard nutritional methods may be harmful to this patient population, mainly because obese patients are especially susceptible to volume overload and glucose intolerance in the setting of a critical illness stress response.[53] Later in this article, special attention is given to the currently available methods to estimate the energy expenditure, the fluid management, the role of hypocaloric feeding, and the methods of vascular and enteral access in the critically ill obese patient.

Estimating Energy Requirements

Indirect calorimetry remains one of the most accurate methods to estimate energy requirements and direct nutritional support in critically ill patients, including the obese and morbidly obese population.[54] However, most of the current equations to estimate energy expenditure were derived from the nonobese, non–critically ill population. These formulas have been repetitively criticized for their inaccuracies, especially in the critically ill patients, and most do not account for obesity as an independent predictor of energy requirements.[55–59] Although the obese patient has both an increased lean body mass and an increased fat mass, the proportion of the two varies widely, and differs significantly from the nonobese patient.[60,61] Using the actual body weight in the energy calculations of the obese patient overestimates the caloric requirements. However, given the larger lean body mass, using the ideal body weight greatly underestimates the caloric requirements of obese patients, thus exposing them to an undesired state of catabolism. Multiple studies have attempted to validate the use of the more than 25 equations (such as the Harris-Benedict or Mifflin calculations) in obese patients, with conflicting results. Most of these studies reported serious inaccuracies of these equations in the morbidly obese population.[62–66] Indirect calorimetry (IC) remains the gold standard method to estimate the energy requirements of the obese and morbidly obese patient in the intensive care unit. IC does not rely on any specific patient characteristic, but relies exclusively on metabolic activity to determine the resting energy expenditure (REE). REE is obtained by measuring oxygen consumption and carbon dioxide generation using a special gas analyzer. As an alternative to the respiratory gas analyzing method, IC can be achieved using thermodilution techniques from measured data such as the cardiac output, arterial oxygen, and mixed venous saturations (using the modified Fick equation). However, in a study by Ogawa and colleagues,[67] thermodilution-based calculation of REE was found to be inaccurate compared with respiratory IC in critically ill patients.

Fluid Management in the Obese Critically Ill Patient

Salt and water retention often accompany the stress response of critical illness. However, obese people often require more fluid volume to maintain homeostasis. The volume administration necessary to maintain nutrition or hemodynamics, in addition to the exaggerated stress-related hyperinsulinemia, put obese patients at a higher risk for total body hypervolemia. Because obesity is closely associated with coronary artery disease, obese ill patients with fluid overload are at a particularly high risk for myocardial infarction, pulmonary edema, and congestive heart failure. Therefore, fluid management of critically ill obese patients is a delicate balance between restricting fluids or nutrition (thus risking malnutrition and dehydration) and excessive fluid administration (risking fluid overload and cardiovascular failure). Accurately estimating the overall volume status and guiding the delicate fluid balance of an obese critically ill obese patient often require measurement of central venous pressure and/or right heart pressure.

Hazards of Standard Nutrition Support in the Obese Critically Ill Patient

Standard or routine nutritional management of critically ill obese patients may be hazardous. In nonobese patients, these standard nutrition formulas usually provide 20 to 35 kcal per kilogram of body weight, 30% to 40% of which is provided as lipids. Administration of 1.0 to 2.0 g of protein per kilogram of body weight is usually recommended. The remainder of the required calories are provided by dextrose (4–7 mg/kg/min).

Dextrose

Concentrated dextrose solutions can result in several unintended consequences, such as hyperglycemia, hyperinsulinemia, lipogenesis, and increased production of carbon dioxide.[53] Contrary to the earlier beliefs that stress hyperglycemia is purely beneficial, hyperglycemia can have dramatic negative consequences, ranging from increased risk of nosocomial infection, depressed immune function, and poor tissue healing to increased overall mortality.[68–73] The obese patient who is often glucose intolerant or even frankly diabetic is especially susceptible to the harmful effects of hyperglycemia. Dextrose loading usually results in an additional substantive risk of hyperinsulinemia. Because insulin is a potent antinatriuretic hormone, salt and water retention follow, increasing the risk for fluid overload and placing the patient at risk for heart failure and pulmonary edema, as discussed earlier. Lipogenesis also results from overzealous dextrose infusions, promoting hepatic steatosis with its increased risk for subsequent liver failure.[74,75] In the patient in intensive care with respiratory failure, increased carbon dioxide production resulting from excessive dextrose administration increases the work of breathing, potentially exacerbating an already compromised respiratory status.[76,77]

Lipids

Lipid infusions are safe but often unnecessary in the obese patient. Because obesity, by definition, is associated with excess body fat and energy storage, lipid administration can occasionally result in overfeeding. However, lipid administration is sometimes necessary to prevent essential fatty acid deficiency in nonobese patients.[60]

The Role of Hypocaloric (or Hypoenergetic) Feeding

Morbidly obese patients have increased insulin levels that contribute to a blunted lipolysis response in the presence of physiologic stress.[78] In the morbidly obese patient, during metabolic stress induced by illness, gluconeogenesis through protein breakdown occurs in an accelerated fashion.[79] Despite the existent excess lipid/calorie storage, protein malnutrition can and does occur in obese and morbidly obese patients in the intensive care unit as the body continues to produce endogenous glucose by protein breakdown. Several studies conducted in obese critically ill patients suggest that protein-rich hypocaloric (or hypoenergetic) feeding may offer nutritional advantages compared with routine or standard feeding strategies.[80–87] The idea of protein-sparing hypoenergetic feeding in obese critically ill patients was inspired by a weight-reduction dietary strategy commonly known as the protein-sparing modified fast (PSMF), and was used to induce weight loss in obese patients who were not ill.[88]

Advantages of hypocaloric feeding

The main advantage of protein-sparing hypocaloric feeding is encouraging endogenous lipid consumption (lipid oxidation) for energy and maintaining protein anabolism through positive nitrogen homeostasis, while simultaneously avoiding the previously discussed complications of excess dextrose administration. With hypocaloric feeding, hyperglycemia rarely occurs, with resultant improved immune function, decreased risk of nosocomial infections, and improved wound healing.[86,87] Although not the primary goal, lipid-based weight loss with maintenance of lean body weight may also be achieved.[52] In a retrospective study by Dickerson[84] in 2002, obese patients treated with hypocaloric feeding had a shorter intensive care unit stay, less need for antibiotics, and a trend toward decreased days of mechanical ventilation.

Optimizing hypocaloric regimens

Hypocaloric feeding is intended to reduce dextrose (and calorie) infusions, while maximizing protein sparing through endogenous fat oxidation. If dextrose is restricted or even excluded altogether from the feedings, the nutritional status of the obese patient can theoretically be improved while avoiding the hazards of glucose. In reality, the availability of nonprotein sources of calories (such as endogenous glucose or exogenous dextrose) is essential to improving the protein-sparing effect of a hypocaloric regimen[89,90] because, in the carbohydrate-deficient patient with exhausted glycogen stores, protein catabolism is needed to fuel gluconeogenesis. The presence of dextrose in the regimen minimizes the need for protein catabolism.[91,92] However, the optimal amount of dextrose to be provided in a hypocaloric regimen is not clear. Protein catabolism and nitrogen wasting are best minimized with higher caloric supply, but the effect plateaus when the amount of calories supplied is greater than 60% of REE.[93] When the amount of caloric administration is less than 50% of REE, protein sparing is suboptimal. Therefore, we recommend that the total energy provided to the obese patient should preferably be between 50% and 60% of REE, as measured by IC.

Complications of hypocaloric regimens

Whether or not endogenous mobilization of fat stores occurs in an efficient manner in obese ill patients is a controversial issue. Jeevanandam and colleagues[79] suggested that poor fat oxidation occurs in stressed obese patients. In a similar patient population, Dickerson and colleagues[86] calculated that fat oxidation accounts for 68% of nonprotein energy use in patients receiving hypocaloric feeding, suggesting a favorable amount of fat oxidation with hypocaloric regimens. Essential fatty acid deficiency, especially linoleic acid, can theoretically occur when patients are fed a hypocaloric fat-free or near fat-free diet. Mobilization of the fat stores releases more than the 2 to 3.5 g of the daily body requirement of linoleic acid, which should be sufficient to prevent deficiencies.[60] However, if fat oxidation or lipolysis in stressed obese patients is suboptimal (as suggested by some studies cited earlier), as in the case of the long-term ill obese patient, a weekly infusion of lipids should be provided to minimize the risk of an essential fatty acid deficiency.

Parenteral versus enteral hypocaloric feeding

Although hypocaloric feeding was initially designed for the parenteral route, enteral feedings are usually preferred in the critically ill patient with ability to tolerate and absorb nutrients through the gastrointestinal tract. Feeding via the gastrointestinal tract is advantageous in part because it helps preserve the gut mucosal integrity and possibly enhances glycemic control. To initiate a hypocaloric enteral feeding regimen, it is often necessary to adjust or modify the standard and currently available tube feeding formulas. Providing 60% of the energy requirements through the standard tube feeds, and then adding protein substrates to achieve 100% of the protein requirements, is one simple way of formulating a hypocaloric protein-sparing regimen. Because the standard formulas approved by the US Food and Drug Administration contain the routine vitamin and mineral requirements based on a 2000-calorie diet, using only 60% of the routine feeding to achieve the hypocaloric goal might place the obese patient at risk for mineral and vitamin deficiencies. Therefore, additional vitamin and mineral administration are warranted with the feeding technique.

Enteral and Central Venous Access in the Obese Patient

Parenteral nutrition in the critically ill obese patient is preferably administered by central vein. However, the body habitus of obese patients is often distorted with short wide necks and an absence of usual anatomic landmarks. Central venous cannulation in this patient population can be hazardous, and associated with both a higher chance of failure and a higher risk of complications. In addition, many obese patients poorly tolerate the Trendelenburg position. Therefore, the challenge of the task of central venous access in the obese patient should never be underestimated. When appropriate, it should be assigned to the more experienced surgeon or surgical resident. Moreover, surgeons should consider central venous line placement in the controlled setting of the operating room, where better illumination and better equipment are immediately available. Ultrasound guidance should be the rule rather than the exception.

Enteral access, such as bedside placement of a nasogastric or nasojejunal tube can also be challenging and carry a higher risk in the obese patient because of increased tissue adiposity and crowdedness at the level of the palate and pharynx.[94] Fluoroscopic guidance for tube placement is preferred, although most fluoroscopic tables cannot tolerate more than 160 or 180 kg of patient weight. Percutaneous endoscopic feeding tube placement in obese patient presents a higher risk of intra-abdominal organ injuries or other complications, because the transillumination part of the procedure is usually suboptimal as a result of the thick, opaque abdominal wall. A laparoscopic-assisted endoscopic tube placement may be safer, but presents the additional risks of laparoscopy, general anesthesia, postoperative pain, and a greater risk for respiratory compromise and wound infections.

SUMMARY

With the dramatic increase in the prevalence of obesity worldwide and in the United States, it is almost certain that the general surgeon (and for that matter, all clinicians) will be dealing with bariatric and obese nonbariatric patients in increasing numbers. This patient population presents several difficulties from the medical and surgical management perspectives. In particular, nutrition of the bariatric patient and critically ill obese patient is challenging. Simply applying the standard nutritional management to these patients might jeopardize their health and possibly their survival. A clear understanding of the nutritional assessment and unique management strategies available for the bariatric and the critically ill obese patients is essential to provide them with the safest and most effective care.

REFERENCES

1. The World Health Organization. Factsheets. Available at: www.who.int/mediacentre/factsheets/fs311/en/index.html. Accessed November 22, 2010.
2. Freedman DS, Khan LK, Serdula MK, et al. Trends and correlates of class 3 obesity in the United States from 1990–2000. JAMA 2002;288:1758–61.
3. Flegal KM, Carroll MD, Ogden CL, et al. Prevalence and trends in obesity among US adults, 1999-2008. JAMA 2010;303(3):235–41.
4. The Centers for Disease Control and Prevention. U.S. obesity trends. Available at: http://www.cdc.gov/obesity/data/trends.html. Accessed November 22, 2010.

5. Mokdad AH, Marks JS, Stroup DF, et al. Actual causes of death in the United States, 2000. JAMA 2004;291(10):1238–45.
6. Cawley J, Meyerhoefer C. The medical care costs of obesity: an instrumental variables approach. NBER Working Paper No. 16467. National Bureau of Economic Research; 2010.
7. Steinbrook R. Surgery for severe obesity. N Engl J Med 2004;350:1075–9.
8. Christou NV, Sampalis JS, Liberman M, et al. Surgery decreases long-term mortality, morbidity, and health care use in morbidly obese patients. Ann Surg 2004;240(3):416–23.
9. Abu-Abeid S, Keidar A, Szold A. Resolution of chronic medical conditions after laparoscopic adjustable silicone gastric banding for the treatment of morbid obesity in the elderly. Surg Endosc 2001;15(2):132–4.
10. Ballantyne GH. Measuring outcomes following bariatric surgery: weight loss parameters, improvement in co-morbid conditions, change in quality of life and patient satisfaction. Obes Surg 2003;13(6):954–64.
11. Dixon JB, Dixon ME, O'Brien PE. Quality of life after lap-band placement: influence of time, weight loss, and comorbidities. Obes Res 2001;9(11):713–21.
12. Dixon JB, O'Brien PE. Changes in comorbidities and improvements in quality of life after LAP-BAND placement. Am J Surg 2002;184(6B):51S–4S.
13. Monk JS Jr, Dia Nagib N, Stehr W. Pharmaceutical savings after gastric bypass surgery. Obes Surg 2004;14(1):13–5.
14. Monteforte MJ, Turkelson CM. Bariatric surgery for morbid obesity. Obes Surg 2000;10(5):391–401.
15. Sjöström CD, Peltonen M, Wedel H, et al. Differentiated long-term effects of intentional weight loss on diabetes and hypertension. Hypertension 2000;36(1):20–5.
16. Fontaine KR, Redden DT, Wang C, et al. Years of life lost due to obesity. JAMA 2003;289(2):187–93.
17. Greenway SE, Greenway FL, Klein S. Effects of obesity surgery on non-insulin-dependent diabetes mellitus. Arch Surg 2002;137:1109.
18. Pories WJ, Swanson MS, MacDonald KG, et al. Who would have thought it? An operation proves to be the most effective therapy for adult-onset diabetes mellitus. Ann Surg 1995;222:339.
19. Sjöström L, Gummesson A, Sjöström CD, et al. Effects of bariatric surgery on mortality in Swedish obese subjects. N Engl J Med 2007;357:741.
20. Adams TD, Gress RE, Smith SC, et al. Long-term mortality after gastric bypass surgery. N Engl J Med 2007;357:753.
21. Pierce J. Bariatric surgery tops list of work units in general surgery. Available at: http://www.generalsurgerynews.com. Accessed December 25, 2010.
22. Karamanakos SN, Vagenas K, Kalfarentzos F, et al. Weight loss, appetite suppression, and changes in fasting and postprandial ghrelin and peptide-YY levels after Roux-en-Y gastric bypass and sleeve gastrectomy: a prospective, double blind study. Ann Surg 2008;247:401.
23. le Roux CW, Aylwin SJ, Batterham RL, et al. Gut hormone profiles following bariatric surgery favor an anorectic state, facilitate weight loss, and improve metabolic parameters. Ann Surg 2006;243:108.
24. Rubino F, Gagner M, Gentileschi P, et al. The early effect of the Roux-en-Y gastric bypass on hormones involved in body weight regulation and glucose metabolism. Ann Surg 2004;240:236.
25. Sugerman HJ, Kellum JM, DeMaria EJ, et al. Conversion of failed or complicated vertical banded gastroplasty to gastric bypass in morbid obesity. Am J Surg 1996;171:263.

26. Laferrère B, Teixeira J, McGinty J, et al. Effect of weight loss by gastric bypass surgery versus hypocaloric diet on glucose and incretin levels in patients with type 2 diabetes. J Clin Endocrinol Metab 2008;93(7):2479–85.
27. Cummings DE, Weigle DS, Frayo RS, et al. Plasma ghrelin levels after diet-induced weight loss or gastric bypass surgery. N Engl J Med 2002;346(21):1623–30.
28. Gluck B, Movitz B, Jansma S, et al. Laparoscopic sleeve gastrectomy is a safe and effective bariatric procedure for the lower BMI (35.0-43.0 kg/m(2)) population. Obes Surg 2010 Dec 3. [Epub ahead of print].
29. Ernst B, Thurnheer M, Schmid SM, et al. Evidence for the necessity to systematically assess micronutrient status prior to bariatric surgery. Obes Surg 2009;19: 66–73.
30. Toh SY, Zarshenas N, Jorgensen J. Prevalence of nutrient deficiencies in bariatric patients. Nutrition 2009;25:1150–6.
31. Mechanick JI, Kushner RF, Sugerman HJ, et al. American Association of Clinical Endocrinologists, The Obesity Society, and American Society for Metabolic & Bariatric Surgery medical guidelines for clinical practice for the perioperative nutritional, metabolic, and nonsurgical support of the bariatric surgery patient. Obesity (Silver Spring) 2009;17:1–70.
32. Bothe A, Bistrian BR, Greenberg I. Energy regulation in morbid obesity by multidisciplinary therapy. Surg Clin North Am 1979;59:1017–31.
33. Avinoah E, Ovnat A, Charuzi I. Nutritional status seven years after Roux-en-Y gastric bypass surgery. Surgery 1992;111:137–42.
34. Halverson JD. Micronutrient deficiencies after gastric bypass for morbid obesity. Am Surg 1986;52:594–8.
35. Smith CD, Herkes SB, Behrns KE, et al. Gastric acid secretion and vitamin B_{12} absorption after vertical Roux-en-Y gastric bypass for morbid obesity. Ann Surg 1993;218:91–6.
36. Poitou Bernert C, Ciangura C, Coupaye M, et al. Nutritional deficiency after gastric bypass: diagnosis, prevention and treatment. Diabetes Metab 2007;33(1):13–24.
37. Brolin RE, Gorman JH, Gorman RC, et al. Are Vitamin B12 and folate deficiency clinically important after Roux-en-Y gastric bypass? J Gastrointest Surg 1998; 2(5):436–42.
38. Sugerman HJ. Bariatric surgery for severe obesity. J Assoc Acad Minor Phys 2001;12:129–36.
39. Skroubis G, Sakellaropoulos G, Pouggouras K, et al. Comparison of nutritional deficiencies after Roux-en-Y gastric bypass and after biliopancreatic diversion with Roux-en-Y gastric bypass. Obes Surg 2002;12:551–8.
40. Brolin RE, Leung M. Survey of vitamin and mineral supplementation after gastric bypass and biliopancreatic diversion for morbid obesity. Obes Surg 1999;9:150–4.
41. Newbury L, Dolan K, Hatzifotis M, et al. Calcium and vitamin D depletion and elevated parathyroid hormone following biliopancreatic diversion. Obes Surg 2003;13:893–5.
42. Halverson JD. Metabolic risk of obesity surgery and long-term follow-up. Am J Clin Nutr 1992;55(Suppl 2):602S–5S.
43. Alverez-Leite JL. Nutrient deficiencies secondary to bariatric surgery. Curr Opin Clin Nutr Metab Care 2004;7:569–75.
44. Goode LR, Brolin RE, Chowdhury HA, et al. Bone and gastric bypass surgery: effects of dietary calcium and vitamin D. Obes Res 2004;12(1):40–7.
45. Coates PS, Fernstrom JD, Fernstrom MH, et al. Gastric bypass surgery for morbid obesity leads to increase in bone turnover and a decrease in bone mass. J Clin Endocrinol Metab 2004;89(3):1061–5.

46. Shaker JL, Norton AJ, Woods MF, et al. Secondary hyperparathyroidism and osteopenia in women following gastric exclusion surgery for obesity. Osteoporos Int 1991;1(3):177–81.
47. Bell NH. Bone loss and gastric bypass surgery for morbid obesity. J Clin Endocrinol Metab 2004;89:1059–60.
48. Pugnale N, Giusti V, Suter M, et al. Bone metabolism and risk of secondary hyperparathyroidism 12 months after gastric banding in obese pre-menopausal women. Int J Obes Relat Metab Disord 2003;27:110–6.
49. Ziegler O, Sirveaux MA, Brunaud L, et al. Medical follow up after bariatric surgery: nutritional and drug issues. General recommendations for the prevention and treatment of nutritional deficiencies. Diabetes Metab 2009;35(6 Pt 2):544–57.
50. Fujioka K. Follow-up of nutritional and metabolic problems after bariatric surgery. Diabetes Care 2005;28:481–4.
51. Nasraway SA, Albert M, Donnelly AM, et al. Morbid obesity is an independent determinant of death among surgical critically ill patients. Crit Care Med 2006; 34:964–70.
52. King DR, Velmahos GC. Difficulties in managing the surgical patient who is morbidly obese. Crit Care Med 2010;38(Suppl 9):S478–82.
53. Shikora SA, Jensen GL. Hypoenergetic nutrition support in hospitalized obese patients. Am J Clin Nutr 1997;66(3):679–80.
54. Cutts ME, Dowdy RP, Ellersieck MR, et al. Predicting energy needs in ventilator dependent critically ill patients: effect of adjusting weight for edema or adiposity. Am J Clin Nutr 1997;66:1250–6.
55. Osborne BJ, Saba AK, Wood SJ, et al. Clinical comparison of three methods to determine resting energy expenditure. Nutr Clin Pract 1994;9:241–6.
56. Daly JM, Heymsfield SB, Head CA, et al. Human energy expenditure: overestimation by widely used prediction equations. Am J Clin Nutr 1985;42:1170–4.
57. Cortes B, Nelson LD. Errors in estimating energy expenditure in critically ill surgical patients. Arch Surg 1989;124:287–90.
58. Ireton-Jones CS. Evaluation of energy expenditure in obese patients. Nutr Clin Pract 1989;4:127–9.
59. Bernstein RS, Thornton JC, Yang MU, et al. Prediction of the resting metabolic rate in obese patients. Am J Clin Nutr 1983;37:595–602.
60. Mascioli EA, Smith MF, Trerice MS, et al. Effect of total parenteral nutrition with cycling on essential fatty acid deficiency. J Parenter Eternal Nutr 1979;3:171–3.
61. Benedetti G, Mingrone G, Marcoccia S, et al. Body composition and energy expenditure after weight loss following bariatric surgery. J Am Coll Nutr 2000; 19:270–4.
62. Weijs PJ. Validity of predictive equations for resting energy expenditure in US and Dutch overweight and obese class I and II adults aged 18-65 y. Am J Clin Nutr 2008;88(4):959–70.
63. Hofsteenge GH, Chinapaw MJ, Delemarre-van de Waal HA, et al. Validation of predictive equations for resting energy expenditure in obese adolescents. Am J Clin Nutr 2010;91(5):1244–54.
64. Weijs PJ, Vansant GA. Validity of predictive equations for resting energy expenditure in Belgian normal weight to morbid obese women. Clin Nutr 2010;29(3):347–51.
65. Frankenfield D, Roth-Yousey L, Compher C. Comparison of predictive equations for resting metabolic rate in healthy nonobese and obese adults: a systematic review. J Am Diet Assoc 2005;105(5):775–89.
66. Boullata J, Williams J, Cottrell F, et al. Accurate determination of energy needs in hospitalized patients. J Am Diet Assoc 2007;107(3):393–401.

67. Ogawa AM, Shikora SA, Burke LM, et al. The thermodilution technique for measuring resting energy expenditure does not agree with indirect calorimetry for the critically ill patient. JPEN J Parenter Enteral Nutr 1998;22(6):347–51.
68. Furnary AP, Wu Y. Clinical effects of hyperglycemia in the cardiac surgery population: the Portland Diabetic Project. Endocr Pract 2006;12(Suppl 3):22–6.
69. Furnary AP, Wu Y. Eliminating the diabetic disadvantage: the Portland Diabetic Project. Semin Thorac Cardiovasc Surg 2006;18:302–8.
70. Zerr KJ, Furnary AP, Grunkemeier GL, et al. Glucose control lowers the risk of wound infection in diabetics after open heart operations. Ann Thorac Surg 1997;63:356–61.
71. McCowen KC, Malhotra A, Bistrian BR. Stress-induced hyperglycemia. Crit Care Clin 2001;17:107–24.
72. Marik PE, Raghavan M. Stress-hyperglycemia, insulin and immunomodulation in sepsis. Intensive Care Med 2004;30:748–56.
73. van den Berghe G, Wouters P, Weekers F, et al. Intensive insulin therapy in the critically ill patients. N Engl J Med 2001;345:1359–67.
74. Baker AL, Rosenberg IH. Hepatic complications of total parenteral nutrition. Am J Med 1987;82:489–97.
75. Raman M, Allard JP. Parenteral nutrition related hepato-biliary disease in adults. Appl Physiol Nutr Metab 2007;32(4):646–54.
76. McMahon MM, Benotti PN, Bistrian BR. A clinical application of exercise physiology and nutritional support for the mechanically ventilated patient. JPEN J Parenter Enteral Nutr 1990;14:538–42.
77. Askanazi J, Rosenbaum SH, Hyman AI, et al. Respiratory changes induced by the large glucose loads of total parenteral nutrition. JAMA 1980;243:1444–7.
78. Ireton-Jones C, Francis C. Obesity: nutrition support practice and application to critical care. Nutr Clin Pract 1995;10:144–9.
79. Jeevanandam M, Young DH, Schiller WR. Obesity and the metabolic response to severe multiple trauma in man. J Clin Invest 1991;87:262–9.
80. Elamin EM. Nutritional care of the obese intensive care unit patient. Curr Opin Crit Care 2005;11:300–3.
81. Port AM, Apovian C. Metabolic support of the obese intensive care unit patient: a current perspective. Curr Opin Clin Nutr Metab Care 2010;13:184–91.
82. Honiden S, McArdle JR. Obesity in the intensive care unit. Clin Chest Med 2009; 30:581–99.
83. Reeds DN. Nutrition support in the obese, diabetic patient: the role of hypocaloric feeding. Curr Opin Gastroenterol 2009;25:151–4.
84. Dickerson RN, Boschert KJ, Kudsk KA, et al. Hypocaloric enteral tube feeding in critically ill obese patients. Nutrition 2002;18:241–6.
85. Baxter JK, Bistrian BR. Moderate hypocaloric parenteral nutrition in the critically ill, obese patient. Nutr Clin Pract 1989;4:133–5.
86. Dickerson RN, Rosato EF, Mullen JL. Net protein anabolism with hypocaloric parenteral nutrition in obese stressed patients. Am J Clin Nutr 1986;44:747–55.
87. Burge JC, Goon A, Choban PS, et al. Efficacy of hypocaloric total parenteral nutrition in hospitalized obese patients: a prospective, double-blind randomized trial. JPEN J Parenter Enteral Nutr 1994;18:203–7.
88. Bistrian BR, Blackburn GL, Flatt JP, et al. Nitrogen metabolism and insulin requirements in obese diabetic adults on a protein-sparing modified fast. Diabetes 1976;25(6):494–504.
89. Greenberg GR, Marliss EB, Anderson GH, et al. Protein sparing therapy in postoperative patients. N Engl J Med 1976;294:1411–6.

90. Young GA, Hill GL. A controlled study of protein-sparing therapy after excision of the rectum. Ann Surg 1980;192:183–91.
91. Hensle TW, Askanazi J. Metabolism and nutrition in the perioperative period. J Urol 1988;139:229–39.
92. Douglas RG, Shaw JH. Metabolic response to sepsis and trauma. Br J Surg 1989; 76:115–22.
93. Elwyn DH, Kinney JM, Askanazi J. Energy expenditure in surgical patients. Surg Clin North Am 1981;61:545–56.
94. Shikora SA. Enteral feeding tube placement in obese patients: considerations for nutrition support. Nutr Clin Pract 1997;12:S9–13.

Nutritional Considerations in Adult Cardiothoracic Surgical Patients

Juan A. Sanchez, MD, MPA[a,b,*], Lise L. Sanchez, RD[c],
Stanley J. Dudrick, MD[a,d]

KEYWORDS

- Cardiac surgery • Thoracic surgery • Nutrition
- Chronic heart failure • Cardiac cachexia
- Malnutrition risk factors

Despite the large volume of scientific research and publications relevant to the nutritional and metabolic considerations of surgical disease states, little attention and investigation have been directed specifically toward patients undergoing cardiovascular or pulmonary surgery. In many respects, it is this group of patients that, perhaps, warrant the most fastidious attention to nutritional detail, given that they are often the most critically ill. Furthermore, a large body of literature has focused on optimizing metabolic conditions to attempt to mitigate the deleterious effects of reperfusion injury on the myocardium and, to a lesser extent, on the lung. Additionally, many of these investigations focus on the effects of a wide variety of nutrients with antioxidant and cardioprotective properties. However, these efforts have often been conducted with the arguably myopic perspective of the heart or the lung as an isolated organ and without apparent consideration of the patients' overall constitutive nutritional and metabolic status or requirements. Nonetheless, the authors review herein the current status of the nutritional aspects of patients who are cardiothoracic and their surgical management, with the overarching goal of focusing attention on the serious

The authors have nothing to disclose.

[a] Department of Surgery, Saint Mary's Hospital/Yale Affiliate, 56 Franklin Street, Waterbury, CT 06706, USA

[b] Department of Surgery, University of Connecticut Health Center, 263 Farmington Avenue, Farmington, CT 06032, USA

[c] Department of Food and Nutrition, Bridgeport Hospital, 267 Grant Street, Bridgeport, CT 06610, USA

[d] Department of Surgery, Yale University School of Medicine, 333 Cedar Street, New Haven, CT 06510, USA

* Corresponding author. Department of Surgery, Saint Mary's Hospital, 56 Franklin Street, Waterbury, CT 06706.

E-mail address: Juan.Sanchez@stmh.org

consequences associated with nutritionally deficient states, either preoperatively or postoperatively, in these complex groups of seriously ill patients.

NUTRITIONAL STATUS OF PATIENTS UNDERGOING CARDIAC SURGERY

Assessing nutritional status in patients prior to cardiac surgery can be quite challenging. Often, these patients come under consideration for treatment by a surgeon during urgent or emergency conditions, mostly after having undergone an extensive series of diagnostic procedures to identify, triage, and stratify their heart disease. Unfortunately, valuable nutrition and metabolic information, which can be of immense importance in the perioperative period, is not always obtained during this phase of investigative assessment. Not only can relevant biochemical and anthropometric studies indicate or identify a compromised nutritional state but basic important information can be derived from a proper history, including recent weight loss, diminished strength or endurance, poor appetite, food allergies, and altered digestion, which can complicate major cardiothoracic operations and the postoperative care, adding considerable risk to the patients' procedure and subsequent management.

Malnutrition had been reported to increase the morbidity and mortality after cardiac operations.[1] Several investigators have correlated poor nutrition with increased complication rates and worse outcomes following heart surgery, many suggesting that nutritional status should be a strong consideration in assessing whether patients should be selected for surgery. Although obesity may be associated with increased but acceptable risks in cardiac surgery, a study by Loop[2] and colleagues has also suggested that thin patients may actually be at a higher risk after coronary operations than obese patients. Although the effect of small body size on the incidence of complications, length of stay, and mortality after cardiac operations has not been extensively studied, current understanding indicates that thin patients with very low fat stores have an elevated risk for surgery.[3,4]

One objective measure of malnutrition is the serum albumin concentration, and preoperative serum albumin levels had been found to be strong independent predictors of morbidity and mortality in a recent large study of patients undergoing noncardiac surgery.[3,5] Accordingly, 5168 consecutive patients undergoing cardiac operations at Brigham and Women's Hospital were studied prospectively to assess the independent contribution of body mass and malnutrition to morbidity and mortality after cardiac operations.[3] The investigators used the preoperative serum albumin level to determine the degree to which hypoalbuminemia contributed to postoperative morbidity and mortality, and they assessed whether any association between body mass index (BMI) and surgical outcome was dependent on the preoperative nutritional status as measured by the serum albumin concentrations.[3] Patients undergoing primary as well as reoperative coronary artery bypass grafting (CABG) or valve surgery, or both, were included in the study.[3] The degree of thinness or obesity was assessed by the BMI, defined as the weight in kilograms divided by the height in meters squared.[3,6] Of all the indexes of obesity, BMI correlates best with more direct measurements of percent body fat, and patients with a BMI of less than 20 were defined as the high-risk thin patient group.[3,7] This designation corresponded to a weight more than 25% below the ideal body weight for an individual's height.[3,8] Patients with a BMI of more than 30 were defined as the high-risk obese group and corresponded to one standard deviation greater than the mean BMI.[3,9] Preoperative serum albumin concentrations were determined in all patients.[3]

Sixty-eight percent of the patients underwent isolated CABG procedures, 18% underwent isolated valve operations, and 14% underwent combined CABG/valve procedures.[3] The median age of the patients was 67 years, with a lower quartile of 59 years and an upper quartile of 74 years. The median BMI was 26.6, with a lower quartile of 23.9 and an upper quartile of 29.7. The median serum albumin level was 3.5 g/dL, with a lower quartile of 2.7 g/dL and an upper quartile of 4.1 g/dL.[3] The overall mortality was 3.8%.[3] Low BMI (<20) and low serum albumin levels (<2.5 g/dL) were each independently associated with increased mortality after cardiopulmonary bypass (p<.0005). Those patients with both low BMIs and low serum albumin levels had the highest mortality (16%). At all levels of BMI, the operative mortality was higher among patients with a serum albumin level of less than 2.5 g/dL. At all serum albumin concentrations, the operative mortality was higher in those with a BMI less than 20. Patients with extremely high BMIs (greater than 35) had a mortality of 4.7%, which was not significantly different from the reference group ($P = .16$).[3] In patients who underwent CABG or CABG/valve procedures, there was no difference in internal thoracic artery usage between patients with a BMI of 20 to 30 and those with a BMI of more than 30. Patients with serum albumin levels less than 2.5 g/dL and a BMI of less than 20 had a greater number of comorbidities and risk factors.[3]

Lower levels of serum albumin were also associated with higher incidences of postoperative complications and longer lengths of hospital stay. The highest prevalence of complications was observed in those patients with serum albumin levels less than 2.5 g/dL. There was no association between preoperative serum albumin levels and saphenous vein harvest site infections. A BMI of less than 20 was also associated with an increased number of postoperative complications. However, patients with BMIs of more than 30 had a significantly increased incidence of deep sternal wound infection and saphenous vein harvest site infections (P<.0005) without any increase in overall length of stay.[3] In multivariable analyses adjusting for potential confounders, patients with serum albumin levels less than 3.5 g/dL had a significantly increased risk of renal failure, postoperative atrial fibrillation, and increased length of stay. Patients with serum albumin levels less than 2.5 g/dL also had increased risks of death, low cardiac output, and re-exploration for postoperative bleeding. Patients with BMIs of less than 20 had increased risks of death, cerebral vascular accidents, transient ischemic attacks, renal failure, pneumonia, and reoperation for bleeding. On the other hand, patients with BMIs of more than 30 had increased risks of atrial arrhythmias, deep sternal wound infections, and saphenous vein harvest site infections. It is remarkable that this cadre of patients also had a significantly decreased risk of re-exploration for bleeding. These findings cannot be explained by differences in internal thoracic artery use, which was nearly identical among patients with a BMI of 20 to 30 and those with a BMI of more than 30.[3] In summary, (1) the mortality results were independent of the type of surgical procedure performed; (2) a low serum albumin level was a better predictor of mortality in isolated valve and combined CABG/valve procedures than in isolated CABG procedures; (3) a BMI of more than 30 or a serum albumin level of 2.5 to 3.5 g/dL was not associated with a significantly increased mortality in any surgical subgroup; and (4) there was no significant interaction between BMI and serum albumin level.[3] In this study, both low BMI and hypoalbuminemia independently predicted increased mortality and postoperative complications after cardiac surgery. Moreover, the thinnest patients were found to have more risk factors for postoperative morbidity and mortality than obese patients, and additionally, women represented a greater percentage of patients in the low BMI group.[3]

Christakos and colleagues[10] suggested a similar relationship between BMI and operative mortality/low cardiac output after isolated CABG procedures. Other studies have similarly implied that patients with smaller body surface areas have a higher mortality independent of other risk factors.[2–4,11,12] Mickleborough and colleagues[3,13] found an increased incidence of perioperative myocardial infarction and low cardiac output in patients with low body surface areas after isolated CABG, but no differences in mortality. Additionally, preoperative unintended weight loss of 10% or greater is associated with serious adverse effects following cardiac surgery independent of body mass.[14] It has been posited that patients with low BMIs (and a lower percentage of body fat) have less nutritional reserve, which may not allow them to employ the usual repertoire of adaptive physiologic responses to complications, resulting in greater mortality.[3]

In the postoperative period, early and aggressive nutritional support efforts should be made to correct or compensate for identified preoperative deficiencies and to meet the anticipated increased metabolic postoperative demands. However, these efforts are often thwarted by several factors and conditions, some of which are unique to this field. For example, it has long been suspected and recently confirmed that taste sensitivity is dramatically altered in patients undergoing cardiac surgery and that recovery of normal taste is slow.[15] Moreover, although the operative risks in preoperatively malnourished patients are high, aggressive use of parenteral nutrition early in the postoperative period has not resulted uniformly in mitigating risks in cardiac surgery patients who were not significantly malnourished preoperatively.[16] However, several investigators are interested in potentially improving the outcomes associated with the uninterrupted administration of enteral and parenteral nutrition in the extended perioperative period by using specific amino acid substrates, which have been shown in the experimental laboratory to be of value in improving myocardial metabolism and reducing the incidence of complications following cardiac surgery.[17–20]

Demographic changes in North America and elsewhere, combined with refinements in technical surgery and with the ability to offer more advanced surgery to the elderly, have resulted in a substantial increase in the geriatric age group that can safely undergo cardiothoracic surgical procedures. It has become apparent, however, that these patients often manifest suboptimal nutritional and metabolic reserves, further compounding the complex technical and management problems in the elderly, particularly when surgical challenges are not straightforward. As such, aggressive and early efforts to assess the nutritional status of those patients is of paramount importance in reducing complications and, thus, improving outcomes in these patients.

HEART FAILURE AND CARDIAC CACHEXIA

Much of the cardiovascular disease burden in the United States and, increasingly, throughout the developed world is not associated with malnutrition, but rather is a product, directly or indirectly, of hypernutrition, a fact corroborated by the obesity epidemic.[21] Through a complex and, as yet, incompletely understood series of biophysical processes and mechanisms involving the body's capacity to handle lipids and carbohydrates, considerable genetic influences, as well as other contributions from the immune system and environmental factors, atherosclerosis variously involves the coronary arteries, the aorta, and its main branches. In addition, patients with long-standing valvular heart disease, either acquired or congenital, and nonischemic diseases of the myocardium resulting in heart failure often exhibit cardiac cachexia, a specific form of protein-calorie malnutrition frequently seen in end-stage or neglected cardiac disease, together with its attendant morbid consequences.

Chronic heart failure has a prevalence of approximately 1% to 2% in the United States.[22,23] Because of the general improvements in health care, an increasing proportion of elderly people in the population, and improved survival after myocardial infarction, the incidence of new patients with chronic heart failure is likely to increase further.[21] Because approximately 10% of the chronic heart failure population manifests cardiac cachexia, as many as 600,000 to 1,200,000 patients may suffer from this condition in North America and Europe.[21] Much more needs to be learned about the pathophysiology of wasting in chronic heart failure, and studies must be undertaken to develop an effective treatment for cardiac cachexia. In the meantime, a reasonable goal is to attempt to predict the development of cardiac cachexia and to try to arrest the wasting process before the onset of significant weight loss.[21] Enhancing the prognosis of cardiac cachexia, or even reversing the cachectic process, will likely have a significant influence on the quality of life of many patients and may improve the long-term prognosis of chronic heart failure overall.[21] This area of cardiac research ranks as one of the most interesting and challenging fields because it requires joint efforts and collaboration of cardiologists, endocrinologists, immunologists, nutritionists, and surgeons, and involves the study of metabolic cardiology and cardiac surgery.

Patients with longstanding heart failure carry inordinately high surgical risks, not only because of the delayed surgical treatment, which is often the case, but also because of the unrecognized, concomitant malnutrition itself. Anker and Coats have pointed out that it has long been recognized that significant weight loss and muscle wasting are important features of severe chronic heart failure, dating back 2300 years to the observations of Hippocrates (about 460–370 BC) on the island of Cos: "The flesh is consumed and becomes water ... the shoulders, clavicles, chest and thighs melt away. This illness is fatal..."[21,24] In 1785, Withering wrote the following about a patient with heart failure: "His countenance was pale, his pulse quick and feeble, his body greatly emaciated, except his belly, which was very large."[21,25] The presence of general weight loss in patients with chronic heart failure has, at times, been somewhat misleadingly termed cardiac cachexia,[21] but whether the process of simple weight loss is ordinarily also accompanied by a loss of cardiac muscle tissue has never been studied comprehensively in such patients. Moreover, whether a distinction between peripheral skeletal cachexia and cardiac cachexia is necessary or useful remains unknown.[21] Thus, the problems of research into cardiac cachexia begin with its definition, and although multiple investigators have extensively investigated a variety of cachectic conditions, there are still no uniformly accepted definitions of cachexia or cardiac cachexia.[21] Approaches to defining cachexia include body composition analysis with body fat and lean tissue estimation, and anthropometric measurements (skin fold thickness, arm muscle circumference); calculations of predicted percent ideal mass matched for age and height; assessment scores, including serum albumin concentrations, cell-mediated immunity changes, weight/height index or BMI; and a history of weight loss.[21] In some heart failure studies, patients have been classified as malnourished when the body fat content was less than 22% in women and less than 15% in men, or when the percentage of ideal body weight was less than 90%.[21,26] Other groups have defined patients with chronic heart failure prospectively as cachectic when the body fat content was less than 29% (women) or less than 27% (men),[27] or when the ideal body weight was less than 85%[28] or even less than 80%.[29] Additionally, it is possible to characterize the lean tissue by studying urinary creatinine excretion rates, skeletal muscle protein turnover (using labeled amino acids), bioelectrical impedance, total body potassium content, or by measuring the skeletal muscle size by means of magnetic resonance imaging (MRI) and computed tomography or body densitometry.[21] It is important to note that the development of the cachectic state in chronic heart failure is a process that can only be proven by a documented weight loss measured in a nonedematous state.[21] Moreover, including weight loss as a criterion excludes patients who constitutionally have a low body weight.[21] Accordingly, Anker and Coats suggest the use of a relatively broad definition of clinical cardiac cachexia, which states: "In patients with chronic heart failure of at least 6 months' duration without signs of other primary cachectic states (eg, cancer, thyroid disease, or severe liver disease), cardiac cachexia can be diagnosed with weight loss of greater than 7.5% of the previous normal weight observed."[21] This weight loss should be observed over a period of greater than 6 months because massive weight loss over a shorter period of time might be cardiac cachexia, but obviously other etiologies of wasting, such as cancer and infection, must also be considered in the differential diagnosis.[21] This definition of cardiac cachexia is simple and readily applicable in theory, but in practice it is necessary to take a very careful and precise weight history to justify the diagnosis.

Three categories of mechanisms are thought to be responsible for the development of cardiac cachexia: (1) malabsorption and metabolic malfunction, (2) dietary deficiency, and (3) loss of nutrients via the urinary or digestive tract.[21] Pittman and Cohen[30] were the first to extensively analyze the pathogenesis of the syndrome of cardiac cachexia, and, in general, they thought that the development of cellular hypoxia was the leading pathogenic factor, causing less efficient intermediary metabolism, therefore, producing increased catabolism (protein loss) and reduced anabolism. Additionally, they suggested that anorexia and increased basal metabolic rate were closely related and possibly the result, in part, of a lack of oxygen.[21,30]

Little is known about the mechanisms of the transition from chronic heart failure to cardiac cachexia.[21] Anorexia can be related to heart failure via its main symptoms (fatigue and dyspnea) or via intestinal edema causing nausea or a protein-losing gastroenteropathy.[21] Additionally, anorexia may be iatrogenic as a side effect of digitalis, sodium-restricted diets, and some angiotensin-converting enzyme (ACE) inhibitors. Thus far, however, multiple studies to test this hypothesis have been equivocal.[31-34]

Simple starvation and anorexia are often considered to be the main causes of cardiac cachexia, but they would lead mainly to a loss of fat tissue while also causing serum albumin levels to decline.[21] However, patients who are cachectic with chronic heart failure suffer from combined fat, muscle, and bone tissue loss (indicating the presence of a general wasting process); and serum albumin and liver enzyme levels are not decreased in these patients.[21,35] This finding would militate against a major contribution of starvation, anorexia, gastrointestinal malabsorption, or liver synthetic dysfunction in the etiology of cachexia in these patients.[21] Physical inactivity and deconditioning have been suggested as potential causes of the muscle atrophy observed in many patients with chronic heart failure, but histologic evidence suggests that the muscle atrophy resulting from states of reduced activity is significantly different from the muscle atrophy observed in chronic heart failure.[21,36-38] Therefore, it seems unlikely that decreased physical activity is of primary importance in the genesis of cardiac cachexia and that the etiology is some other agnogenic mechanism.[21]

NUTRITIONAL SUPPORT OF CARDIAC CACHEXIA

When cardiac cachexia is detected in patients with chronic heart failure, 18-month survival is only approximately 50%, primarily because no specific therapy for patients who are cachectic with chronic heart failure exists.[21] Theoretically, it appears clear that the nutritional status must be improved to regain energy reserves (fat tissue), the muscle tissue must be increased to improve exercise capacity, and anticytokine therapy might be feasible and useful.[21] At the present time, except for judicious preoperative and postoperative nutritional support of patients with cardiac cachexia, there are no other controlled therapeutic strategies for improving outcomes in cardiac cachexia.[21] In stable patients with chronic heart failure and no signs of severe malnutrition, nutritional support alone has had no significant effect on the clinical status of the heart failure.[21,39] Although intensive nutritional support could further increase the oxidative demands of the body, it has nonetheless been shown that appropriate adequate nutritional support is safe in patients with cardiac cachexia and can indeed lead to the accrual of an increased amount of lean tissue.[21,40] This strategy is of great importance in the preoperative and postoperative periods if surgery is required.[21] Immediate postoperative total parenteral nutrition alone did not improve survival in one cardiac study,[16] whereas, in another study, patients with cachexia with heart failure who received preoperative support (5–8 weeks duration intravenously (IV) with up to 1200 kcal/d) had lower mortality than did patients who were not given nutritional support (17% versus 57%; $P<0.05$).[21,29] Others have suggested a feeding regimen of 40 to 50 $kcal/m^2$ body surface per hour, including 1.5 to 2.0 g/kg/h protein, and the restriction of sodium (2 g/d) and fluid (1000–1500 mL/d) using high-density continuous IV nutrient infusion.[16,21] In any case, but especially for patients who are ambulatory cachectic but stable, dietary consultation with a nutritional support team can be very helpful.[21]

CHRONIC HEART FAILURE

Chronic heart failure is a significant problem that affects more than 2% of the United States population (about 5 million people), and 30% to 40% of patients die of heart failure within 1 year after diagnosis.[41,42] Moreover, heart failure can be disabling and severely compromise patients' quality of life. On the other hand, in the past 2 decades, considerable progress has been made in the treatment of chronic heart failure with ACE inhibitors,[43,44] aldosterone antagonists,[45] beta-receptor blockers,[46,47] and resynchronization therapy.[41,48,49] Despite these advances, chronic heart failure is still associated with an annual mortality of 10%, and the search for better treatments is a major challenge for cardiologists and cardiac surgeons.[41,49] In a comprehensive review, Neubauer[41] has pointed out the many reasons why a human heart can fail, but that the available evidence suggests that "the failing heart is an engine out of fuel," and that altered energetics play an important role in the mechanisms of heart failure.[41,50] Accordingly, the modulation of cardiac nutrition and metabolism has promise as a new approach to the treatment of heart failure.[41] The concept that the failing heart is an energy-starved engine that has run out of fuel is decades old, having first been proposed in 1939 by Herrmann and Dechard[41,51] who described a significantly reduced creatine content in failing myocardium. During the next 20 years, the energy-depletion hypothesis was pursued by various groups, and energy metabolism in the heart (myocardial energetics) is still a topic of considerable interest today.[41,52–63] An explanation or justification of the attention to this area of research is that any energy-sparing treatment for heart failure, such as the previously mentioned beta-receptor blockers,[46,47] ACE inhibitors,[43,44] or angiotensin II blockers,[64,65] improves the prognosis of patients.[41] Another analogy advanced is that the failing heart resembles a weak, tired horse, and if the horse is nourished optimally, it can recover and work, but at a reduced capacity.[41,66]

Deprivation of cardiac energy plays a major role in chronic heart failure.[41,57] The heart consumes more energy than any other organ in the body, cycling about 6 kg of ATP daily, equivalent to about 20 to 30 times its own weight.[41] Each day, it beats about 100,000 times and pumps approximately 10 tons of blood throughout the body, thus performing an enormous amount of work.[41] To acquire the energy necessary to carry out its function, the heart converts chemical energy stored in fatty acids and glucose into the mechanical energy of the actin-myosin contractile interaction of the myofibrils.[41] Failure to produce an adequate amount of energy to provide the heart with its required needs causes mechanical failure.[41]

NUTRITIONAL SUPPORT OF THE FAILING HEART

Neubauer summarized the complex subject of cardiac energy metabolism thusly:

The metabolic machinery has three main components. The first is substrate utilization – the use of fuel that comes from food. This process entails the cellular uptake of mainly three fatty acids and glucose, the breakdown of these components by beta-oxidation and glycolysis, and the entry of the resulting intermediary metabolites into the Krebs cycle. The second component is oxidative phosphorylation – the production of energy by the mitochondrial respiratory chain. The phosphorylation of ADP (adenosine diphosphate) by this mechanism produces the high-energy phosphate compound ATP, which is the final direct source of energy for all energy-consuming reactions in the heart. The third component is ATP transfer and utilization transfer – the transport of energy to, and its consumption by, the heart's motor, the myofibrils. This process entails an energy-transfer mechanism termed the creatine kinase energy shuttle.[67–69] In the third component of cardiac energy metabolism, ATP transfer and utilization, mitochondrial creatine kinase catalyzes the transfer of the high-energy phosphate bond in ATP to creatinine to form phosphocreatine and ADP. Phosphocreatine, a smaller molecule than ATP, rapidly diffuses from the mitochondria to the myofibrils where myofibrillar creatine kinase catalyzes the reformation of ATP from phosphocreatine. The free creatine, formed by the removal of phosphate from phosphocreatine, then diffuses back to the mitochondrium... A small amount of creatine is constantly lost from the heart by passive diffusion across the sarcolemma.[70] An important function of the creatine kinase system is to act as an energy buffer. When the energy demand outstrips the energy supply, the phosphocreatine level falls, keeping ATP at a normal level, but the free ADP level rises.[68] The increased level of free ADP inhibits the function of many intracellular enzymes, causing failure of the heart's contraction mechanism. Thus, a metabolic derangement in the cardiac myocyte can occur when phosphocreatine levels fall and free ADP levels rise, even if ATP levels remain unchanged. The various components of energy metabolism in the heart can be measured with the use of standard methods in myocardial specimens obtained during a biopsy or at the time of transplantation, or in cardiac tissue from animals. The analysis of ATP and phosphocreatine in tissue samples is problematic, however, because of the instability of these molecules.[68] For this reason, the principal method for measuring ATP and phosphocreatine is phosphorus-31 magnetic resonance spectroscopy.[71–74] The MRI system can obtain cine images of the heart at the same time for quantification of cardiac function. The most powerful method for assessing energy metabolism in heart failure entails the in vivo assessment of turnover rates of glucose and fatty acids[75–78] and rates of oxidative phosphorylation[79] and ATP transfer.[72–74] An important methodologic consideration is intracellular compartmentalization.[80] Whether a cardiac myocyte functions normally cannot be determined by measuring the average cellular levels of ATP, phosphocreatine, or ADP, but instead is determined by their concentration in the perimyofibrillar space and near the sarcoplasmic reticulum and sarcolemmal ion pumps. No method is currently available to make such measurements; therefore, they have to be extrapolated from global measurements.[41]

NUTRITIONAL SUPPORT OF CARDIOTHORACIC SURGICAL PATIENTS

Randomized, controlled clinical studies have been reported in patients undergoing cardiac surgery in whom arginine,[17,81–83] aspartate,[84] or glutamate[85] was administered, and have shown improved cardiac flow,[82,83] cardiac function measured as plasma troponin T, creatine kinase (CK), and CK-MB,[81,84,85] or cardiac metabolism measured as myocardial acidosis, ATP, and lactate in myocardial biopsies.[17,84,85] Amino acid supplementation minimized apoptosis in cardiomyocytes by increasing ATP production and myocardial oxygen consumption,[86] by reducing myocardial ischemic damage, and by increasing diastolic pressure, in animal laboratory studies.[17,87] In cardiac surgery patients, parenteral amino acid supplementation increased esophageal core temperature; shortened duration of postoperative mechanical ventilation, intensive care unit stay, and hospitalization; and speeded tracheal extubation in patients undergoing CABG.[17,18] Enteral nutrition in cardiac surgical patients repleted cardiomyocytes with nutrients, improved left ventricular end-diastolic volume preoperatively,[19] improved preoperative host defense, reduced the number of postoperative infections, and preserved renal function.[17,20] The results of all of these studies have shown favorable effects of nutritional support on cardiac function. However, the effects of uninterrupted, perioperative supplementation of amino acids, glucose, vitamins, and minerals on cardiac amino acid profile, cardiomyocyte structure, cardiac perfusion, left ventricular function, and metabolism of cardiac surgical patients have never been investigated to this day. This unfortunate truth provides the opportunities for the next generation of cardiothoracic surgeons and their nutritional scientist colleagues to attempt to achieve a level of nutritional and metabolic support perfection comparable to that which the current generation of cardiovascular surgeons has achieved technically.

RATIONALE FOR NUTRIENT ADMINISTRATION IN CARDIAC SURGERY PATIENTS

Both enteral and parenteral nutrition formulations contain amino acids, glucose, vitamins, and minerals, which function together as precursors for protein synthesis. Additionally, amino acids are available to replenish components of the tricarboxylic acid cycle, which can increase ATP production in heart cells, with resultant positive effects on cardiomyocyte metabolism.[17,21] Many of the amino acids are essential amino acids, such as histidine, isoleucine, leucine, lysine, methionine, phenylalanine, threonine, tryptophan, and valine, which cannot be synthesized in the human body and, therefore, must be supplied exogenously as essential nutrients.[17] Two of the nonessential amino acids, glutamate and aspartate, are important components of the nutrient regimen because they are present abundantly intracellularly as free amino acids in the heart, and have been shown to have a cardioprotective effect by enhancing ATP production.[17,88,89] Furthermore, depleted levels of aspartate and glutamate in cardiomyocytes and low plasma levels of arginine have been found in patients with heart failure.[17,90,91] Additionally, the semiessential amino acid arginine is the precursor of nitric oxide (NO), a dominant active compound that influences blood flow and endothelial function, is involved in myocardial relaxation and distensibility, and might improve left ventricular function.[17,92] Moreover, arginine supplementation might improve the arginine/asymmetric dimethylarginine ratio, an indicator of potential NO production.[17] Exogenous glucose provided in enteral or parenteral nutrition can avoid conversion of the administered amino acids into glucose via gluconeogenesis and can prevent or minimize protein catabolism.[17,93] Finally, the vitamins and minerals in parenteral and enteral nutrient formulations are essential ingredients of the nutritional regimen of the cardiac surgery patient because several of them have antioxidant properties and all of them can prevent micronutrient deficiencies from occurring.[17,94]

CURRENT AND FUTURE CHALLENGES FOR CARDIAC NUTRITIONAL AND METABOLIC SUPPORT

A promising strategy for metabolic intervention in chronic heart failure is to modulate substrate utilization, which is feasible, for example, with the use of partial inhibitors of fatty acid oxidation or carnitine palmitoyl transferase 1 inhibitors. These compounds have complex actions, but they all partially inhibit fatty acid utilization and promote glucose utilization.[41,58,60,62] Whether the suppression of fatty acid oxidation is beneficial or detrimental in heart disease is highly controversial, and the cause or stage of heart failure may dictate the outcome of this type of treatment. Several recent clinical studies have suggested that partial inhibition of fatty acid oxidation is promising therapeutically.[41] A second potential strategy for metabolic therapy for heart failure is direct stimulation of oxidative phosphorylation; however, no effective stimulators of oxidative phosphorylation currently exist.[41] An alternative approach is to reduce free fatty acid levels, which should suppress mitochondrial uncoupling proteins, thereby increasing ATP synthesis.[41] A third strategy for metabolic intervention is the direct manipulation of high-energy phosphate stores or manipulating the availability or efficiency of their utilization.[41] Creatine and phosphocreatine levels can be augmented by increasing the creatine transporter function.[41,95] Because a substantially supernormal creatine level increases the free ADP level, massive increases in the creatine transporter function would be detrimental, but moderate stimulation of creatine transporter activity is likely to be beneficial in heart failure.[41] Finally, it may be feasible to improve the myofibrillar efficiency of ATP utilization with new calcium-sensitizing or myosin activator compounds.[41,96]

The current status of nutritional and metabolic treatment of patients with cardiovascular disease has been summarized concisely and eloquently by Neubauer[41]:

> Metabolic therapy is a promising new avenue for the treatment of heart failure, and suitable targets for therapy are substrate utilization, oxidative phosphorylation, and the availability of high-energy phosphates. A multipronged effort is needed to fully investigate this concept. Experimental studies will, for example, further clarify the mechanisms leading to energetic derangement and will suggest new molecular targets for therapeutic intervention. New metabolic modulator compounds need to be developed by academia and industry. Proof-of-principle clinical studies may use the myocardial phosphocreatine/ATP ratio of the heart to monitor metabolic therapy, and this method may provide a surrogate marker of long-term prognostic effects. Finally, large-scale clinical trials will have to prove or disprove the clinical efficacy of metabolic modulators. There is substantial hope that such a combined effort will lead to new therapies targeted at cardiac energetics. These therapies may improve the symptoms and prognosis of patients with the life-threatening illness of chronic heart failure.[41]

The challenges to discover and develop the optimal nutritional, metabolic, and pharmacologic management of surgical patients with compromised heart function will test the mettle not only of the cardiothoracic surgeon but of all health care clinicians and scientists interested in supporting optimal myocardial performance. The heart is a most remarkable and unique organ that works constantly throughout life to support the body cell mass, and it is dependent upon a special array of energetic and metabolic molecular substrates that must be available in a timely, qualitative, and quantitative manner for maintenance of its vital life-sustaining function. All surgeons must maintain a keen interest in maintaining optimal, precisely responsive cardiac function in all of their patients if the best outcomes of therapeutic surgical approaches are to be realized. To state the obvious for emphasis, when cardiothoracic function is compromised, all bodily functions are compromised, and when the heart stops, life stops.

INFECTIOUS COMPLICATIONS AND HYPERGLYCEMIA

Open heart operations are associated with several infrequent, but life-threatening complications. Sepsis (particularly in the setting of myocardial infarction), heart failure, and emergency bypass surgery are accompanied by increases in the incidence of postoperative infections and are independent risk factors for deep sternal wound infection along with diabetes, obesity, and other comorbid factors. The magnitude of these complications imposes enormous caloric requirements on patients and results in an extended catabolic state, which, in turn, increases susceptibility to other, more common, complications, such as pneumonia. In these patients, the heightened level of critical illness and the focus on the cardiovascular system can divert the health care team's attention away from the consequent accentuated nutritional needs that are central to ultimate successful outcomes.

Maintaining normal glucose levels in the postoperative state in individuals undergoing cardiac surgery has been shown to be associated with a statistically significant reduction in deep sternal wound infections, whether patients are diabetic or not.[97] Large-scale efforts to control postoperative glucose levels through intensive insulin therapy during and following surgery have generally been successful, but may somewhat hinder early optimal nutrition in patients with diabetes because of the concern that providing adequate calories early might induce hyperglycemia and attendant complications. This conundrum can be obviated by conscientious administration and monitoring of the nutrient infusion by a competent nutrition support team.

VENTRICULAR ASSISTANCE AND NUTRITION

Although transplantation of the heart and lungs carries considerable nutritional and metabolic consequences, these transplants are not dissimilar from other solid organ procedures and are not discussed directly in this article. However, the enhanced metabolic demands following the institution of long-term mechanical circulatory support, whether as a bridge to transplantation, to myocardial recovery, or as destination therapy, are underappreciated. It is well-known that, despite the usual extreme catabolic and malnourished state of these patients at the time of device implantation as previously described, most are able to be restored to normal metabolic and nutritional status with judicious nutritional support and sufficient time.[98,99] This restoration requires a dedicated, multidisciplinary approach to patient care, including considerable attention to nutritional intake, particularly early after incorporation of the device when continued catabolism, ongoing subclinical activation of fibrinolysis, and a repertoire of chemokine and cytokine activating events persist unabated as the host becomes acclimated to the mechanically supported circulation.[100–102] Dang,[103] for example, reported that outcomes of patients receiving an implantable left ventricular assist device with low preoperative serum albumin, total protein, or absolute lymphocyte levels were inferior to those of better-nourished cohorts, primarily because of the higher rates of infectious complications, lower rates of successful bridging to transplantation, and worse posttransplant survival.

NUTRITIONAL STATUS OF PATIENTS UNDERGOING PULMONARY SURGERY

Cancer involving major organs and systems is closely associated with nutritional deficiencies, and patients with malignant neoplasms are often thought of as being malnourished virtually by definition. Moreover, nutritional status is often correlated not only with operative survival but also with long-term prognosis. Pulmonary complications following lung surgery are also associated with poor nutritional status.

Several studies have examined the effects of age on postoperative complications following thoracic surgery.[104,105] Most stratagems for identifying those individuals at high risk included not only an assessment of nutritional status beyond BMI but also measures of visceral protein stores and, increasingly, anthropometric measurements.[106] Isowa[107] examined preoperative risk factors for a prolonged air leak following anatomic pulmonary resections and found that, besides diabetes mellitus, both preoperative low serum albumin and cholinesterase levels correlated with an increased air leak. With a much shorter half-life, cholinesterase can identify potentially malnourished patients earlier than serum albumin levels.[108]

Patients with poor pulmonary reserve, such as those with chronic obstructive lung disease, manifest a considerably increased amount of energy expended in the work of breathing. Combined with the metabolic demands of a major thoracic procedure, malnutrition in these patients can result in an increased risk for postoperative respiratory failure. Minimally invasive techniques employing video-assisted thoracic surgery, however, have improved the ability of these patients to tolerate major intrathoracic procedures. However, hypoventilation and CO_2 retention can often be vexing problems in the postoperative period, and high caloric enteral and parenteral formulations should be modulated to reduce the respiratory quotient and improve ventilation while providing sufficient nutritional support in these challenging fragile patients.

CHYLOTHORAX

Chylous pleural effusions are found in a wide variety of disease states, and surgical procedures involving the mediastinal structures can infrequently result in chyle leakage. Chyle, or intestinal lymphatic fluid, is unique in that it is enriched with fat, in the form of triglycerides and chylomicrons, along with fat-soluble vitamins, lymphocytes, and albumin.[109,110] Disruption of the main thoracic duct or its tributaries can result in persistent leakage with significant consequences related to protein and fluid losses, immune suppression, and an increasing caloric deficit.

The incidence of chylothorax after surgery is highest with esophagectomy, particularly with a transthoracic approach, and is commonly associated with the more advanced stages of cancer.[111,112] These patients have increased rates of pulmonary complications, including pneumonia and prolonged intensive care unit and hospital stays. Chyle leakage is often not recognized early, but becomes apparent once patients are taking oral or enteral feedings. The characteristic milky white fluid observed in the pleural drainage may require confirmation as chyle by analyzing the fluid for triglyceride levels, lymphocyte count, fat stain, and other diagnostic methods. Occasionally, observation of the response to oral intake of pure cream is necessary to confirm the diagnosis. The volume of drainage is often dramatic and at times is greater than 2 L/d.

Preferably, chylous leakage is initially managed conservatively. Cessation of oral intake and initiation of total parenteral nutrition results in successful resolution of the leak in as many as 80% of patients.[111] On the other hand, early intervention with right thoracoscopy and ligation of the thoracic duct near the diaphragm is increasingly being employed, particularly in patients who are frail and malnourished and are at an increased risk for serious complications from a protracted hospitalization and parenteral nutrition. Early diagnosis and treatment are essential in this condition, and the impact of any delay in restoring normal nutrition, fluid balance, and the immune system in chylothorax cannot be overstated.

SUMMARY

Cardiothoracic surgical patients are often critically ill, and the magnitude of cardiothoracic procedures often results in a severe assault on normal physiology with increased catabolism and augmented nutritional requirements. These adverse effects are compounded by the fact that, increasingly, these patients are older and present the surgeon with a panoply of comorbid conditions, including malnutrition, which increases the risk of postoperative complications. Accordingly, it is incumbent upon the surgical team to identify those patients who are poorly nourished preoperatively and, whenever possible, improve their nutritional status prior to the surgery. In the setting of unstable angina and other acute coronary syndromes, delay is not always prudent, and, in these situations, early, aggressive provision of adequate nutrition should be a major focus in the postoperative period. Currently clinical trials are underway to provide safe, systematic, uninterrupted, optimally combined enteral and parenteral nutritional support throughout the perioperative period while diligently maintaining normoglycemia. Another important research goal is to develop energetic and metabolic molecular substrates specially formulated to enhance the function of the myocardium sufficiently to reverse chronic heart failure and cardiac cachexia and to promote optimal recovery and performance following major cardiac operations. Finally, supporting adequate nutritional status of all cardiothoracic surgical patients judiciously will likely yield the best operative results and outcomes.

REFERENCES

1. Rich MW, Keller AJ, Schechtman KB, et al. Increased complications and prolonged hospital stay in elderly cardiac surgical patients with low serum albumen. Am J Cardiol 1989;63:714–8.
2. Loop FD, Golding LR, Macmillan JP, et al. Coronary artery surgery in women compared to men: analyses of risks and long-term results. J Am Coll Cardiol 1983;1:383–90.
3. Engelman DT, Adams DH, Burne JG, et al. Impact of body mass index and albumin on morbidity and mortality after cardiac surgery. J Thorac Cardiovasc Surg 1999;118:866–73.
4. Habib RH, Zacharias A, Schwann TA, et al. Effects of obesity and small body size on operative and long-term outcomes of coronary artery bypass surgery: a propensity-matched analysis. Ann Thorac Surg 2005;79(6):1976–86.
5. Gibbs J, Cull W, Henderson W, et al. Preoperative serum albumin level as a predictor of operative mortality and morbidity. Arch Surg 1999;134:36–42.
6. Keys A, Fidanza F, Karvonen MJ, et al. Indices of relative weight and obesity. J Chronic Dis 1972;25:329–43.

7. Criqui MH, Klauber MR, Barrett-Conner EL, et al. Adjustment for obesity in studies of cardiovascular disease. Am J Epidemiol 1982;116:685–91.
8. Rady MY, Ryan T, Starr NJ. Clinical characteristics of preoperative hypoalbuminemia predict outcome of cardiovascular surgery. JPEN J Parenter Enteral Nutr 1997;21:81–90.
9. Moulton MJ, Cresswell LL, Mackey ME, et al. Obesity is not a risk factor for significant adverse outcomes after cardiac surgery. Circulation 1996;94(Suppl):II87–92.
10. Christakis GT, Weisel RD, Buth KJ, et al. Is body size the cause for poor outcomes of coronary artery bypass operations in women? J Thorac Cardiovasc Surg 1995;110:1344–58.
11. Fisher LD, Kennedy JW, Davis KB, et al. Association of sex, physical size, and operative mortality after coronary artery bypass in the Coronary Artery Surgery Study (CASS). J Thorac Cardiovasc Surg 1982;84:334–41.
12. O'Conner GT, Morton JR, Diehl MJ, et al. Differences between men and women in hospital mortality associated with coronary artery bypass graft surgery. Circulation 1993;88:2104–10.
13. Mickleborough LL, Takagi Y, Maruyama H, et al. Is sex a factor in determining operative risk for aortocoronary bypass graft surgery? Circulation 1995;92(Suppl):II80–4.
14. van Venrooij LM, de Vos R, Borgmeijer-Hoelen MM, et al. Preoperative unintended weight loss and low body mass index in relation to complications and length of stay after cardiac surgery. Am J Clin Nutr 2008;87(6):1656–61.
15. Keith M, Mokbel R, San Emeterio M, et al. Evaluation of taste sensitivity in patients undergoing coronary artery bypass graft surgery. J Am Diet Assoc 2010;110(7):1072–7.
16. Abel RM, Fischer JE, Buckley MJ, et al. Malnutrition in cardiac surgery patients. Arch Surg 1976;111:45–50.
17. Visser M, Davids M, Verberne HJ, et al. Rationale and design of a proof-of-concept trial investigating the effect of uninterrupted perioperative (par)enteral nutrition on amino acid profile, cardiomyocytes structure, and cardiac perfusion and metabolism of patients undergoing coronary artery bypass grafting. J Cardiothorac Surg 2011;6:36–43.
18. Umenai T, Nakajima Y, Sessler DI, et al. Perioperative amino acid infusion improves recovery and shortens the duration of off-pump coronary artery bypass grafting. Anesth Analg 2006;103(6):1386–93.
19. Jeejeebhoy F, Keith M, Freeman M, et al. Nutrition supplementation with MyoVive repletes essential cardiac myocyte nutrients and reduces left ventricular size in patients with left ventricular dysfunction. Am Heart J 2002;143(6):1092–100.
20. Tepaske R, Velthius H, Oudemans-van Straaten HM, et al. Effect of preoperative oral immune enhancing nutritional supplement on patients at high risk of infection after cardiac surgery: a randomised placebo controlled trial. Lancet 2001;358(9283):696–701.
21. Anker SD, Coates AJS. Cardiac cachexia: a syndrome with impaired survival and immune and neuroendocrine activation. Chest 1999;115:836–47.
22. Kannel WB, Belanger AJ. Epidemiology of heart failure. Am Heart J 1991;121:951–7.
23. Cowie MR, Mosterd AA, Wood DA, et al. The epidemiology of heart failure. Eur Heart J 1997;18:208–25.
24. Katz AM, Katz PB. Diseases of the heart in works of Hippocrates. Br Heart J 1962;24:257–64.

25. Aronson JK. An account of the foxglove and its medical uses. London: Oxford University Press; 1985. p. 11–100.
26. Carr JG, Stevenson LW, Walden JA, et al. Prevalence and hemodynamic correlates of malnutrition in severe congestive heart failure secondary to ischemic or idiopathic dilated cardiomyopathy. Am J Cardiol 1989;63:709–13.
27. McMurray J, Abdullah I, Dargie HJ, et al. Increased concentrations of tumor necrosis factor in "cachectic" patients with severe chronic heart failure. Br Heart J 1991;66:356–8.
28. Levine B, Kalman J, Mayer L, et al. Elevated circulating levels of tumor necrosis factor in severe chronic heart failure. N Engl J Med 1990;323:236–41.
29. Otaki M. Surgical treatment of patients with cardiac cachexia: an analysis of factors affecting operative mortality. Chest 1994;105:1347–51.
30. Pittman JG, Cohen P. The pathogenesis of cardiac cachexia. N Engl J Med 1964;271:403–9.
31. King D, Smith ML, Chapman TJ, et al. Fat malabsorption in elderly patients with cardiac cachexia. Age Ageing 1996;25:144–9.
32. King D, Smith ML, Lye M. Gastro-intestinal protein loss in elderly patients with cardiac cachexia. Age Ageing 1996;25:221–3.
33. Braunwald E. Clinical manifestation of heart failure. In: Heart disease. A textbook of cardiovascular medicine, vol. 1. Philadelpha: WB Saunders; 1984. p. 499.
34. MacGowan GA, Mann DL, Kormos RL, et al. Circulation IL-6 in severe heart failure. Am J Cardiol 1997;79:1128–31.
35. Anker SD, Chua TP, Swan JW, et al. Hormonal changes and catabolic/anabolic imbalance in chronic heart failure: the importance for cardiac cachexia. Circulation 1997;96:526–34.
36. Mancini DM, Walter G, Reichek N, et al. Contribution of skeletal muscle atrophy to exercise intolerance and altered muscle metabolism in heart failure. Circulation 1992;85:1364–73.
37. Vescovo G, Serafini F, Facchin L, et al. Specific changes in skeletal muscle myosin heavy chains composition in cardiac failure: differences compared with disuse atrophy as assessed on microbiopsies by high resolution electrophoresis. Heart 1996;76:337–43.
38. Simonini A, Long CS, Dudley GA, et al. Heart failure in rats causes changes in skeletal muscle morphology and gene expression that are not explained by reduced activity. Circ Res 1996;79(1):128–36.
39. Broqvist M, Arnqvist H, Dahlstrom U, et al. Nutritional assessment and muscle energy metabolism in severe congestive heart failure: effects of long-term dietary supplementation. Eur Heart J 1994;15:1641–50.
40. Heymsfield SB, Casper K. Congestive heart failure: clinical management by use of continuous nasoenteric feeding. Am J Clin Nutr 1989;50:539–44.
41. Neubauer S. The failing heart – an engine out of fuel. N Engl J Med 2007;356: 1140–51.
42. McMurray JJ, Pfeffer MA. Heart failure. Lancet 2005;365:1877–89.
43. The CONSENSUS Trial Study Group. Effects of enalapril on mortality in severe congestive heart failure: results of the Cooperative North Scandinavian Enalapril Survival Study (CONSENSUS). N Engl J Med 1987;316:1429–35.
44. Pfeffer MA, Braunwald E, Moye LA, et al. Effect of captopril on mortality and morbidity in patients with left ventricular dysfunction after myocardial infarction: results of the survival and ventricular enlargement trial. N Engl J Med 1992;327: 669–77.

45. Pitt B, Zannad F, Remme WJ, et al. The effect of spironolactone on morbidity and mortality in patients with severe heart failure. N Engl J Med 1999;341: 709–17.

46. CIBIS Investigators and Committees. A randomized trial β-blockade in heart failure: the Cardiac Bisoprolol Insufficiency Study (CIBIS). Circulation 1994;90: 1765–73.

47. Packer M, Bristow MR, Cohen JN, et al. The effect of carvedilol on morbidity and mortality on patients with chronic heart failure. N Engl J Med 1996;334: 1349–55.

48. Bristow MR, Saxon LA, Boehmer J, et al. Cardiac-resynchronization therapy with or without an implantable defibrillator in advanced chronic heart failure. N Engl J Med 2004;350:2140–50.

49. Cleland JG, Daubert JC, Erdmann E, et al. The effect of cardiac resynchronization on morbidity and mortality in heart failure. N Engl J Med 2005;352: 1539–49.

50. Mann DL, Bristow MR. Mechanisms and models in heart failure: the biomechanical model and beyond. Circulation 2005;111:2837–49.

51. Hermann G, Decherd GM. The chemical nature of heart failure. Ann Intern Med 1939;12:1233–44.

52. Wollenberger A. On the energy-rich phosphate supply of the failing heart. Am J Physiol 1947;150:733–6.

53. Olson RE, Schwartz WB. Myocardial metabolism in congestive failure. Medicine (Baltimore) 1951;30:21–41.

54. Olson RE. Myocardial metabolism in congestive heart failure. J Chronic Dis 1959;9:442–64.

55. Ingwall JS, Weiss RG. Is the failing heart energy starved? On using the chemical energy to support cardiac function. Circ Res 2004;95:135–45.

56. Taegtmeyer H. Metabolism – the lost child of cardiology. J Am Coll Cardiol 2000; 36:1386–8.

57. Taegtmeyer H. Cardiac metabolism as a target for the treatment of heart failure. Circulation 2004;110:894–6.

58. Stanley WC, Recchia FA, Lopaschuk GD. Myocardial substrate metabolism in the normal and failing heart. Physiol Rev 2005;85:1093–129.

59. Ventura-Clapier R, Garnier A, Veksler V. Energy metabolism in heart failure. J Physiol 2004;556:1–13.

60. Morrow DA, Givertz MM. Modulation of myocardial energetics; emerging evidence for a therapeutic target in cardiovascular disease. Circulation 2005; 112:3218–21.

61. Lopaschuk GD, Rebeyka IM, Allard MF. Metabolic modulation: a means to mend a broken heart. Circulation 2002;105:140–2.

62. Essop MF, Opie LH. Metabolic therapy for heart failure. Eur Heart J 2004;25: 1765–8.

63. van Bilsen M, Smeets PJ, Gilde AJ, et al. Metabolic remodeling of the failing heart: the cardiac burn-out syndrome? Cardiovasc Res 2004;61:218–26.

64. Cohn JM, Tognoni G. A randomized trial of angiotensin-receptor blocker valsartan in chronic heart failure. N Engl J Med 2001;345:1667–75.

65. Pfeffer MA, Swedberg K, Granger CB, et al. Effects of candesartan on mortality and morbidity in patients with chronic heart failure: the CHARM-Overall programme. Lancet 2003;362:759–66.

66. Katz AM. Heart failure: Pathophysiology, molecular biology and clinical management. Philadelphia: Lippincott Williams & Wilkins; 2000.

67. Bessman SP, Geiger PJ. Transport of energy and muscle: the phosphorylcrea-tine shuttle. Science 1981;211:448–52.
68. Ingwall JS. ATP and the heart. Norwell (MA): Kluwer Academic; 2002.
69. Wallimann T, Wyss M, Brdiczka D, et al. Intracellular compartmentation, structure and function of creatine kinase isoenzymes in tissues with high and fluctuating energy demands: the "phosphocreatine circuit" for cellular energy homeostasis. Biochem J 1992;281:21–40.
70. Wyss M, Wallimann T. Creatine metabolism and the consequences of creatine depletion in muscle. Mol Cell Biochem 1994;133:51–66.
71. Garlick PB, Radda GK, Selly PJ. Phosphorus NMR studies on perfused heart. Biochem Biophys Res Commun 1977;74:1256–62.
72. Inwall JS. Phosphorus nuclear magnetic resonance spectroscopy of cardiac and skeletal muscles. Am J Physiol 1982;242:H729–44.
73. Bottomley PA. MR spectroscopy of the human heart: the status and the chal-lenges. Radiology 1994;191:593–612.
74. Neubauer S. Cardiac magnetic resonance spectroscopy. In: Lardo AC, Fayad ZA, Chronos NA, et al, editors. Cardiovascular magnetic resonance: established and emerging applications. London: Martin Dunitz; 2003. p. 39–60.
75. Vitale GD, deKemp RA, Ruddy TD, et al. Myocardial glucose utilization and opti-mization of (18)FDG PET imaging in patients non-insulin-dependent diabetes mellitus, coronary artery disease, and left ventricular dysfunction. J Nucl Med 2001;42:1730–6.
76. Wallhus TR, Taylor M, DeGrado TR, et al. Myocardial free fatty acid and glucose use after carvedilol treatment in patients with congestive heart failure. Circula-tion 2001;103:2441–6.
77. Davila-Roman VG, Vedala G, Herrero P, et al. Altered myocardial fatty acid and glucose metabolism in idiopathic dilated cardiomyopathy. J Am Coll Cardiol 2002;40:271–7.
78. Lewandowski ED. Cardiac carbon 13 magnetic resonance spectroscopy: on the horizon or over the rainbow? J Nucl Cardiol 2002;9:419–28.
79. Ning XH, Zhang J, Liu J, et al. Signaling and expression for mitochondrial membrane proteins during left ventricular remodeling and contractile failure after myocardial infarction. J Am Coll Cardiol 2000;36:282–7.
80. Gudbjarnason S, Mathes P, Ravens KG. Functional compartmentation of ATP and creatine phosphate in heart muscle. J Mol Cell Cardiol 1970;1:325–39.
81. Colagrande L, Formica F, Porta F, et al. L-arginine effects on myocardial stress in cardiac surgery: preliminary results. Ital Heart J 2005;6:904–10.
82. Quyyumi AA, Dakak N, Dodati JG, et al. Effect of L-arginine on human coronary endothelium-dependent and physiologic vasodilation. J Am Coll Cardiol 1997; 30:1220–7.
83. Wallace AW, Ratcliffe MB, Galindez D, et al. L-arginine infusion dilates coronary vasculature in patients undergoing coronary bypass surgery. Anesthesiology 1999;90:1577–86.
84. Uyar I, Mansuroglu D, Kirali K, et al. Aspartate and glutamate-enriched cardio-plegia in left ventricular dysfunction. J Card Surg 2005;20:337–44.
85. Bitzikas G, Papakonstantinou C, Lazou A, et al. The supportive value of pre-bypass L-glutamate loading in patients undergoing coronary artery bypass grafting. J Cardiovasc Surg (Torino) 2005;46:551–7.
86. Scarabelli TM, Pasini E, Stephanou A, et al. Nutritional supplementation with mixed essential amino acids enhances myocyte survival preserving mitochondrial func-tional capacity during ischemia-reperfusion injury. Am J Cardiol 2004;93:35A–40A.

87. Pasini E, Scarabelli TM, D'Antona G, et al. Effect of amino acid mixture on the isolated ischemic heart. Am J Cardiol 2004;93:30A–4A.
88. Venturini A, Ascioni R, Lin H, et al. The importance of myocardial amino acids during ischemia and reperfusion in dilated left ventricle of patients with degenerative mitral valve disease. Mol Cell Biochem 2009;330:63–70.
89. Taegtmeyer H, Harinstein ME, Gheorghiade M. More than bricks and mortar: comments on protein and amino acid protein in the heart. Am J Cardiol 2008; 101:3E–7E.
90. Suleiman MS, Fernando HC, Dihmis WC, et al. A loss of taurine and other amino acids from ventricles of patients undergoing bypass surgery. Br Heart J 1993; 69:241–5.
91. Kaye DM, Ahlers BA, Autelitano DJ, et al. In vivo and in vitro evidence for impaired arginine transport in human heart failure. Circulation 2000;102:2707–12.
92. Visser M, Paulus WJ, Vermeulen MA, et al. The role of asymmetric dimethylarginine and arginine in the failing heart and its vasculature. Eur J Heart Fail 2010; 12:1274–81.
93. Wolfe BM. Substrate-endocrine interactions and protein metabolism. JPEN J Parenter Enteral Nutr 1980;4:188–94.
94. Witte KK, Clark AL, Cleland JG. Chronic heart failure and micronutrients. J Am Coll Cardiol 2001;37:1765–74.
95. Wallis J, Lygate CA, Fischer A, et al. Supranormal myocardial creatine and phosphocreatine concentrations lead to cardiac hypertrophy and heart failure: insights from creatine transporter-overexpressing transgenic mice. Circulation 2005;112:3131–9.
96. Ng TM. Levosimendan, a new calcium-sensitizing inotrope for heart failure. Pharmacotherapy 2004;24:1366–84.
97. Zerr KJ, Furnary AP, Grunkemeier GL, et al. Glucose control lowers the risk of wound infection in diabetics after open heart operations. Ann Thorac Surg 1997;63(2):356–61.
98. Aquilani R, Opasich C, Verri M, et al. Is nutritional intake adequate in chronic heart failure patients? J Am Coll Cardiol 2003;42:1218–23.
99. Vega JD, Poindexter SM, Radovancevic B, et al. Nutritional assessment of patients with extended left ventricular assist device support. ASAIO Trans 1990;36:M555–8.
100. Loebe M, Koster A, Sänger S, et al. Inflammatory response after implantation of a left ventricular assist device comparison between the axial flow MicroMed DeBakey VAD and the pulsatile Novacor device. ASAIO J 2001;47(3):272–4.
101. Koster A, Loebe M, Hansen R, et al. Alterations in coagulation after implantation of a pulsatile Novacor LVAD and the axial flow MicroMed DeBakey LVAD. Ann Thorac Surg 2000;70(2):533–7.
102. Itescu S, Ankersmit JH, Kocher AA, et al. Immunobiology of left ventricular assist devices. Prog Cardiovasc Dis 2000;43(1):67–80.
103. Dang NC, Topkara VK, Kim BT, et al. Nutritional status in patients on left ventricular assist device support. J Thorac Cardiovasc Surg 2005;230(5):e3–4.
104. Machado AN, Sitta Mdo C, Jacob Filho W, et al. Prognostic factors for mortality among patients above the 6th decade undergoing non-cardiac surgery: CARES–clinical assessment and research in elderly surgical patients. Clinics (Sao Paulo) 2008;63(2):151–6.
105. Fukuse T, Satoda N, Hijiya K, et al. Importance of a comprehensive geriatric assessment in prediction of complications following thoracic surgery in elderly patients. Chest 2005;127:886–91.

106. Carney DE, Meguid MM. Current concepts in nutritional assessment. Arch Surg 2002;137:42–5.
107. Isowa N, Hasegawa S, Bando T, et al. Preoperative risk factors for prolonged air leak following lobectomy or segmentectomy for primary lung cancer. Eur J Cardiothorac Surg 2002;21:951.
108. Ollenschlager G, Schrappe-Bacher M, Steffan M, et al. Assessment of nutritional status – a part of routine clinical diagnosis: cholinesterase activity as a nutritional indicator. Klin Wochenschr 1989;67(21):1101–7 [in German].
109. Merrigan BA, Winter DC, O'Sullivan GC. Chylothorax. Br J Surg 1997;84:15–20.
110. Machleder HI, Paulus H. Clinical and immunological alterations observed in patients undergoing long-term thoracic duct drainage. Surgery 1978;84: 157–65.
111. Lagarde SM, Omloo JM, de Jong K, et al. Incidence and management of chyle leakage after esophagectomy. Ann Thorac Surg 2005;80:449–54.
112. Bolger C, Walsh TN, Tanner WA, et al. Chylothorax after oesophagectomy. Br J Surg 1991;78:587–8.

Nutrition Management of Geriatric Surgical Patients

Stanley J. Dudrick, MD[a,b,*]

KEYWORDS

- Geriatric nutrition • Geriatric surgery • Geriatric assessment
- Frailty syndrome • Elderly surgical risks
- Geriatric demographics • Geriatric nutritional assessment

The common physiologic and chronologic goal of the traditionalists, baby boomers, Xers, Yers, and Nexters is, despite their many differences in their approaches to life, for the vast majority of them to become elderly, barring premature interruptions by untoward life-threatening incidents or pathophysiologic processes. Thus, the double-edged sword of the steadily increasing life expectancy of these groups or segments of the population consists of the usual trade-off for extended longevity, that is, the longer one lives, the more likely one is to experience pathophysiologic disorders, diseases, or trauma which will probably require hospitalization and significant medical and/or surgical interventions. This is the "bottom line" or common denominator for those who comprise the geriatric age group. As the older adult population in the United States, and in most Western nations, continues to expand rapidly, their unique characteristics and demographic trends present increasing challenges to those attempting to provide them with optimal nutritional support. In 1900, the average life expectancy in the United States was approximately 48 years, and throughout the twentieth century, it had climbed steadily to approximately 76 years by 1995.[1] At present, approximately 34 million Americans are 65 years of age or older, and they constitute approximately 12% of the United States population. By 2030, it is predicted that this segment of the population will increase to 22% of the total census.[2] Indeed, Americans 85 years and older are actually the fastest growing segment of the US population! By the year 2050, an estimated 79 million Americans will be 65 years or older,

The author has nothing to disclose.
[a] Department of Surgery, Yale University School of Medicine, 333 Cedar Street, New Haven, CT 06510, USA
[b] Department of Surgery, Saint Mary's Hospital, 56 Franklin Street, Waterbury, CT 06706, USA
* Department of Surgery, Saint Mary's Hospital/Yale Affiliate, 56 Franklin Street, Waterbury, CT 06706.
E-mail address: sdudrick@stmh.org

Surg Clin N Am 91 (2011) 877–896
doi:10.1016/j.suc.2011.05.003
0039-6109/11/$ – see front matter © 2011 Elsevier Inc. All rights reserved.

and of these approximately 18 million will be 85 years or older.[2] In absolute numbers, the size of the elderly population in the United States has increased by about 50% in the past 20 years, and now totals more than 25 million.[1,2] Comparable geriatric growth rate predictions have been made for Canada, and even greater relative increases are predicted for Europe.[3,4]

The elderly experience and endure substantially more diseases and health challenges than the younger population groups.[5] The elderly are hospitalized more frequently, and for longer durations.[5,6] Eighty-five percent of the elderly have one or more chronic illnesses, and 30% have 3 or more; this high prevalence of illness contributes to increased risk for primary and secondary malnutrition.[6,7] It is estimated that approximately 85% of noninstitutionalized elderly persons suffer from at least one condition that could be improved by proper nutrition,[8] and although the elderly comprise about 12% of the total population, is it estimated that at least 30% of the nation's total health care expenditures are generated by this age group.[3,6] Therefore, nutrition screening and intervention in selected settings have been proposed recently as appropriate cost-effective measures.[9] Information on the health and nutritional status of the elderly in America from the National Health and Nutritional Examination Survey (NHANES III) suggests that diet plays a major role in the health and disease of adults aged 65 years and older; and for many low-income and minority elders, it may be the most important factor.[10] Appropriate nutrition contributes to maintenance of vital functional status, whereas nutritional deficiencies have been associated with impairment in mobility and independence.[11] Malnutrition may also predispose community-dwelling elderly individuals to acute illness and hospitalization,[12] and an estimated 5% to 10% prevalence of protein-energy malnutrition (PEM) has been reported among the community-dwelling elderly.[13] Unfortunately, in many cases PEM remains unrecognized by most clinicians in their ambulatory elderly patients[14,15]; and, furthermore, some clinicians also fail to recognize functional deficits that may reflect underlying malnutrition in the elderly.[2,16] Older adults inherently are at increased risk of consuming an inadequate diet due to the presence of disease, physical disability, inability to chew food adequately, polypharmacy, social isolation, and poverty.[1] Indeed, as a real-time indicator of the magnitude of the problems of providing adequate diet, 44.2 million people depend on government-supplied food stamps in 2011, or 1 of every 7 persons living in the United States today. Nutrient intake tends to decline as age increases; and total calories and protein, and intakes of calcium, vitamin B12, vitamin D, and folate fall well below those suggested by the Recommended Dietary Allowances (RDA) and the Dietary Reference Intakes (DRI) published by the National Academy of Sciences Food and Nutrition Board.[17]

SURGERY AND MALNUTRITION IN GERIATRIC PATIENTS

The numbers of institutionalized elderly increase as the total elderly population grows and grows older. Only 1% of those younger than 74 years resides in institutions, but the number is substantially increased to 22% of those elderly who are older than 85 years. In a recent review of malnutrition in nursing homes, an alarmingly high rate of 30% to 50% PEM was noted in nursing home patients who were, in turn, associated with increased mortality rates.[18] Moreover, the investigators provided convincing evidence that much of the malnutrition in institutionalized elderly is preventable or reversible, although some wasting and nutrient deficiencies result from disease and cannot be easily prevented or reversed. However, numerous studies have demonstrated that malnutrition is neither integral to aging, nor is it inevitable in illness.[2] It is clear that appropriate nutritional interventions have resulted in improvements in quality of life and in nutritional status in the community-dwelling elderly, the chronically institutionalized elderly, and the acutely ill elderly.[18–24] It is now obvious that much better efforts must be made to prevent and to treat malnutrition in the elderly, especially those elderly patients who require, or who have undergone, surgical procedures. The elderly should not be regarded as a homogeneous group, primarily because of the wide diversity in age, the presence of one or more illnesses, and the differences in functional levels, which are significant factors contributing to the diversity of the elderly population, and cause the development of a comprehensive screening or assessment to be somewhat difficult. Therefore their nutritional needs, and therapeutic strategies, must be crafted in a manner that reflects the unique characteristics of the various subgroups of the elderly. Ample research during the past several decades regarding the perioperative risks in elderly patients suggests that advanced age itself only minimally increases the operative risks.[25] The more important risk factors are associated with underlying chronic diseases, such as hypertension, heart disease, generalized atherosclerosis, malignancies, and so forth, which are more prevalent in the elderly patient but represent pathologic alterations rather than normal physiologic changes associated with aging.[26–29] On the other hand, emergency surgical procedures greatly increase the operative risk in the elderly from approximately 1% for elective cases up to 45% for emergency procedures.[26,28] This incidence is likely secondary to the diminished functional (physiologic) reserve capacity that accompanies aging, and declines rather steadily as age advances, both globally and in the individual organs and systems. In addition to the anticipated large increase in the elderly as a result of the entry of the baby-boomer generation into this age group, it is projected that patients currently 80 years of age will live at least 4 more years, and patients who reach 100 years of age will live another 3 years, thus emphasizing the fact that as the mean age of the population increases, more surgical procedures are likely to be performed in the very elderly.[30] Despite these facts, there are clinicians among us who continue to "write off" geriatric patients and deny them optimal care simply because they are elderly. This most unprofessional, disrespectful, demeaning, and ignorant attitude is already creeping insidiously and increasingly into our culture and society, and is beginning to corrupt not only our current and proposed health care system, but our morals, ethics, and core values as individuals and as a society. Physicians and surgeons are obligated to treat all patients, especially geriatric patients, as individuals and with respect, dignity, and compassion rather than as inanimate entry items in a computerized health care management algorithm. Moreover, with improved medical care delivery and effectiveness, and with people living longer, the population of patients with whom surgeons will be interacting to provide both nutritional support and operative therapies is progressively aging at an unprecedented rate.

From 1980 to 2000, the percentage of operations performed on elderly patients older than 65 years increased from 19% to 38% of the total operations performed in all age groups.[31] As the elderly segment of the population continues to grow, an ever-increasing need and demand for surgical care in this age group is predicted and anticipated. Caring for these individuals requires an awareness and understanding by surgeons of the global changes that take place as an individual ages, as well as a clinical acumen and ability to assess accurately their relative needs, both as inpatients and as outpatients. Maintenance of good nutritional status is essential for optimal geriatric surgical care, particularly in acute situations, in which malnutrition is clearly associated with increased complications and other adverse health outcomes. Geriatric epidemiologic studies of malnutrition have indicated that 40% to 50% of noninstitutionalized older adults ingest diets that are deficient in 3 or more nutrients.[10] Furthermore, it has been shown that one or more nutritional inadequacies are present in 9% to 15% of elderly adults in outpatient clinics, in 12% to 50% of hospitalized elderly patients, and in 25% to 85% of elderly patients residing in extended-care institutions.[7,8,32]

PEM is the most common nutritional inadequacy found in the geriatric population, and it exists when insufficient energy and/or protein is available to meet the metabolic needs of the body. The clinical significance of PEM, a serious form of poor nutritional status in elderly adults, is that it is associated with altered immunity, impaired wound healing, reduced functional status, increased health care use, and increased morbidity and mortality. An inverse age-energy relationship has been recognized in older adults: lean body mass decreases with aging, physical activity decreases with aging, mean daily energy intake of elderly men is only 70% of the recommended daily allowance (1600 kcal), mean daily energy intake of elderly women is only 63% of the recommended daily allowance (1200 kcal), and greater than 15% of the elderly studied consume less than 1000 kcal per day.[33,34] Thus, it is obvious that chronic undernutrition occurs commonly in older adults, and that simply not having access to adequate food intake can be a problem for many free-living, noninstitutionalized elderly people.[10]

FACTORS CONTRIBUTING TO GERIATRIC MALNUTRITION

Although confounding effects of nonnutritional factors cannot be completely ruled out, many studies have shown that poor nutrition is an independent determinant of increased morbidity and mortality after adjusting for nonnutritional factors. Socioeconomic factors contributing to inadequate nutrition in older adults include: fixed income; reduced access to food secondary to social isolation, inadequate storage, and cooking facilities; poor knowledge of nutrition; and dependence on others, including caretakers and institutions. The psychological factors contributing to inadequate nutrition in older patients include, but are not limited to, depression, bereavement, anxiety, paranoia, and dementia. Physiologic factors contributing to inadequate nutrition in elderly adults include: impaired strength and aerobic capacity; impaired mobility and dexterity (arthritis, stroke); chewing and swallowing difficulties; dementia, Parkinson disease, stroke, amyotrophic lateral sclerosis, and other neurologic conditions; impaired sensory input (smell, taste, sight); poor dentition (missing or loose teeth, oral mucosal lesions or infections, edentulous condition); malabsorption; chronic illness (associated anorexia, altered metabolism); alcohol abuse and medications (serotonin reuptake inhibitors, digoxin, narcotics, antibiotics, xanthines, nonsteroidal anti-inflammatory drugs, and others). Factors related to hospitalization for acute illness, which contribute to inadequate nutrition in elderly adults, include (1) failure to monitor dietary intake and to obtain and record daily weights, (2) failure to consider the increased metabolic requirements associated with illness, (3) iatrogenic starvation (frequent and/or prolonged periods of nothing-by-mouth as prerequisites for test purposes), and (4) delay in instituting reasonable or adequate nutritional support.

NUTRITIONAL ASSESSMENT OF GERIATRIC PATIENTS

Although the efficacy of nutritional support has been difficult to prove statistically or establish unequivocally in many circumstances, data are available to suggest that clinical outcomes can be improved by interventions to correct or prevent most nutritional deficits. Recognition by physicians or surgeons of malnutrition in the elderly is often lacking, despite its obvious clinical importance, and several studies suggest that even when malnutrition is recognized, appropriate attempts to correct the conditions are not always made. Optimally, effective care of the frail or ill elderly patient mandates evaluation of nutritional status for early recognition and consideration of appropriate supportive nutritional interventions. The key components of nutritional assessment of elderly patients include: (1) careful history taking and physical examination; (2) proportional weight change (usual to current); (3) serum total protein and albumin concentrations; (4) total lymphocyte counts; and (5) anthropometrics mid-arm muscle circumference, triceps skin-fold, and body mass index. Indicators of severe malnutrition in the geriatric patient consist of the following: weight loss exceeding 20% of pre-morbid weight, serum albumin level less than 21 g/L, serum transferrin level less than 1 g/L, and a total lymphocyte count less than 800/µL.

Although elderly patients may appear to have worse outcomes following operations as compared with younger patients, age itself is not an independent risk factor for increased mortality, and when corrected for comorbid disorders, age alone has little influence on prognosis. Despite aggressive perioperative nutritional support (oral, enteral, parenteral) of the elderly surgical patient, it is often difficult to attenuate the catabolic response to illness or injury. Anthropometric measurements indicate that when body weight does increase with nutritional support of the elderly patient, gains are made mostly in fat and extracellular water, whereas gains in lean body mass might result in better functional and clinical outcomes. When undertaking surgical interventions in the elderly patient, consideration must be taken into account that mortality rates for emergency operations of all types are at least 3 times greater than those for comparable surgical procedures performed under elective conditions. Nutritional status predictors of mortality in geriatric patients that have proven valuable include the Katz Index of Activities of Daily Living (ADL) Score,[35] serum albumin concentration, usual weight percentage, presence of decubitus ulcers, dysphagia, and mid-arm muscle circumference. The Katz Index of Independence in ADL quantifies an individual's overall performance in primary biological and psychosocial functions, specifically bathing, dressing, going to the toilet, transferring, continence, and feeding[35] (**Table 1**). The Instrumental Activities of Daily Living (IADL) is a somewhat more complex set of behaviors, such as telephoning, shopping, food preparation, housekeeping, laundering, use of medicine, use of transportation, and financial behavior, which are aids not only in assessment but also in formulation implementation, and evaluation of treatment plans.[36]

Preoperative assessment of the elderly patient must be global. Cardiac complications in this population are among the most common postoperative problems, and an effort must be made to reduce the risk of these serious complications by effectively optimizing the condition of the patient before operation. An electrocardiogram should be obtained, cardiopathology must have a full preoperative assessment, hypertension must be controlled, and cardiac output must be optimized.

Pulmonary function must also be accurately assessed and improved to optimal levels. A history of dyspnea, chronic bronchitis, asthma, or of chronic bronchodilator use, as well as aspiration risk, must be examined. Occult disease should be assessed by chest radiograms and, at times, also by appropriate computed tomography scans. Smokers should be encouraged to stop smoking at least 6 weeks before elective surgical procedures if feasible.

Nutritional status should include accurate weight and height measurements as well as serum albumin levels, because an individual with poor nutrition indices will likely have impaired wound healing and a longer, more complicated postoperative recovery and hospital stay. Alcohol use should be investigated thoroughly because the risk for postoperative delirium tremens can significantly increase both postoperative morbidity and mortality. Pretreatment with benzodiazepines and thiamine should be

Table 1
Katz Index of Independence in Activities of Daily Living

Activities	Independence (1 Point) No Supervision, Direction, or Personal Assistance	Dependence (0 Points) With Supervision, Direction, Personal Assistance, or Total Care
Bathing Point: —	(1 Point) Bathes self completely or needs help in bathing only a single part of the body such as the back, genital area, or disabled extremity	(0 Points) Needs help in bathing more than one part of the body getting out of the tub or shower. Requires total bathing
Dressing Point: —	(1 Point) Gets clothes from closets and drawers and puts on clothes and other garments complete with fasteners. May have help tying shoes	(0 Points) Needs help with dressing self or needs to be completely dressed
Toileting Point: —	(1 Point) Goes to toilet, gets on and off, arranges clothes, cleans genital area without help	(0 Points) Needs help transferring to the toilet, cleaning self, or uses bedpan or commode
Transferring Point: —	(1 Point) Moves in and out of bed or chair unassisted. Mechanical transferring aides are acceptable	(0 Points) Needs help in moving from bed to chair or requires a complete transfer
Continence Point: —	(1 Point) Exercises complete self control over urination and defecation	(0 Points) Is partially or totally incontinent of bowel or bladder
Feeding Point: —	(1 Point) Gets food from plate into mouth without help. Preparation of food may be done by another person	(0 Points) Needs partial or total help with feeding or requires parenteral feeding
Total points = —	6 = High (patient independent)	0 = Low (patient very dependent)

Data from Katz S, Ford AB, Moskowitz RW, et al. Studies of illness in the aged: the index of ADL: a standard measure of biological and psychosocial function. JAMA 1963;185(12):914–9.

strongly considered in those patients with a history of alcohol abuse, and should be continued postoperatively for a few days.

The most basic laboratory tests that should be obtained in the elderly surgical patient include a complete blood count with differential, hemoglobin A_{1C}, serum glucose levels, serum electrolytes, blood urea nitrogen, creatinine clearance, electrocardiogram, and chest radiograph. For those who require them, as dictated by their disease and medication histories, arterial blood gas determination, prothrombin time, and partial thromboplastin time should also be obtained.

POSTOPERATIVE CONSIDERATIONS IN THE ELDERLY

Postoperatively the patient should be aggressively encouraged to ambulate as soon as possible, even on the day of surgery, unless contraindicated by other factors. Early mobilization will decrease significantly the risk of pulmonary embolus, deep vein thrombosis, and pneumonia in this susceptible population. Patient-controlled analgesia should be used to assist with early mobilization and to minimize the total dose of opiates administered. The patient should also be given prophylactic laxatives and/or a stool softener as early as feasible to minimize constipation and its sequelae. Blood pressure should be controlled aggressively and appropriately to avoid both hypotension and hypertension. Volume status should be monitored assiduously, as it is integral to controlling the diastolic cardiac dysfunction manifested in many elderly patients. Volume overload should be avoided conscientiously, and rehydration should be accomplished gently and gradually rather than by infusing a bolus of fluid, in order to avoid taxing an already tenuous cardiovascular system. β-Blockers should be used, especially in those patients with a history of coronary artery disease. Care must also be taken when reinstating preoperative medications postoperatively so as to avoid drug interactions, relative overdosages, and redundancies.

One must bear in mind that fear of loss of independence weighs heavily on the minds of the elderly, and that the goal of a successful discharge from the hospital is to return the patient to home or to an environment that closely approximates home. Surgeons should not make decisions to send their elderly patient to an extended-care facility just because they are old. A detailed assessment of their preoperative independence and ability should be performed, and every effort to return them to their previous "norm" of habitat and functionality should be made during their hospital course.

OPERATIVE RISK ASSESSMENT IN FRAIL GERIATRIC PATIENTS

It is well known that older patients are at increased risk for postoperative complications, and that if a complication occurs, it can lead to a cascade of events resulting in disability, loss of independence, diminished quality of life, high health care costs, and increased mortality.[37,38] Surgical decision making in this population is particularly challenging because of the heterogeneity of health status in the elderly and the paucity of metrics for predicting operative risk.[39] The commonly used predictors of postoperative complications have considerable limitations, most are based on a single organ system, or are subjective; and none estimate the physiologic reserves of the patient.[40] For example, the criteria developed by Lee and colleagues[41] and Eagle and colleagues[42] account for cardiac function only, and the commonly used American Society of Anesthesiologists (ASA) score is determined by a subjective estimate of organ system disease and the likelihood of survival.[43] Thus, despite the widespread adoption of these useful scoring systems, complications in elderly patients have remained difficult to predict accurately.[39]

Recognizing that preoperative risk assessment is important, yet inexact, in elderly patients because physiologic reserves are difficult to measure, Makary and colleagues[39] recently reported the results of a study to determine whether frailty predicts surgical complications and enhances current perioperative risks. Frailty is thought to estimate physiologic reserves, although its use had not been previously evaluated in surgical patients.[39] Conceptually, decrements in reserves can determine the resilience of an elderly surgical patient in recovering from an operation. Frailty is also increasingly recognized as a unique domain of health status that can be a marker of decreased reserves and resultant increased vulnerability in older patients. Moreover, it has been thought to represent a global phenotype of physiologic reserves and resistance to stressors.[44,45] In nonsurgical populations, the frailty phenotype has been associated with adverse health outcomes[44,46–48]; however, implications of frailty for surgical patients had not been previously studied. The investigators hypothesized that frailty predicts operative risk in older surgical patients, and that the addition of frailty to other risk models will enhance the ability of surgeons to identify patients at risk for complications.[39] Frailty based on a validated scoring system[44,45] that characterizes frailty as an age-associated decline was evaluated in 5 areas: shrinking, weakness, exhaustion, low physical activity, and slow walking speed.[39] Each of these areas was assigned a dichotomous score of 0 or 1, based on the following criteria: (1) shrinking (weight loss) was defined as unintentional weight loss of about 10 pounds in the past year, (2) decreased grip strength (weakness) was measured by having the patient squeeze a hand-held dynamometer, with the strength measurement being adjusted for gender and body mass index,[44,45] (3) exhaustion was measured by responses to questions about effort and motivation,[49] (4) low physical activity was ascertained by inquiring about leisure-time activities, and (5) slowed walking speed was measured by the speed at which a patient could walk 15 feet.[39] Information was also collected on other potentially confounding variables including age, race, gender, comorbidity (history of myocardial infarction, angina, congestive heart failure, claudication, arthritis, cancer, hypertension, diabetes, chronic obstructive lung disease, or smoking),[48] current procedure for cancer (any malignancy on a pathology report), and preoperative residence (home, nursing home, or skilled care facility).[39] The investigators also assessed variables regarding the operation category: major versus minor procedure (major, procedure typically requiring hospitalization; minor, procedure typically performed the same day); open versus percutaneous or minimally invasive; and intra-abdominal versus non–intra-abdominal.[39] The patients in the study were evaluated on the basis of the study of the 4 risk models: the frailty index, ASA score, Lee's revised cardiac risk index, and Eagle score.[39] The results of their study indicated that among the 594 participants, 62 (10.4%) were frail, 186 (31.3%) were intermediately frail, and 346 (58.3%) were nonfrail, when applying these multiple risk indices. Of the 62 frail patients, 83.9% were Caucasian and 41.9% were female.[39] The unadjusted incidence of complications following minor procedures was 3.9% in the nonfrail, 7.3% in the intermediately frail, and 11.4% in the frail patients; after major procedures, the unadjusted incidence of complications was 19.5% in nonfrail patients, 33.7% in intermediately frail patients, and 43.5% in frail patients.[39] After adjusting for known risk factors and relevant patient factors, frailty remained an independent predictor of surgical complications.[39] Intermediately frail patients had 2.06 times higher odds (95% confidence interval [CI], 1.18–3.60) of complications, and frail patients had a 2.54 times higher odds (95% CI, 1.12–5.77) of complications when compared with nonfrail patients. In various adjusted models, the odds ratio for intermediately frail patients ranged from 1.78 to 2.13, and for frail patients ranged from 2.48 to 3.15.[39] The predictive ability of the 3 risk models *without* the inclusion of the frailty index were 63% (ASA score), 62% (Lee score), and 68% (Eagle score), as estimated by the AUC (area under the curve); these increased to 70%, 67%, and 71%, respectively, when the frailty index was added to the other 3 risk models ($P<.01$).[39]

The mean length of stay (LOS) after minor procedures was 0.7 days for nonfrail, 1.2 days for intermediately frail, and 1.5 days for frail patients; after major procedures, mean LOS was 4.2 days for nonfrail, 6.2 days for intermediately frail, and 7.7 days for frail patients.[39] Moreover, intermediately frail patients had 44% to 53% longer hospital stays, and frail patients had 65% to 89% longer hospital stays. The association between frailty and LOS remained significant ($P<.001$) when frailty was compared directly with each of the other risk indices individually.[39] The unadjusted incidence of being discharged to a skilled or assisted living facility after a minor procedure was 0.8% in nonfrail, 0% in intermediately frail, and 17.4% in frail patients; after major procedures, the unadjusted incidence was 2.9% in nonfrail, 12.2% in intermediately frail, and 42.1% in frail patients.[39]

Makary and colleagues[39] posit that for years, it had been recognized subjectively that some elderly patients might not have the physiologic reserve to withstand an operation; however, physicians have lacked a standardized definition for this risk domain. As a result, the science of this vulnerability had not been advanced. Using their validated scoring system, the investigating team found that their preoperative characterization of frailty predicted surgical outcomes and augmented other risk assessment models.

The concept of frailty might help to explain why some older patients recover better than expected, and others fair worse than expected. Walston and colleagues[50] believe this phenomenon to be related to a phenotype that identifies those with decreased physiologic reserves in multiple organ systems. This phenotype has been associated with dysregulation of multiple physiologic systems, including a generalized increased inflammatory state, dysregulated cortisol,[51] altered heart variability, changes in hormonal status,[52] and decreased immune function.[53,54] It has further been posited that each criterion of the phenotype is related in a vicious cycle of dysregulated energetics,[44] a cycle that spirals downward with decreasing adaptive capacity. Their work identifies the frailty syndrome as a clinically apparent, and now measurable, manifestation of these changes after a certain threshold point is crossed.[39]

The Makary study demonstrates clearly that frailty is common in older surgical patients, and is independently associated with a greater risk for postoperative complications, increased LOS, and an increased likelihood for discharge to an assisted or skilled nursing facility rather than to home.[39] In addition, the frailty index strengthened the predictive ability of other commonly used operative risk models, and it is predicted that broad use of the frailty index can help inform the clinical decisions among patients and their medical and surgical clinicians.[39]

THE FRAILTY SYNDROME, SARCOPENIA, AND OSTEOPOROSIS

The frailty syndrome can be characterized as a combination of various symptoms or assessment markers, primarily secondary to the age-related losses and dysfunction of skeletal muscle and bone that occur mostly in the elderly and place them at increased risk for adverse events such as disability, institutionalization, and death. Sarcopenia results from the loss of muscle mass that occurs commensurate with the aging process, and is characterized initially by a decrease in the mass of the muscle (about 1% per year, usually starting at age 50 years and continuing throughout life), which is a direct cause of weakness and ensuing frailty. Muscle atrophy, which is characterized by shrinkage in the size of individual muscle cells (myocytes) is different from sarcopenia, in which there is actual loss of muscle cells and a replacement of them with fat and fibrosis. Muscle weakness, which is also referred to as muscle fatigue or lack of strength, is the inability to exert force by the effective contraction of skeletal muscles; and it often follows muscle atrophy and a decrease in activity such as that associated with long periods of bed rest secondary to an illness. Sarcopenia can also be associated with muscle weakness, which is usually gradual in onset and secondary to the age-related loss of skeletal muscle mass.

Osteoporosis is an age-related disease of bone that can lead to an increased risk of fracture and is a primary component of the frailty syndrome. The bone mineral density is reduced, the bone microarchitecture is disrupted, and the amount and variety of protein in bone is altered. Osteoporosis occurs most commonly in women after menopause, but it can also develop in men, and may be manifested in anyone secondary to specific hormonal disorders and other chronic diseases, or as a result of medications, especially glucocorticoids. Because of its profound influence on the risk of a fragility fracture, osteoporosis can significantly affect quality of life, life expectancy, and mortality. The establishment of frailty as a predictor of surgical outcomes in older patients by Makary and colleagues[39] in 2010 was the first formal study demonstrating the association of frailty and surgical outcomes, as has been discussed previously here. Frailty has also been associated with morbidity, mortality, falls, disability related to ADL, and hospitalization in the nonsurgical elderly populations.[44–47] In addition, cardiovascular disease, insulin resistance, and female gender have been associated with the frailty syndrome.[39,44,55–57] Finally, these findings support the concept of frailty as an inherent capacity to adapt to stressors.[39,44,58]

At present, approximately one-half of all surgical operations in the United States are performed in patients older than 65 years.[39] Based on recent projections, it is estimated that the average surgical volume will increase by 14% to 47% from the year 2000 to 2020, primarily because of the increased number of procedures performed in elderly patients.[59] The elderly are at high risk for morbidity, mortality, and increased costs, and it has been demonstrated that postoperative complications are more predictive than preoperative risk factors in determining survival.[39,60] Accordingly, health care providers, especially surgeons, should be alerted to the special needs and risks of older surgical patients.[39,46,61–64] It might be possible to decrease the risk of complications in frail patients in the postoperative period by closer monitoring and attention to hydration, nutrition, and early mobilization.[39] Reducing postoperative complications in older patients is particularly important because complications have been shown to increase the 30-day mortality by 26% in patients 80 years of age and older.[63] Well-designed, specific clinical studies are needed to develop targeted risk-reduction strategies for frail elderly patients.[39] In 1965, Bernard Isaacs, known as a "hero of geriatrics" in Great Britain, described the "geriatric giants" as the 4 major categories of impairment that appear in elderly people, especially as they begin to become frail. The 4 "giants" are immobility, instability, incontinence, and impaired intellect/memory, and Isaacs asserted that if examined sufficiently closely, all common problems with the elderly ultimately relate back to one or more of these "giants."[65] Diminishing functional and organ capacity accompany the aging process, and problems in the function of one organ or system can result in a cascading effect on others, much more commonly in the elderly than in other age groups. Impaired vision and hearing loss are common chronic problems among the elderly, and hearing problems can lead to social isolation, depression, and dependence as the patient can no longer communicate effectively with other people, receive information over the telephone, or engage in simple transactions such as talking to a person at a bank or store. Vision problems can lead to falls from tripping over unseen objects, taking medicine incorrectly because the written instructions cannot be read accurately, and financial transactions being undertaken or managed inappropriately.

MINI NUTRITIONAL ASSESSMENT IN THE ELDERLY

As has been demonstrated in many elderly surgical patients, an association has been established between malnutrition and important outcomes in hospitalized patients such as mortality, LOS, readmission rate, and discharge destination.[66–73] Assessment of nutritional status in most of these studies was based primarily on serum albumin concentrations or anthropometric measurements, which can particularly be influenced by confounding factors. Accordingly, clinical assessment tools have been developed such as the Mini Nutritional Assessment (MNA), which is a simple clinical scale for the evaluation of the nutritional status of elderly patients, especially the frail. It has been validated previously in older patients by comparing it with clinical assessments performed by expert geriatric nutritionists.[74,75] The MNA is an inexpensive and relatively easy protocol for screening aged individuals, primarily to identify those who are at increased risk of developing complications related to malnutrition.[76] The MNA is composed of 18 items, including anthropometric measurements (weight, height, and weight loss), a global assessment (6 questions related to lifestyle, medications, and mobility), a dietary questionnaire (8 questions related to meals, food, and fluid intake), and a subjective assessment (self-perception of health and nutrition).[76] Maximum score achievable is 30 points, and the risk for malnutrition increases with lower scores. The MNA score is used to classify patients as well-nourished (a score of 25–30), at risk for malnutrition (a score of 17–24), or malnourished (a score of <17).[74–77] In a study of 1319 patients having a mean age of 84.2 years and a gender composition of 70% female, MNA scores ranged from 8.0 to a maximum of 27.5, with a median of 20.5.[76] A strong relationship between mortality and MNA scores was established, with a threefold increase in death rate in the malnourished individuals having an MNA score less than 17, compared with those in the well-nourished group having an MNA score greater than 24; there was no relation to age or gender. The median length of hospital stay was also closely related to the MNA, and increased from 30.5 days in those with a score greater than 24 to 42.0 days in those with a score less than 17.[76] In listing the components of the MNA, the anthropometric assessment consists of: (1) body mass index, (2) mid-arm circumference, (3) calf circumference, and (4) weight loss during the last 3 months; the general assessment items of information consist of: (1) lives independently, (2) takes more than 3 medications a day, (3) experienced recent emotional event or acute disease, (4) level of mobility, (5) neuropsychological problems such as severe dementia and/or depression, (6) pressure sores; the dietary assessment includes the following: (1) number of meals per day, (2) eats dairy products, (3) eats legumes or eggs, meat, fish, and/or poultry every day, (3) eats fruits or vegetables twice a day, (4) loss of appetite, (5) daily fluid consumption, (6) mode and difficulty of feeding; and the self-assessment by the patient consists of: (1) self-assessed malnutrition status and (2) perceived health status compared with peers.[76]

Nutritional evaluation is a key component of comprehensive geriatric assessment.[76,78–80] The MNA is a validated nutritional assessment tool that does not rely on laboratory tests. It can easily be administered by any competent health professional and has been shown to be closely associated with outcomes in older hospitalized populations. Patients with a low MNA score are more likely to die or to be discharged to a nursing home, and to have a longer LOS. Whether the MNA is able to identify patients likely to benefit from nutritional support, especially elderly surgical patients, and consequently to have a more favorable outcome, deserves further investigation.[76] However, nutritional intervention studies to date have shown that nutritional support can shorten hospital stay and improve outcomes in specific studies of older hip fracture patients, suggesting that comparable results in other surgical patients are highly likely to occur.[76–78]

NUTRITIONAL REQUIREMENTS OF THE ELDERLY

The specific nutritional requirements of older patients are difficult to quantify exactly or consistently because of the physiologic diversity and heterogeneity of this population and the high prevalence of chronic disease and/or disability. Signs and symptoms of nutritional deficiencies are perceived uncommonly in the elderly who are able to live freely in the community, but are occasionally seen in elderly who are frail, homebound, institutionalized, and/or who must rely on others to meet their basic nutritional needs and ADL. In general, the nutrient needs in the elderly appear to be similar to those for middle-aged adult patients; however, for some nutrients, clear evidence of increased needs exist for the elderly, particularly those stressed by injury, surgical operations, sepsis, and/or other pathophysiologic processes. Osteoporosis is an obvious major health risk, especially for older women but also for older men. Because bones that are calcium rich are known to be less susceptible to fracture, calcium recommendations have been set at levels associated with maximum retention of body calcium.

Thus, the daily recommended intake for persons in the sixth decade of life and upward is 1200 mg/d with the upper tolerable level of calcium intake set at 2500 mg/d. For vitamin D, the daily recommended intake for this population group has recently been increased by the Institute of Medicine from 400 IU to 600 IU (15 μg) per day. The upper limit for vitamin D intake for adults is 2000 IU (50 μg per day, but doses above this level should be considered for frail homebound or institutionalized elderly whose exposure to sunlight is limited, or in those in whom osteomalacia or osteoporosis is documented. The determination of serum vitamin D levels is highly recommended in establishing the diagnosis of hypovitaminosis D and in monitoring its response to nutritional therapy. The DRI for folic acid (folate) in the geriatric population aged 50 years and older is 400 mg/d, with the upper limit for folate intake set at 1000 mg/d. It has been shown that the consumption of folate in recommended amounts can reduce the levels of homocysteine in the blood, which has been linked to an increased risk of cardiovascular disease; it has also been suggested that adequate intakes of folate may protect against the development of colorectal cancer. The DRI for vitamin B12 for the elderly has been set at 2.4 mg/d and vitamin B6 at 1.5 mg/d (with an upper limit set at 100 mg/d), and both of these requirements can be met through ordinary dietary means. However, 10% to 30% of older people can manifest deficiencies in these vitamins. As a general rule, in a malnourished elderly patient requiring therapeutic nutritional rehabilitation, the daily multivitamin dosage can be doubled safely until normal nutritional status has been restored.[1]

As with all other patients, planning nutritional intervention begins with estimating the nutrient balance of the patient, that is, nutrient intake plotted against nutrient losses. Nutrient intake is estimated by obtaining a directed dietary history and then calculating the calorie and protein intake, whereas nutrient losses are estimated by calculating the basal energy expenditure (BEE) and then adding any abnormal nutrient losses, such as those from external fistula output, diarrhea, or proteinuria. BEE can be estimated by applying the Harris-Benedict equations and adding a correction factor depending on the degree of metabolic stress in the patient.[7,81]

Men 66.47 + 13.75 (W) + 5.0 (H) − 6.76 (A)
Women 665.1 + 9.56 (W) + 1.85 (H) − 4.68 (A)
where W = weight in kilograms, H = height in centimeters, A = age in years.

The BEE result obtained from these equations is expressed in kilocalories per day. Resting energy expenditure (REE) can be measured at the patient's bedside by indirect calorimetry using a portable metabolic cart. Most indirect calorimeters calculate only oxygen consumption, whereas some also measure carbon dioxide production.[7] The measurement of oxygen consumption alone provides a reliable calculation for the REE; however, the measurement of carbon dioxide production also allows for the calculation of the respiratory quotient (RQ = CO_2 production/O_2 consumption). The RQ measurement can be very helpful with monitoring nutritional intervention in critically ill patients because a high RQ greater than 1, for example, is suggestive of lipogenesis secondary to excessive calorie intake, which can lead to liver dysfunction, especially in patients receiving excessive or unbalanced TPN.[82] Finally, the use of indirect calorimetry is not necessary in every elderly patient, and for most a simple calculation of the BEE is sufficient to initiate nutritional therapy.[7] Modifications in the nutritional regimen can then be made judiciously as the patient responds and reacts to the nutritional rehabilitation therapy.

The primary nutrient substrate required by the surgical patient, especially the elderly patient, is protein, which plays an essential role in the metabolic response to stress.[7]

The acute-phase proteins are synthesized in response to stress, whereas amino acids are ordinarily mobilized from endogenous muscle to provide precursors for hepatic gluconeogenesis. Elderly patients have a lower tolerance for this virtual autocannibalism than younger patients because of their reduced capacity to resynthesize protein. Therefore, it is essential to maintain an adequate supply of exogenous protein or amino acids in elderly patients experiencing severe metabolic stress. The exact quantities of protein moieties to be administered can be calculated by measuring nitrogen losses. Because the main route for nitrogen loss is the urine, a measurement of the 24-hour urinary urea nitrogen (UUN) allows calculation of the total nitrogen excreted. A more accurate formula has been derived, which accounts for urinary nitrogen excreted in forms other than urea (20%) together with fecal and cutaneous losses (2 g/d):

Total nitrogen losses = 24 h UUN (g/d) + 0.20 × 24 h UUN + 2 g/d

Protein requirements for the elderly can also be estimated without making measurements of losses. Under basal conditions, an adult patient requires approximately 0.8 g/kg body weight daily. Elderly patients have a slightly higher requirement of 1 to 1.2 g/kg body weight, because of their age-related impaired capacity for protein synthesis.[7,83] On the other hand, compromised renal and/or hepatic function, especially in the elderly, mandates caution and conscientious monitoring in order not to exceed the capacities of those organs to metabolize the protein optimally.

Baseline fluid requirements of elderly patients without renal and/or cardiac insufficiency are usually estimated at 25 mL/kg/d.[7,84] Fluid requirements may be increased by losses from vomiting, diarrhea, enterocutaneous fistula, polyuria, or excess perspiration, whereas on the other hand, fluid intake may require restriction because of chronic renal insufficiency, pulmonary insufficiency, or congestive heart failure. The risk of both dehydration and fluid overload is also high in the elderly because of their fairly common use of diuretics. Moreover, these fluid imbalances can be accompanied by electrolyte aberrations, which can cause significant problems. Finally, when initiating and advancing nutritional support in a severely malnourished elderly patient, the risk of refeeding syndrome is even higher than in the general population. This situation can be dangerously life threatening, and should be assiduously avoided by meticulous, conscientious attention to details in the formulation and administration of any and all forms of nutritional support in the elderly surgical patient. The principles and practices of optimal nutritional support in surgical patients have been described and discussed throughout this 2-volume issue, and must be applied meticulously to the elderly as well, with an extra dose of patience, persistence, prudence, and caution.

PERIOPERATIVE NUTRITIONAL SUPPORT OF THE ELDERLY

Axiom I—Maintenance of good nutritional status is essential for optimal geriatric surgical care, particularly in acute situations in which malnutrition is clearly associated with increased complications and other adverse health outcomes. This point is especially important considering that 40% to 50% of institutionalized older adults are at moderate to high risk for nutritional problems, and that 40% of noninstitutionalized older adults ingest diets that are deficient in 3 or more nutrients.[10] Moreover, the prevalence of geriatric malnutrition is underscored by data confirming that one or more nutritional inadequacies exist in all of the following: 9% to15% of older adults in outpatient clinics; 12% to 50% of hospitalized elderly patients; and 25% to 85% of older adults residing in institutions. PEM is the most common nutritional inadequacy in the geriatric population, and occurs or exists when insufficient energy and/or protein is available to meet the metabolic needs of the body. The clinical significance to the surgeon of PEM in the elderly is that poor nutritional status and PEM are associated with altered immunity, impaired wound healing, reduced functional status, increased health care use, and increased morbidity and mortality.

Axiom II—Although confounding effects of nonnutritional factors cannot completely be ruled out, many studies have shown that poor nutrition is an independent determinant of increased morbidity and mortality after adjusting for nonnutritional factors.

Axiom III—Although the efficacy of nutritional support is unproven unequivocally in many circumstances, data are available to suggest that clinical outcomes can be improved by interventions to correct or prevent nutritional deficits.

Axiom IV—Physician recognition of malnutrition in the elderly is often lacking, despite its apparent clinical importance, and several studies suggest that even when malnutrition is recognized, appropriate attempts to correct the condition are not made.

Axiom V—Optimally effective care of frail or ill elderly patients mandates evaluation of nutritional status for early recognition of malnutrition and consideration of appropriate supportive nutritional interventions. The importance of comprehensive nutritional assessment in elderly patients and the significant adverse effects of severe malnutrition in geriatric surgical patients have been discussed earlier.

Axiom VI—Although elderly patients appear to have worse outcomes following operations than younger patients, age itself is not an independent risk factor for increased mortality, and when corrected for comorbid disorders, including malnutrition, age alone has little influence on prognosis.

Axiom VII—Despite aggressive nutritional support (oral, enteral, parenteral) of the elderly patient, it is often difficult to attenuate, and virtually impossible to reverse, the catabolic response to illness, injury, surgical operation, and/or sepsis.

Axiom VIII—Anthropometric measurements indicate that when body weight does increase with nutritional support of the elderly patient, the initial gains are mostly in fat and extracellular water, whereas gains in lean body mass might result in better functional and clinical outcomes.

Axiom IX—Mortality for emergency operations of all types in elderly patients is at least 3 times greater than for comparable procedures performed under elective conditions, and the presence and severity of malnutrition is a highly significant comorbid factor in these outcomes.

Axiom X—Unfortunately, and regrettably, decisions regarding surgery and nutritional support in elderly patients are still often made on the basis of ignorance, speculation, and unfounded prejudice, instead of judicious assessment based on scientifically derived knowledge, data, experience, judgment, and wisdom.

SUMMARY

Comprehensive geriatric health care should include the maintenance of normal nutritional status in those who are in good health and provision of adequate nutritional support for the sick or injured, especially the frail. The elderly may be at risk for development of malnutrition because of a variety of physiologic and socioeconomic factors. Hospitalized elderly patients are a heterogeneous and diverse population, but they are at significant risk for presenting to the hospital with, or subsequently developing, both PEM and micronutrient deficiencies. Nutritional assessment should be routine and comprehensive at admission and at regular intervals thereafter during hospitalization. However, assessment of nutritional status of older geriatric patients (ages 65–100 years) remains a challenging task because of the lack of adequate specific reference data in this broad age group. In elderly patients requiring nutritional support, parenteral nutrition is indicated when the early establishment of effective oral or enteral nutrition is not, or cannot be, reliable in meeting nutritional and metabolic needs, and parenteral nutrition should be initiated early in the hospital course for optimal results. Peripheral parenteral nutrition can be a valuable short-term interim solution when the clinical course and volitional or enteral intake are uncertain, or the feedings are inadequate to meet target goals. Dietary counseling and more aggressive nutritional support with central venous total parenteral nutrition are just 2 of the many interventions required for the optimal care of the elderly segment of our society. Further research in basic and clinical areas is indicated and necessary to define more clearly the many nutritional and metabolic changes that occur with aging and to define the indications and nutritional support techniques for optimal management of these changes. Issues in overall geriatric management and in geriatric surgery and nutritional support specifically will continue to challenge surgeons in the future and must be addressed expeditiously. The most compelling reality is that the geriatric population will continue to grow in number and increase in longevity. This trend will require a major sea change in the manner in which their health, fitness, and function will be supported, literally on an individual basis; and the means by which the fundamental social, professional, medical, ethical, financial, and other costs thereof will be embraced and met by our society. The acceptance of elective surgery in elderly patients, especially the frail, will continue to increase and gain favor as better understanding of indications and outcomes are obtained, and as the risks incurred by comorbidities, including malnutrition, are further limited by judicious perioperative management and development of new nutritional support technologies. Surgeons must develop and carry out relevant, meticulously controlled study protocols specifically designed for the various cohorts of the geriatric populations, especially in the frail, to provide the data essential to understanding and solving their unique nutritional, functional, and surgical problems. We must recognize and allow for the difficulties associated with performing studies in aged patients with seemingly inevitable comorbidities. Moreover, we must understand that the physiologic changes that accompany the normal aging process, especially those related to nutritional needs, occur at different rates and times among human beings. The difference between chronologic age and physiologic age in elderly patients must be determined clinically in a scientific manner to help guide prudent decision making in their management. Although the old adage is that the chronologic age of the patient is not an independent risk factor for surgical procedures or actions, the age of the elderly patient can indeed become an independent risk factor in some elderly, in whom a great disparity exists between their chronologic age and their physiologic age. Finally, establishing age-specific nutrient requirements for the heterogeneous geriatric population will not be an easy task even when the group is healthy, much less when accompanied by wide variations of health conditions, comorbidities, fitness, deficiencies, disabilities, nutritional status, resources, support, and multiple other more specific or unique individual factors. Nutritional management of geriatric surgical patients will continue to challenge the patience, skills, ingenuity, and resilience of surgeons for quite some time into the future if surgical optimal outcomes are to be achieved in this special age group of our population.

REFERENCES

1. White J, Ham RJ. Older adults. In: Morrison GM, Hark L, editors. Medical nutrition and disease. Malden (MA): Blackwell Science; 1999. p. 134–47.

 2. Saltzman E, Mason JB. Enteral nutrition in the elderly. In: Rambeau JL, Rolandelli RH, editors. Clinical nutrition: enteral and tube feeding. Philadelphia: WB Saunders; 1997. p. 385–402.
 3. Chandra RJ, Imbach A, Moore C, et al. Nutrition of the elderly. Can Med Assoc J 1991;145(11):1475–87.
 4. Dall JL. The greying of Europe. Br Med J 1994;309:1282–5.
 5. Public Health Service. Centers for disease control, National Center for health statistics: health United States 1993 chartbook. DHHS Pub. No. (PHS) 94-1232-1. Hyattsville (MD): US Department of Health and Human Services; 1994.
 6. Katz MS, Gerety MB, Lichenstein MJ. Gerontology and geriatric medicine. In: Stein JH, editor. Internal medicine. St Louis (MO): Mosby; 1994. p. 2825.
 7. Rolandelli RH, Ullrich JR. Nutritional support in the frail elderly surgical patient. Surg Clin North Am 1994;74(1):79–92.
 8. U.S. Senate Committee on Education and Labor. Incorporating nutrition screening and interventions into medical practice: a monograph for physicians. Washington, DC: Nutrition Screening Initiative; 1994.
 9. Carey M, Gillespie S. Position of the American dietetic association: little cost-effectiveness of medical nutrition therapy. J Am Diet Assoc 1995;95(1):88–91.
10. Marwick C. NHANES III health data relevant for aging population. JAMA 1997; 277:100–2.
11. Galanos AN, Pieper CF, Cornoni-Huntley JC, et al. Nutrition and function: is there a relationship between body mass index and the functional capabilities of community-dwelling elderly? J Am Geriatr Soc 1994;42:368–73.
12. Mowe M, Bohmer T, Kindt E. Reduced nutritional status in an elderly population (>70y) is probable before disease and possibly contributes to the development of disease. Am J Clin Nutr 1994;59:317–24.
13. Fiatorone M. Nutrition in the geriatric patient. Hosp Pract 1990;30:38–40.
14. Morley JE. Why do physicians fail to recognize and treat malnutrition in older persons? J Am Geriatr Soc 1991;39:1139–40.
15. Manson A, Shea S. Malnutrition in elderly ambulatory medical patients. Am J Public Health 1991;81(9):1195–7.
16. Calkins DR, Rubenstein LV, Cleary PD, et al. Failure of physicians to recognize functional disability in ambulatory patients. Ann Intern Med 1991; 114(6):451–4.
17. Yates AA, Schlicker SA, Suitor CW. Dietary reference intakes: the new basis for recommendations for calcium and related nutrients, B vitamins, and choline. J Am Diet Assoc 1998;98:699–706.
18. Abbasi AA, Rudman DR. Undernutrition in the nursing home: prevalence, consequences, causes and prevention. Nutr Rev 1994;52(4):113–22.
19. ASPEN board of directors: geriatric conditions. JPEN J Parenter Enteral Nutr 1993;17(4):24SA.
20. Kaminski MV, Nasr NJ, Freed BA, et al. The efficacy of nutritional support in the elderly. J Am Coll Nutr 1982;1:35–40.
21. Lipschitz DA, Mitchell CO. The correctability of the nutritional, immune, and hematopoietic manifestations of protein calorie malnutrition in the elderly. J Am Coll Nutr 1982;1:17–25.
22. Winograd CH, Brown EM. Aggressive oral feeding in hospitalized patients. Am J Clin Nutr 1990;52:967–8.
23. Schiffman SS, Warwick ZS. Effect of flavor enhancement of foods for the elderly on nutritional status, food intake, biochemical indices, and anthropometric measures. Physiol Behav 1993;53(2):395–402.

24. Gray-Donald K, Payette H, Boutier V, et al. Evaluation of the dietary intake of homebound elderly and the feasibility of dietary supplementation. J Am Coll Nutr 1994;13(3):277–84.
25. Evers BM, Townsend CM Jr, Thompson JC. Organ physiology of aging. Surg Clin North Am 1994;74(1):23–39.
26. Adkins R, Scott H. Surgical procedures in patients aged 90 years and older. South Med J 1984;77:1357–64.
27. Goldman L, Caldera D, Southwick F, et al. Cardiac risk factors and complications in non-cardiac surgery. Medicine 1978;57:357–70.
28. Greenburg A, Saik R, Farris J, et al. Operative mortality in general surgery. Am J Surg 1982;144(1):22–8.
29. Linn B, Linn M, Wallen N. Evaluation of results of surgical procedures in the elderly. Ann Surg 1982;195:90–6.
30. Koruda MJ, Sheldon GF. Surgery in the aging. Adv Surg 1991;24:293–331.
31. Katlic MR. Principles of geriatric surgery. In: Rosenthal RA, Zenilman ME, Katlic MR, editors. Principles and practice of geriatric surgery. New York: Springer-Verlage; 2001. p. 92–104.
32. Nutrition. In: Abram WB, Beers MH, Berkow R, editors. The Merck manual of geriatrics. Whitehouse Station (NJ): Merck Research Laboratories; 1996. p. 7–16.
33. Elahi VK, Elahi D, Andres R, et al. A longitudinal study of nutritional intake in men. J Gerontol 1983;38:162–80.
34. Roberts SB. Energy requirements of older individuals. Eur J Clin Nutr 1996; 50(Suppl 1):S112–8.
35. Katz S, Ford AB, Moskowitz RW, et al. Studies of illness in the aged: the index of ADL: a standard measure of biological and psychosocial function. JAMA 1963; 185(12):914–9.
36. Lawton MP, Brody EM. Assessment of older people: self-maintaining and instrumental activities of daily living. Gerontologist 1969;9(3):179–86.
37. Polanczyk CA, Marcantonio E, Goldman L, et al. Impact of age on perioperative complications and length of stay in patients undergoing noncardiac surgery. Ann Intern Med 2001;134:637–43.
38. Hamel MB, Henderson WG, Khuri SF, et al. Surgical outcomes for patients aged 80 and older: morbidity and mortality from major noncardiac surgery. J Am Geriatr Soc 2005;53:424–9.
39. Makary MA, Segev DL, Pronovost PJ, et al. Frailty as a predictor of surgical outcomes in older patients. J Am Coll Surg 2010;210(6):901–8.
40. Davenport DL, Bowe EA, Henderson WG, et al. National surgical quality improvement program (NSQIP): risk factors can be used to validate American Society of Anesthesiologist Physical Status classification (ASA PS) levels. Ann Surg 2006; 243:636–44.
41. Lee TH, Marcantonio ER, Mangione CM, et al. Derivation and prospective validation of a simple index for prediction of cardiac risk of major noncardiac surgery. Circulation 1999;100:1043–9.
42. Eagle KA, Berger PB, Calkins H, et al. ACC/AHA guideline update for perioperative cardiovascular evaluation for noncardiac surgery—executive summary: a report of the American College of Cardiology/American Heart Association task force on practice guidelines. J Am Coll Cardiol 2000;39:542–53.
43. Saklad M. Grading of patients for surgical procedures. Anesthesiology 1941;2: 281–4.
44. Fried LP, Tangen CM, Walston J, et al. Frailty in older adults: evidence for a phenotype. J Gerontol A Biol Sci Med Sci 2001;56:M146–56.

45. Bandeen-Roche K, Xue QL, Ferrucci L, et al. Phenotype of frailty: characterization in the women's health and aging studies. J Gerontol A Biol Sci Med Sci 2006;61: 262–6.
46. Boyd CM, Darer J, Boult C, et al. Clinical practice guidelines and quality of care for older patients with multiple comorbid diseases: implications for pay for performance. JAMA 2005;294:716–24.
47. Woods NF, LaCroix AZ, Gray SL, et al. Frailty: emergence and consequences in women aged 65 and older in the women's health initiative observational study. J Am Geriatr Soc 2005;53:1321–30.
48. Fried LP, Kronmal RA, Newman AB, et al. Risk factors for 5-year mortality in older adults: the cardiovascular health study. JAMA 1998;279:585–92.
49. Radloff LS. The CES-D scale: a self-report depression scale for research in the general population. Appl Psychol Meas 1977;1:401.
50. Walston J, McBurnie MA, Newman A, et al. Frailty and activation of the inflammation and coagulation systems with and without clinical comorbidities: results from the cardiovascular health study. Arch Intern Med 2002;162:2333–41.
51. Varadhan R, Walston J, Cappola AR, et al. Higher levels and blunted diurnal variation of cortisol in frail older women. J Gerontol A Biol Sci Med Sci 2008; 63:190–5.
52. Cappola AR, Bandeen-Roche K, Wand GS, et al. Association of IGF-I levels with muscle strength and mobility in older women. J Clin Endocrinol Metab 2001;87: 4139–46.
53. Leng SX, Cappola AR, Andersen RE, et al. Serum levels of insulin-like growth factor-I (IGF-I) and dehydroepiandrosterone sulfate (DHEA-S), and their relationships with serum interleukin-6, in the geriatric syndrome of frailty. Aging Clin Exp Res 2004;16:153–7.
54. Leng SX, Yang H, Walston JD. Decreased cell proliferation and altered cytokine production in frail older adults. Aging Clin Exp Res 2004;16:249–52.
55. Newman AB, Gottdiener JS, McBurnie MA, et al. Associations of subclinical cardiovascular disease with frailty. J Gerontol A Biol Sci Med Sci 2001;56: M158–66.
56. Purser JL, Kuchibhatla MN, Fillenbaum GG, et al. Identifying frailty in hospitalized older adults with significant coronary artery disease. J Am Geriatr Soc 2006;54: 1674–81.
57. Barzilay JI, Blaum C, Moore T, et al. Insulin resistance and inflammation as precursors of frailty: the cardiovascular health study. Arch Intern Med 2007; 167:635–41.
58. Bortz WM 2nd. A conceptual framework of frailty: a review. J Gerontol A Biol Sci Med Sci 2002;57:M283–8.
59. Etzioni DA, Liu JH, O'Connell JB, et al. Elderly patients in surgical workloads: a population-based analysis. Am Surg 2003;69:961–5.
60. Khuri SF, Henderson WG, DePalma RG, et al. Determinants of long-term survival after major surgery and the adverse effect of postoperative complications. Ann Surg 2005;242:326–43.
61. Bartali B, Semba RD, Frongillo EA, et al. Low micronutrient levels as a predictor of incident disability in older women. Arch Intern Med 2006;166:2335–40.
62. Gill TM, Baker DI, Gottschalk M, et al. A prehabilitation program for physically frail community-living older persons. Arch Phys Med Rehabil 2003;84:394–404.
63. Semba RD, Blaum CS, Bartali B, et al. Denture use, malnutrition, frailty, and mortality among older women living in the community. J Nutr Health Aging 2006;10:161–7.

64. Gill TM, Allore HG, Holford TR, et al. Hospitalization, restricted activity, and the development of disability among older persons. JAMA 2004;292:2115–24.
65. Isaacs B. Prognostic factors in elderly patients in a geriatric institution. Gerontol Clin (Basel) 1965;7(4):202–15.
66. Burness R, Horne G, Purdi G. Albumin levels and mortality in patients with hip fractures. N Z Med J 1996;109:56–7.
67. Anderson MD, Collins G, Davis G, et al. Malnutrition and length of stay: a relationship? Henry Ford Hosp Med J 1985;33:190–3.
68. Bernstein LH. Relationship of nutritional markers to length of hospital stay. Nutrition 1995;11:205–9.
69. Sullivan DH. Risk factors for early hospital readmission in a select population of geriatric rehabilitation patients: the significance of nutritional status. J Am Geriatr Soc 1992;40:792–8.
70. Herrmann FR, Safran C, Levkoff SD, et al. Serum albumin level on admission as a predictor of death, length of stay and readmission. Arch Intern Med 1992;152: 125–30.
71. Friedmann JM, Jensen GL, Smiciklas-Wright H, et al. Predicting early nonelective hospital readmission in nutritionally compromised older adults. Am J Clin Nutr 1997;65:1714–20.
72. Potter J, Klipstein K, Reilly JJ, et al. The nutritional status and clinical course of acute admissions to a geriatric unit. Age Ageing 1995;24:131–6.
73. Chima CS, Barco K, Dewitt ML, et al. Relationship of nutritional status to length of stay, hospital costs and discharge status of patients hospitalized in the medicine service. J Am Diet Assoc 1997;97:975–8.
74. Guigoz Y, Vellas B, Garry PJ. Mini nutritional assessment: a practical assessment tool for grading the nutritional status of elderly patients. Facts and research in gerontology. Paris: Serdi Publishing; 1994. p. 15–9.
75. Vellas B, Guigoz Y, Garry PJ, et al. The mini nutritional assessment (MNA) and its use in grading the nutritional state of elderly patients. Nutrition 1999;15: 116–22.
76. Van Nes M-C, Herrmann FR, Gold G, et al. Does the mini nutritional assessment predict hospitalization outcomes in older people? Age Ageing 2001;30: 221–6.
77. Lauque S, Arnaud-Battandier F, Mansourian R, et al. Protein-energy oral supplementation in malnourish nursing-home residents. A controlled trial. Age Ageing 2000;29:51–6.
78. Antonelli Incalzi R, Landi F, Cipriani L, et al. Nutritional assessment: a primary component of multidimensional geriatric assessment in the acute care setting. J Am Geriatr Soc 1996;44(2):166–74.
79. Rubenstein LZ, Harker J, Guigoz Y, et al. Comprehensive Geriatric Assessment (CGA) and the MNA: an overview of CGA, Nutritional Assessment, and Development of a shortened version of the MNA. In: Vellas B, Garry PJ, Guigoz Y, editors. Mini Nutritional Assessment (MNA): research and practice in the elderly. Basel (Switzerland): Karger; 1999. p. 101–16.
80. Vellas BJ, Guigoz Y. Nutritional assessment as part of the geriatric evaluation. In: Rubenstein LZ, Wielan D, Bernabei R, editors. Geriatric assessment technology: the state of the art. Milan (Italy): Kurtis; 1995. p. 179–84.
81. Harris J, Benedict F. A biometric study of basal metabolism in man: publication #279. Washington, DC: Carnegie Institution; 1919.
82. Elwyn DH, Askanazi J, Kinney JM, et al. Kinetics of energy substrates. Acta Chir Scand 1981;507(Suppl):209–19.

83. Gersovitz M, Motil K, Munro HN, et al. Human protein requirements: assessment of the adequacy of the current recommended dietary allowance for dietary protein in elderly men and women. Am J Clin Nutr 1982;35:6–14.

84. Randall HT. Fluid, electrolyte, and fluid base balance. Surg Clin North Am 1976; 56:1019–58.

Overview of Enteral and Parenteral Feeding Access Techniques: Principles and Practice

Melissa S. Phillips, MD*, Jeffrey L. Ponsky, MD

KEYWORDS

• Enteral access • Parenteral access • Nutrition

The importance of adequate nutritional support has long been appreciated in both critically ill patients and those undergoing routine surgical intervention. Malnutrition results in decreased immunocompetence and a negative impact on wound healing, leading to increased infectious complications and diminished postoperative recovery. Severe malnutrition increases overall morbidity and mortality associated with surgical intervention. Nutritional assessments should be performed on all patients, and those who are at risk for complications of malnutrition should be given adequate nutritional and metabolic supplemental support.

The enteral route of alimentation should be used in patients with a normal functioning gastrointestinal (GI) tract who require nutritional support. Enteral nutrition is considered safer because it results in fewer infectious complications when compared with parenteral nutrition.[1,2] There is also a clear cost advantage of enteral nutrition in both direct and indirect costs. In addition, there are metabolic and immunity-related advantages of enteral feedings.[3,4] However, all patients are not suitable for enteral nutritional support, and thus practitioners must have knowledge of, and competence in, the options for parenteral feeding access.

ENTERAL ACCESS
General Indications

Neurologic diseases constitute the most common indication for enteral access and nutritional support. Many different neurologic conditions result in dysphagia, aspiration, lack of coordination in swallowing, or a combination of these symptoms.

The authors have no relevant financial disclosures or conflicts of interest.

Department of Surgery, University Hospitals Case Medical Center, Case Western Reserve University 11100 Euclid Avenue, Lakeside 7, Mailstop 5047, Cleveland, OH 44106, USA

* Corresponding author.

E-mail address: Phillips.Melissa@gmail.com

Surg Clin N Am 91 (2011) 897–911

doi:10.1016/j.suc.2011.04.006

surgical.theclinics.com

0039-6109/11/$ – see front matter © 2011 Elsevier Inc. All rights reserved.

Cerebrovascular accidents, often resulting in severe deficits or coma, are a common indication for enteric feeding tube placement. Hypoxic encephalopathy, pseudobulbar paralysis, and severe dementia can also be indications for placement of a feeding tube for enteral support. Other neurologic indications for access include myasthenia gravis, multiple sclerosis, and amyotrophic lateral sclerosis.

Multisystem trauma may also be a frequent indication for enteral access. Catabolic states associated with trauma, such as patients with large total body surface area burns, especially require nutritional support. Severe facial, neck, neurologic, and chest trauma may also result in anatomic and/or functional limitations to oral intake that require enteral access.

Neoplastic processes of the head, neck, and esophagus are other common indications for enteral access. Patients having dysphagia or other oral intake problems related to the primary lesion or who have undergone a major curative resection frequently require feeding tube placement. Maintaining adequate nutritional support during surgical, chemotherapeutic, and radiation therapy is important for optimal healing and survival.[5] These patients, especially those with partially or completely obstructing lesions, may present a challenge for endoscopic access placement.

Pediatric patients have multiple needs for enteral access, including congenital neurologic syndromes, birth asphyxia, cerebral palsy, seizure disorders, and neuromotor retardation. Congenital lesions such as tracheomalacia, tracheoesophageal fistula, or maxillofacial abnormalities comprise absolute indications for enteral access until the anatomic lesion can be corrected. Enzymatic deficiencies and other childhood illnesses associated with malnutrition and failure to thrive may also respond favorably to enteral support.

Enteral access may be indicated not only for feeding but also for decompression of the GI tract. Patients with unresectable malignancies causing bowel obstruction, carcinomatosis, or severe radiation enteritis may benefit from gastrostomy tube placement for palliation, or in combination with parenteral nutrition support, as part of a comprehensive treatment plan including chemotherapy, radiation therapy, and/or surgical debulking.

Other less common indications for placement of enteral access include patients who would benefit from refeeding of externalized biliary drainage, treatment of gastric volvulus, and administration of unpalatable medications. Patients with inflammatory bowel disease may also benefit from enteral access for supplemental nocturnal feedings.

Patients with significant gastroesophageal reflux or aspiration pneumonitis should be considered for jejunal access rather than gastric access. An additional indication for jejunal access is poor gastric emptying or gastric outlet obstruction. This type of access is also considered in patients with pancreatitis who are unable to tolerate gastric feeds. Jejunal access can be accomplished through a jejunal extension of gastric access or as a separate jejunal access site, as detailed later.

Contraindications

Absolute contraindications to enteral access include a GI tract that is not functional. Patients with limited life expectancy, generally accepted as less than 4 weeks, should be managed with nasoenteral tube access, given the cost, risk, and impracticality of a more permanent access site. A discussion should be held with the patient or appointed surrogate regarding all treatment options, including the indications, risks, and potential benefits related to enteral access, before a decision is made to proceed with invasive placement.

Relative contraindications include massive ascites or severe malnutrition because formation of the intended gastrocutaneous fistula may be impaired and result in leakage of enteral contents. Other relative contraindications include overall clinical decompensation such as sepsis or fevers of unknown origin. In addition to the medical considerations outlined earlier, patients with psychologically based eating disorders, such as anorexia nervosa, or those at risk for exploitation, must have all ethical considerations evaluated before an enteral access is established. Previous surgical intervention is not an absolute contraindication although attention must be given to postsurgical anatomic modifications and the presence of adhesions in the choice of the ideal procedure. Consideration must also be given to the presence of coagulopathy, portal hypertension, history of peritoneal dialysis, hiatal hernia, and morbid obesity when choosing the type of enteral access. There is no justification for an emergent percutaneous endoscopic gastrostomy (PEG), because feedings may be accomplished in patients through nasoenteral access until definitive surgical access can be obtained safely.

Temporary Access

The use of nasal or oral enteric tubes is a common practice in hospitals to provide temporary or bridging nutritional support. Nasogastric or nasojejunal tubes provide the easiest enteral access for nutritional support. Feedings can be administered by bolus or continuous infusion. The use of these tubes can augment oral intake in the form of nocturnal support during acute recovery, or can provide full caloric support in patients unable to eat. This technique has a low cost and low morbidity. However, concerning long-term nutritional support, nasoenteric tubes are associated with many complications. Large-bore tubes may cause erosion of the nasal cartilage and are associated with sinusitis.[6] The presence of the tube across the lower esophageal sphincter may disrupt its integrity and lead to gastroesophageal reflux, which may contribute to aspiration and consequently to pneumonitis and or pneumonia. Patient discomfort also limits the long-term applicability of nasoenteric tubes.

Softer, smaller-diameter tubes have modestly improved patient discomfort, but often become blocked and require replacement. In addition, nasoenteric tubes are often inadvertently removed. This option for enteral access in the short-term provides many benefits, but long-term enteral nutrition is best accomplished by a permanent gastrostomy or jejunostomy.

ENDOSCOPIC APPROACH

In 1980, Gauderer and colleagues[7] introduced a technique of gastrostomy tube placement that did not require laparotomy. This technique revolutionized access to the GI tract, offering a less invasive, relatively safe procedure though which enteral nutritional support can be given. Over the years since the first description of a PEG, variations have been described, including the pull technique, push technique, and the Russell or introducer technique.[8] These approaches have yielded equivalent or improved results and lower costs when compared with surgical gastrostomy.

Specific Indications

Absolute contraindications for endoscopic enteral access include limited life expectancy, nonfunctional GI tract, and anorexia nervosa. The presence of peritonitis is an absolute contraindication for the endoscopic approach, and surgical treatment should be performed. Inability to pass the endoscope is an obvious absolute contraindication. Severe esophageal stricture, head or neck cancer, trauma of the face or oropharynx, and various other causes may limit the endoscopic options, and other techniques for access should be evaluated.

Relative contraindications specifically related to the endoscopic approach include portal hypertension with esophageal and gastric varices, peritoneal dialysis, hepatomegaly, large hiatal hernia, previous subtotal gastrectomy, and morbid obesity.

Technique

The patient is prepared by discontinuation of enteral feedings and a fasting period for 8 hours before the proposed endoscopic access procedure. A complete blood count including platelet count and prothrombin time are reviewed. A preoperative antibiotic, usually a cephalosporin, is administered within 1 hour of the procedure to decrease the risk of associated wound infection in the abdominal wall. Antibiotics should be tailored for coverage of skin flora.

Intravenous access is obtained for the administration of analgesia and sedation. The patient is placed in the supine position, and stepwise titration of medications, commonly a narcotic and benzodiazepam, are administered.[9] Topical anesthesia may also be sprayed on the mucosal surfaces of the oropharynx. Patients should be monitored for respiratory rate, blood pressure, heart rate, and oxygen saturation throughout the procedure.[10]

General anesthesia should be considered for all patients with increased risk for aspiration or for patients in whom concern for inability to maintain airway protection exist, such as those with advanced head or neck neoplasms or who are morbidly obese. Patients with the inability to comprehend and participate in their care, such as children or the delirious patient, may also be considered as candidates for general anesthesia.

The first step in placement of endoscopic enteral access is to perform a full upper endoscopy. The gastroscope is introduced into the patient's esophagus. If difficulty is encountered in the supine position, the patient may be rotated to the left lateral decubitus position temporarily to facilitate passage of the endoscope. The stomach and duodenum should be evaluated for disease and to rule out pyloric obstruction.[11] The endoscope is then withdrawn into the body of the stomach, and the stomach is insufflated, resulting in better opposition of the anterior gastric and abdominal walls. A point is chosen in the midepigastrium where maximal transillumination of the endoscope is visualized. This task may be facilitated by darkening the room. Direct external palpation of the abdominal wall should be visualized simultaneously by the gastroscope. Multiple sites may be palpated until the best location for transillumination and gastric indentation are achieved. These techniques help decrease the risk of intervening tissue being present between the gastric and abdominal walls, avoiding inadvertent puncture of adjacent organs. Morbid obesity or previous abdominal surgeries may limit the endoscopic visualization of palpation and/or transillumination, leading some practitioners to prefer palpation in combination with the safe tract approach.

The safe tract technique is then performed.[12] In this method, the best site for puncture is identified by the techniques described earlier, and a small caliber needle attached to a syringe filled with fluid is introduced through the anterior abdominal wall while negative pressure is applied to the plunger. The syringe is slowly advanced through the abdominal wall, and the needle is visualized by the gastroscope. Any air seen in the syringe before visualization of the needle in the gastric lumen implies that the needle is within an unintended loop of bowel. Aspiration of blood implies that the left segment of the liver is interposed between the gastric and abdominal wall. If either of these possibilities occurs, the needle is then removed, an alternative site chosen, and the technique is repeated.

Local anesthetic is then infiltrated into the skin and subcutaneous tissue at the chosen site, and a 1-cm incision is made in the transverse direction. A needle angiocatheter is then introduced into the gastric lumen under direct visualization by the endoscope. A polypectomy snare is passed through the working channel of the endoscope and used to grasp the angiocatheter. The needle component of the angiocatheter is then removed, and a guidewire is passed through the abdominal wall via the catheter. After several centimeters of guidewire have been passed, the snare is loosened and the guidewire is grasped. The endoscope is then withdrawn, while advancing the proximal end of the guidewire through the esophagus and mouth.

In the pull method, the tapered gastrostomy tube is attached to the guidewire outside the patient's mouth. Gentle tension is applied to the guidewire from the abdominal side to introduce the gastrostomy tube/guidewire unit into the esophagus and then into the stomach.

In the push method, the gastrostomy tube is passed over the guidewire, and the endoscope is used to grasp and stabilize the end of the wire beyond the gastrostomy tube. The gastrostomy tube is then pushed through the abdominal wall into the stomach using the endoscope while tension is applied to both ends of the guidewire.

In both methods, the endoscope may be reintroduced to confirm optimal placement of the internal bumper against the gastric mucosa but without undue tension. The literature supports the lack of reintroduction of the gastroscope, showing equivalent results, reduced time, and reduced patient discomfort.[13] However, repeat gastroscopy should be performed in all cases in which there is a concern for internal bumper location. An external bumper is then used to secure the PEG in place, with care taken to avoid undue pressure on the skin. A distance of 1 to 2 mm between the bolster and skin is advisable to decrease ischemic necrosis and subsequent infection.

The Russell or introducer method uses the Seldinger technique for placement of a balloon-tipped PEG tube. This technique provides significant benefit for patients with an oropharyngeal or upper GI narrowing because the gastrostomy tube is not passed through the oral cavity. It also offers the advantage that there is no contamination of the gastrostomy tube by oral flora. In patients with head and neck neoplasms, the pull method of PEG placement has been associated with malignant seeding of the gastrostomy tract.[14] Implications of this research are that the introducer technique may offer a potential benefit in this population to decrease the seeding risk, but definitive conclusions have yet to be established.

Preparation is similar to the push and pull techniques detailed earlier through the performance of the complete upper endoscopy and identification of the site, including safe tract technique. A 1-cm incision is made over the selected area on the abdominal wall. An angiocatheter is introduced through the incision into the stomach under direct visualization via the gastroscope, and a guidewire is passed several centimeters into the stomach. The angiocatheter is removed, leaving the guidewire in place. A dilator with a peel-away introducer is passed over the guidewire, dilating the tract into the stomach in accordance with the Seldinger technique. Care must be taken to follow the curve of the guidewire and avoid kinking, which could lead to the inability to complete the procedure. The gastroscope is used to verify that both the introducer and dilator are clearly seen in the gastric lumen. The wire and dilator are both removed, leaving the peel-away introducer in place. A lubricated balloon-tipped gastrostomy tube is inserted through the introducer until several centimeters of it are seen in the stomach. The balloon is then insufflated with saline, and the tube is secured to the skin. Modifications of the introducer method have been described, for example, the SLiC approach,[15] which uses standard laparoscopic ports to provide dilation under endoscopic visualization as a means of introducing the gastrostomy tube.

Jejunal Access

Patients experiencing aspiration and reflux often fare better with a jejunostomy than a gastrostomy for feedings. Jejunostomy feeding may also be more practical and effective in patients with severe gastroparesis, gastric atony, or other gastric emptying problems. Contraindications to percutaneous endoscopic jejunostomy (PEJ) placement include mechanical obstruction of the small bowel in addition to the general endoscopic contraindications discussed earlier.

One option for jejunal feeding is a jejunal extension, or J-arm, which is placed through a standard PEG. A standard 24-French PEG accommodates up to a 12.5-French J-tube, and a 20-French PEG accommodates up to an 8.5-French J-tube. After adequate sedation and complete upper endoscopy to evaluate for gastric outlet obstruction or pyloric stenosis, a gastroscope is returned to the stomach. The J-tube is passed through the existing PEG, and the suture on the distal end of the J-tube is grasped using an endoscopic clip applicator passed through the working channel of the endoscope. The gastroscope and jejunal tube are then passed through the pylorus and into the small bowel under direct visualization. The suture loop is then secured to the small bowel mucosa by firing the endoscopic clip. Although the clip often dislodges within the first week or two, this technique allows for easier removal of the endoscope from the small bowel and decreases the risk for inadvertent dislodgement of the jejunal feeding tube during placement.

Direct PEJ tube placement provides direct feeding access distal to the ligament of Treitz. This technique has been shown to yield superior results when compared with gastrostomy feedings in patients with GI reflux-related aspiration, although aspiration of oropharyngeal secretions is unchanged.[16] However, direct PEJ has a higher documented rate of bleeding, inadvertent visceral injury, and leakage when compared with PEG. After sedation and appropriate antibiotic administration, a pediatric colonoscope is advanced into the small bowel. Fluoroscopy is used to confirm scope positioning within the small bowel. Palpation of the abdominal wall is used to identify this loop and the safe tract technique described earlier is used to facilitate access into the identified small bowel loop. Using a pull technique, the PEJ tube, usually 16-French or 20-French, is then introduced via the method described earlier for a pull PEG. The pediatric colonoscope is then reintroduced into the small bowel to confirm satisfactory final positioning of the PEJ bumper at the completion of the procedure.

Complications

Early dislodgement of the feeding tube (within the first 7 days) is a feared complication after endoscopic placement. Because there is no direct attachment of the stomach to the anterior abdominal wall, dislodgement before maturation and fixation of gastrocutaneous fistula formation may lead to spillage of gastric contents and peritonitis, requiring expedient laparotomy for repair. An attempt may be made to replace the tube at the bedside, and a water-soluble contrast study should be obtained to confirm accurate intraluminal placement. If the tube is unable to be replaced, successful conservative management with bowel rest, nasogastric decompression, and antibiotics has been described, but should only be attempted in patients in whom serial reliable abdominal examinations disclose no signs of an acute abdomen.[17] If the patient remains stable, conservative management is continued for 5 to 7 days, at which time a repeat percutaneous endoscopic approach may be performed. Any patient with increasing abdominal pain, signs or symptoms of peritonitis, or clinical decompensation requires emergent laparotomy.

Dislodgement of the gastrostomy tube more than 7 days after placement requires reinsertion of a new tube through the mature gastrocutaneous tract. This process must be performed in a timely manner because the tract may close within a few hours after tube removal. If an appropriate replacement gastrostomy tube is not available, a standard Foley catheter may be used as a temporary substitute. A water-soluble contrast study should be performed to confirm accurate intraluminal replacement of the tube.

Wound problems are common with percutaneous tube placement and are often associated with excessive tension on the tube, leading to tissue ischemia and necrosis. A little drainage around the tube is expected and is part of the normal reaction of the body to a foreign body. Ensuring tension-free tube placement and providing local wound care with soap and water are the best management options. Occlusive dressings may aggravate skin reaction by trapping moisture in the area. Excessive tension on the tube may also result in buried bumper syndrome, a condition in which the head of the tube is extruded from the gastric lumen into the subcutaneous tissue. Tension on the tube may also lead to progressive enlargement of the stoma. Minimizing tube mobility and reducing tension on the tube should allow healing to proceed normally around the tract.

Although wound problems are common, true wound infections such as those associated with major surgical operations are rare after PEG placement. Focal areas of associated redness or fluctuance may represent a peritubal abscess that requires incision and drainage for resolution. A minimal skin incision at the time of the initial PEG placement that encircles the tube tightly fails to allow free egress of bacteria-laden secretions and can lead to higher postplacement infection rates. The incidence of wound infection is significantly decreased by a single timely preoperative prophylactic dose of antibiotics that have activity against common skin flora. Yeast infections are best managed by application of antifungal powders or creams to the affected skin.

Clogging of the tube is a common complication, is more common with smaller-diameter tubes, and is often associated with medication administration. Prevention is the best treatment. Gastrostomy tubes should be flushed with tap water after each use to ensure patency. If the tube is clogged, instilling soda or commercially available enzymatic agents may be adequate. If these measures are unsuccessful, passage of a guidewire or smaller catheter through the tube may restore patency. In worst-case scenarios, the gastrostomy tube may require removal and reinsertion following the guidelines detailed earlier.

Perforation during routine upper endoscopy occurs in 0.03% of cases,[18] most commonly at the pharynx and upper esophagus. This risk can be decreased by ensuring patient cooperation and avoiding forceful insertion of the endoscope. Perforation of a viscus related to PEG placement is also a rare complication. Transillumination, direct palpation, and the safe tract technique can decrease, but not completely eliminate, the risk of unintentionally puncturing a viscus during PEG placement.

Hemorrhage is an uncommon complication after PEG placement. Massive bleeding requires an emergent operative intervention, but most cases can be managed conservatively. Gastric puncture and dilation may lead to hemorrhage of the gastric wall at the site of PEG insertion. In addition, introduction of the PEG through the mouth, especially in the setting of oropharyngeal or esophageal cancers, may cause mucosal lacerations with resultant hemorrhage. Upper endoscopy may be helpful in identification and treatment of bleeding after PEG placement.

Cardiopulmonary abnormalities are not uncommon during upper endoscopy and PEG placement, although the incidence of severe complications of this type is rare. Vigilant electrocardiogram and oxygen saturation monitoring of patients while they are undergoing this procedure is essential to minimize the incidence of cardiopulmonary events. As many as 10% of patients undergoing upper endoscopy experience hypoxemia with desaturation, as a result of oversedation or procedural encroachment on the airway. Most of these episodes are transient, responding to a jaw lift maneuver or to verbal direction to the patient to take a deep breath. Bradycardia and hypotension, often signs of a vasovagal reflex from gastric distention, can be treated with decompression of gastric distension or, if the patient is unresponsive to that maneuver, atropine administration.

Aspiration is a known complication of upper endoscopy. During PEG placement, this risk is potentially worsened by the predisposing condition, such as neurologic impairment or severe dysphagia, that necessitated this feeding access intervention. The supine position is preferred for PEG placement, but this position does not encourage expectoration of secretions and, thus, special attention must be paid to maintaining the patient's upper airway during PEG placement.

Benign pneumoperitoneum may be seen in up to 20% of patients undergoing routine imaging after endoscopic gastrostomy tube placement, but is often of no clinical significance.[19,20] The overall clinical appearance of the patient must be considered. If the patient has a benign abdominal examination, this condition may be watched without laparotomy. If the clinical picture is unclear, pathologic causes for pneumoperitoneum must be evaluated. This finding on routine imaging may persist for up to 5 weeks after PEG placement.

Other complications, such as parotitis, esophageal reflux, diarrhea, abdominal cramping, hyperglycemia, and essential fatty acid deficiencies, are rare. Neoplastic seeding has been reported after PEG placement for oropharyngeal and esophageal cancers and should be kept in mind in situations in which tubes are not placed for palliation. The introducer technique may offer an advantage in obviating this complication, but this has not been studied adequately to justify definitive conclusions.

SURGICAL APPROACH

Before the introduction of percutaneous techniques for gastrostomy tube placement, surgical gastrostomy was the mainstay for access to the GI tract. This procedure carries a historical significance as it was one of the earliest performed surgical interventions. Dating back to 1849, Sedillot performed the first gastrostomy, pulling the anterior gastric wall through the abdominal wall, forming a cone.[21] Amputation of the point of the cone then produced access to the stomach. This technique was complicated by external leakage, and modifications were subsequently attempted. The formation of a serosal lined channel from the anterior gastric wall to the abdominal wall became the next style of gastrostomy tube placement, exemplified by the Witzel and Stamm techniques that are still in use today. This approach decreased external drainage, but required that a gastrostomy tube be kept in place at all times to avoid tract obliteration. Another approach was the formation of a full-thickness gastric tube, most notably Depage-Janeway gastrostomy, to allow intermittent catheterization with permanent access to the stomach.

Specific Indications

However, since the introduction of endoscopic approaches, surgical gastrostomy tube placements have been reserved for patients in whom a PEG cannot be performed or is contraindicated. Specifically, this includes patients with an obstructing or nearly obstructing oropharyngeal or esophageal lesion that precludes passage of the endoscope. An open surgical approach may also be indicated in patients in whom the concern for additional structures such as colon, omentum, or liver overlying the stomach precludes percutaneous access through a blind approach, specifically in patients in whom a safe tract technique did not confirm intragastric placement. Often, patients have gastrostomy tubes placed surgically during surgical intervention for another intra-abdominal process.

Technique

There are many and varied open and laparoscopic approaches to surgically placed gastrostomy tubes. The operative approach must be carefully chosen to meet the specific needs of the patient. Specifically, 2 commonly used options exist: either formation of a serosal lined tract from the anterior gastric wall to abdominal wall through which a gastrostomy tube remains in place, or fixation of a full-thickness segment of gastric wall to the surface of the skin through which a catheter can be introduced intermittently for feeding. To exemplify these techniques, Stamm and Janeway techniques are described.

Both procedures begin similarly. Patients are positioned in the supine position in the operating room. Preoperative prophylactic antibiotics are administered. Cooperative patients may have this procedure performed under local anesthesia, but general or regional anesthesia is often needed for access to the peritoneal cavity. A small upper vertical midline or small left upper quadrant transverse incision allows access to the anterior wall of the stomach.

The Stamm technique begins with the placement of inner and outer purse-string sutures on the anterior gastric wall, and a small gastrostomy is then made inside these sutures. A balloon-type or mushroom-type catheter is then introduced through the anterior abdominal wall and through the gastrostomy. The purse-string sutures are sequentially tied, inverting the seromuscular gastric wall around the catheter. The anterior gastric wall is then secured to the posterior aspect of the abdominal wall using 4-quadrant fixation with absorbable suture. The catheter is then secured externally to the skin at the exit site, and the laparotomy site is closed in standard fashion.

The Janeway approach requires additional exposure of the stomach when compared with the Stamm technique, and thus a longer incision is required. The anterior gastric wall is elevated in the direction of the proposed tube, in either the transverse or oblique direction. A standard bowel stapler with multiple rows of staples and a contained knife is then applied to the anterior gastric wall and fired to create a full-thickness gastric tube. If a bowel stapler is not available, this technique may be performed by a hand-sewn process. The gastric tube is then brought through the rectus muscle and anterior abdominal wall. The laparotomy incision is then closed in standard fashion. The tip of the gastric tube, which resembles a diverticulum, is then amputated, and the full-thickness tube is secured to the skin in a circumferential manner using absorbable suture. Gastric decompression is maintained with a catheter until postoperative ileus resolves.

Laparoscopic approaches are available as modifications of both the Stamm and Janeway procedures. The construction of a simple gastrostomy without a mucosal lined tube is appropriate for most indications.[22] Two ports are required: one at the umbilicus for a 30° laparoscope and one in the right upper quadrant for use as a working port. An atraumatic grasper is used to elevate the anterior abdominal wall, selecting an appropriate location for gastrostomy tube placement. Four T-fasteners are then introduced through the anterior abdominal wall and through the anterior gastric wall, securing the stomach. A 1-cm skin incision is then made to allow for passage of the gastrostomy tube. A 14-gauge needle is introduced through this incision into the stomach, and a guidewire is passed into the gastric lumen. The tract is then serially dilated until the gastrostomy tube can be introduced using the Seldinger technique. The gastrostomy tube is then secured to the skin, and the laparoscopic port sites are closed in standard fashion.

Surgical jejunal access for feeding is also an alternative. Both open and laparoscopic approaches exist and are generally performed in a manner similar to that already described for gastrostomy tube placement. Similar considerations apply for the placement of open and endoscopic jejunal access, as discussed earlier.

Complications

Complications of surgically placed gastrostomy and jejunostomy tubes include wound complications, tube dislodgement, missed enterotomy, intra-abdominal leakage of feedings, aspiration, and cardiopulmonary complications. These complications are detailed in the endoscopic approach section, but apply to both the percutaneous and surgical approaches to tube placement. Specific complications related to surgical placement include incisional wound complications, bleeding, dehiscence, and hernia formation. Compared with percutaneous approaches, surgical interventions often require general anesthesia, which carries with it a low, but real morbidity. This morbidity includes, but is not limited to, allergic reactions, aspiration, cardiac arrhythmias, myocardial infarctions, loss of airway, and death.

PARENTERAL APPROACH

In patients who do not have a functional GI tract, parenteral nutrition becomes the treatment of choice to provide adequate caloric intake and hydration. This type of nutritional support should again be reserved for patients who cannot be fed using any of the approaches described earlier.

Specific Indications

Indications for parenteral support include situations in which the GI tract is unavailable or inadequate. These situations include short bowel syndrome, enterocutaneous and enteroenteral fistulas, necrotizing enterocolitis, and malabsorption syndromes such as celiac sprue, hypoproteinemia, granulomatous colitis, or regional enteritis. Additional indications include supplemental feedings for patients with cystic fibrosis, inflammatory bowel disease, chemotherapy, and hyperemesis gravidarum. Infants with intestinal atresia, gastroschisis, or omphalocele may require parenteral support until surgical repair is undertaken and enteral feeds can be started. Temporary parenteral support is needed during prolonged paralytic ileus secondary to both surgical and nonsurgical causes. It is also used for support in acute pancreatitis before enteral feedings can be started. Patients with intractable diarrhea may also benefit from temporary support while measures to diagnose and treat the diarrhea are addressed. Patients in whom enteral feeding was attempted but failed secondary to inadequate caloric intake or high gastric residuals should be considered for parenteral support.

Technique

Temporary percutaneous central lines are the mainstay for parenteral access, especially in the acute setting. These lines can be placed in the femoral, jugular, and subclavian veins, with each having advantages and disadvantages. Because of the hypertonicity of parenteral nutrition, the tip of each catheter should be positioned in the superior vena cava (SVC) or inferior vena cava so that adequate dilution can occur.

The preferred site of access when balancing all involved factors is the subclavian vein. This site carries the lowest infection risk and an overall complication rate similar to internal jugular vein access. Internal jugular vein access has been reported to have the lowest rate of placement-related complications[23] but with a slightly higher infectious risk than the subclavian position. Femoral vein lines allow for easy access to the central venous system in emergency situations, but are less desirable for access for parenteral nutrition. Femoral sites have a higher rate of associated infectious complications because of their location and contamination risk. They also carry a higher associated risk for venous thrombosis, making this location less than ideal.[24]

Ultrasound guided venipuncture is strongly recommended for all central lines. The use of ultrasound is associated with a lower incidence of placement-related complications and a higher success rate in achieving central venous access.[25,26] The use of ultrasound guidance also shortens the time required for central line insertion and offers a cost saving of greater than $300 per central line placement.[27]

In patients who require a more permanent access route for parenteral support, options beyond placement of a temporary central line include placement of a peripherally introduced central catheter, a tunneled cuffed catheter, or a completely implanted device. A peripherally introduced central catheter (PICC) is introduced into a vein in the antecubital area or upper forearm and advanced intravascularly into the SVC, allowing peripherally initiated solutions to be delivered to the central venous system. PICCs are well tolerated and easy to care for because of their location in an upper extremity. There is literature to support that PICCs may be preferable to central catheters[28,29] because of fewer mechanical complications at placement and lower costs of insertion. Lower rates of infection with PICC compared with central catheters have been reported, although the data are under debate.[30]

Tunneled, cuffed catheters, such as a Hickman, Broviac, Hohn, or Groshong, allow for longer-term use of the subclavian and internal jugular access sites. These catheters are tunneled through the subcutaneous tissue from their venous insertion sites to decrease the infectious risk of the catheter. A completely implanted device for access, such as a port, provides another alternative for longer-term central vein access. The choice between a tunneled, cuffed catheter and port depends on many factors, including patient choice, nursing staff experience, and frequency of access. In patients who require continuous or frequent access, a tunneled line may be preferable to a completely implanted device, although the supporting evidence is lacking.

The technique for all central line placements is similar, although slight modifications must be made based on anatomic location or the type of line to be placed. Selection of the site should include consideration of the factors listed earlier. Once appropriate anatomic landmarks have been identified, the vein of choice is accessed using a large-bore needle. A guidewire is passed through the needle to obtain further access to the vein. Contact between the myocardium and guidewire may lead to cardiac irritability and arrhythmias if the wire is advanced too far. Monitoring by means of telemetry should be considered in patients undergoing central line placement by inexperienced personnel. The skin is then incised to allow for passage of the catheter. Serial dilation over the guidewire is then used to enlarge the tract to allow for catheter introduction. The catheter is then introduced using the Seldinger technique and secured in place. A postprocedure chest radiograph is mandatory both to confirm catheter tip placement and to exclude complications, including pneumothorax.

Complications

Complications related to parenteral access can broadly be divided into those that are insertion related and those that occur during maintenance therapy. Insertion-related complications include arterial injury or hematoma formation at the site of catheter placement. These complications are more common when using the femoral and internal jugular approach, and have been reported in up to 10% of central lines.[31] Most injuries resolve with direct pressure but, in rare circumstances, angiography or surgery is necessary. Care must be taken during identification of landmarks to decrease the risk of inadvertent arterial injury. Routine use of ultrasound guidance in line placement has decreased this risk substantially.

Pneumothorax occurrence rates range from 2% to 5% for both the internal jugular and subclavian vein approaches.[32] If the patient is clinically stable and has a small (<15%) pneumothorax, conservative management with supplemental oxygen can be attempted. Larger pneumothoraces or unstable patients require tube thoracostomy placement. Any patient who develops subcutaneous emphysema after central line placement should be reevaluated by chest radiograph, because delayed onset (24–48 hours after the procedure) of pneumothorax has been reported.

Arrhythmias, most frequently premature ventricular contractions, are commonly seen during placement of central venous lines. The metal guidewire can cause cardiac irritability when it comes in contact with the myocardial surface of the right heart. Most arrhythmias resolve with withdrawal of the guidewire into the SVC. In rare circumstances, cardiac arrest may occur.

Air embolism is a rare but feared complication of central line placement because it may be fatal. An air embolism occurs when the negative intrathoracic pressure draws air into the central vein via an open catheter or needle. Onset of hypotension, respiratory distress, and a cogwheel murmur herald the diagnosis. If an air embolism is suspected, the patient should be placed in the left lateral decubitus position (Trendelenburg). This procedure helps trap the air in the right atrium while allowing blood to continue to flow through the outflow tract, and aspiration can then be attempted through the central venous line. Prevention is accomplished by adherence to good technique in line placement.

Additional complications of central venous line insertion include hemothorax, SVC or cardiac perforations, and cardiac tamponade. Nerve injury and development of arterial and venous pseudoaneurysms have also been reported. Thoracic duct laceration is another rare complication after central venous line insertion.

Infectious complications are a common threat associated with parenteral feeding. Infections of the catheter insertion site manifest as purulent drainage and erythema of the surrounding skin. Local wound care can reduce catheter site infection rates. Catheter-related infections occur in up to 15% of patients[33] with central venous lines and are associated with significant morbidity and mortality as well as health care costs.[34,35] Offending microbes are often skin flora (eg, *Staphylococcus epidermis* and *Staphylococcus aureus*). Line infection must be considered in any patient who develops fever, hyperglycemia, or leukocystosis. In this setting, the catheter should be removed and the catheter tip sent for bacterial and fungal culture. In patients with documented positive blood cultures or in patients with catheter cultures revealing more than 15 colony-forming units, the catheter should be removed and a line holiday attempted with peripheral access. A new central venous catheter can then be inserted at a separate site once bacteremia has resolved.

Prevention of infection can be accomplished by meticulous care both at the time of insertion and each time the line is accessed for therapy to maintain sterile technique and avoid introduction of contamination.[36] Maximal barrier precautions have been shown in randomized series to decrease infectious complications.[37] The location of the central venous catheter also affects infectious risk, with the subclavian vein having the lowest rate and the femoral vein the highest. The use of chlorhexidine for cutaneous antisepsis has been shown to decrease catheter infection and catheter-related bacteremia when compared with iodine and alcohol preparations.[38] Routine exchange of central venous catheters is not recommended because it has not been shown to decrease infectious complications. The use of multilumen catheters may be associated with a slight increase in infectious risk. The impact of greater manipulation and increased use of the catheter for nonfeeding interventions may confound these results.

Catheter occlusion usually presents as increased resistance to infusion or inability to aspirate blood. Common causes include kinking of the catheter or intraluminal obstruction. Adequate line care, including secure positioning and routine flushing of the catheter, may decrease this risk. Instillation of thrombolytic agents into the catheter may help salvage a clotted catheter.

Central venous thrombosis may be increased at the site of central catheters because of damage to the intima of the vessel. Catheter-related thrombosis may also predispose to the formation of venous stricture. For subclavian lines, this may present as a spectrum ranging from asymptomatic neck vein distension to severe SVC syndrome. Patients who develop venous congestion or swelling associated with a central catheter should have the line removed. In patients requiring hemodialysis, the risk of venous stricturing must be considered in the choice of access site to avoid any potential negative interaction with the hemodialysis access.

SUMMARY

Nutritional support of patients who are critically ill or undergoing elective surgical intervention has been well documented in the literature. Common indications for enteral access include neurologic injury, trauma-induced dysphagia, and neoplastic processes. In patients who have a functioning GI tract, enteral access is the preferred means through which to provide alimentation. Endoscopic options for enteral access include PEG, percutaneous endoscopic gastrojejunostomy (PEG-J), and PEJ, with multiple variations for placement. Surgical approaches are reserved for patients undergoing concomitant intra-abdominal surgery or for those who are not candidates for an endoscopic approach. In patients who have contraindications to enteral support, parenteral support provides needed nutrition, but carries risks from access insertion and infectious complications. In evaluating a patient for nutritional support, the specific needs of the patients must be considered in choosing the best treatment pathway. Having knowledge of available options and understanding of the risk and benefits of each allows a practitioner to offer the most effective, customized access for nutritional support.

REFERENCES

1. DeLegge M. Enteral access–the foundation of feeding. JPEN J Parenter Enteral Nutr 2001;25:58.
2. Mazaki T, Ebisawa K. Enteral versus parenteral nutrition after gastrointestinal surgery: a systematic review and meta-analysis of randomized controlled trials in the English literature. J Gastrointest Surg 2008;12(4):739–55.
3. Braunschweig C, Levy P, Sheean P, et al. Enteral compared with parenteral nutrition: a meta-analysis. Am J Clin Nutr 2001;74:534.
4. Moore FA, Feliciano DV, Andrassy RJ, et al. Early enteral feeding, compared with parenteral, reduces postoperative septic complications. The results of a meta-analysis. Ann Surg 1992;216(2):172–83.
5. Bozzetti F, Braga M, Gavazzi C, et al. Postoperative enteral versus parenteral nutrition in malnourished patients with gastrointestinal cancer: a randomised multicentre trial. Lancet 2001;358:1487.

6. George D, Falk P, Umberto Meduri G, et al. Nosocomial sinusitis in patients in the medical intensive care unit: a prospective epidemiological study. Clin Infect Dis 1998;27(3):463–70.
7. Gauderer M, Ponsky J, Izant R Jr. Gastrostomy without laparotomy: a percutaneous endoscopic technique. J Pediatr Surg 1980;15:872–5.
8. Russell T, Brotman M, Norris F. Percutaneous endoscopic gastrostomy: a new simplified and cost effective technique. Am J Surg 1984;148:132–7.
9. Arrowsmith J, Gertsman B, Fleischer D, et al. Results from the American Society for Gastrointestinal Endoscopy/US Food and Drug Administration collaborative study on complication rates and drug use during gastrointestinal endoscopy. Gastrointest Endosc 1991;37:421–7.
10. Holzman R, Cullen D, Eichhorn J, et al. Guidelines for sedation by nonanesthesiologists during diagnostic and therapeutic procedures. J Clin Anesth 1994;6:265–76.
11. Jane P. Technique of upper gastrointestinal endoscopy. Gastrointest Endosc Clin N Am 1994;4:501–21.
12. Foutch P, Talbert G, Waring J, et al. Percutaneous endoscopic gastrostomy in patients with prior abdominal surgery: virtues of the safe tract. Am J Gastroenterol 1988;83:147–50.
13. Sartori S, Trevisani L, Nielsen I, et al. Percutaneous endoscopic gastrostomy placement using the pull-through or push-through techniques: is the second pass of the gastroscope necessary? Endoscopy 1996;28(8):686–8.
14. Cappell M. Risk factors and risk reduction of malignant seeding of the percutaneous endoscopic gastrostomy track from pharyngoesophageal malignancy: a review of all 44 known reported cases. Am J Gastroenterol 2007;102(6):1307–11.
15. Sabnis A, Liu R, Chand B, et al. SLiC technique. A novel approach to percutaneous gastrostomy. Surg Endosc 2006;20(2):256–62.
16. Kadakia S, O'Sullivan H, Starnes E, et al. Percutaneous endoscopic gastrostomy or jejunostomy and the incidence of aspiration in 79 patients. Am J Surg 1992;164:114–7.
17. Pofahl W, Ringold F. Management of early dislodgment of percutaneous endoscopic gastrostomy tubes. Surg Laparosc Endosc Percutan Tech 1999;9(4):253–6.
18. Bhatia N, Collins J, Nguyen C, et al. Esophageal perforation as a complication of esophagogastroduodenoscopy. J Hosp Med 2008;3(3):256–62.
19. Wiesen A, Sideridis K, Fernandes A, et al. True incidence and clinical significance of pneumoperitoneum after PEG placement: a prospective study. Gastrointest Endosc 2006;64(6):886–9.
20. Blum C, Selander C, Ruddy J, et al. The incidence and clinical significance of pneumoperitoneum after percutaneous endoscopic gastrostomy: a review of 722 cases. Am Surg 2009;75(1):39–43.
21. Gauderer M, Stellato T. Gastrostomies: evolution, techniques, indications, and complications. Curr Probl Surg 1986;23(9):657–719.
22. Duh Q, Way L. Laparoscopic gastrostomy using T-fasteners as retractors and anchors. Surg Endosc 1993;7:60–3.
23. Macdonald S, Watt A, McNally D, et al. Comparison of technical success and outcomes of tunneled catheters inserted via the jugular and subclavian approaches. J Vasc Interv Radiol 2000;11:225–31.
24. Merrer J, DeJonghe B, Golliot F, et al. Complications of femoral and subclavian venous catheterization in critically ill patients: a randomized, controlled trial. JAMA 2001;286(6):700–7.

25. Keenan S. Use of ultrasound to place central lines. J Crit Care 2002;17(2): 126–37.
26. Hind D, Calvert N, McWilliams R, et al. Ultrasonic locating devices for central venous cannulation: meta-analysis. BMJ 2003;327(7411):361.
27. Calvert N, Hind D, McWilliams R, et al. Ultrasound for central venous cannulation: economic evaluation of cost-effectiveness. Anaesthesia 2004;59(11):1116–20.
28. Raad I, Davis S, Becker M, et al. Low infection rate and long durability of nontunneled silastic catheters. A safe cost effective alternative for long-term venous access. Arch Intern Med 1993;153:1791–6.
29. Ryder M. Peripheral access options. Surg Oncol Clin N Am 1995;4:395–427.
30. Safdar N, Maki D. Risk of catheter-related bloodstream infection with peripherally inserted central venous catheters used in hospitalized patients. Chest 2005;128: 489–95.
31. Ruesch S, Walder B, Tramer M. Complications of central venous catheters: internal jugular versus subclavian access–a systematic review. Crit Care Med 2002;30(2):454–60.
32. Giacomini M, Iapichino G, Armani S, et al. How to avoid and manage a pneumothorax. J Vasc Access 2006;7(1):7–14.
33. Lorente L, Henry C, Martín M, et al. Central venous catheter-related infection in a prospective and observational study of 2,595 catheters. Crit Care 2005;9(6): R631–5.
34. Kohn L, Corrigan J, Donaldson M, editors. To err is human: building a safer health system. Committee on Quality of Health Care in America. Institute of Medicine. Washington, DC: National Academy Press; 2000.
35. Veenstra D, Saint S, Sullivan S. Cost-effectiveness of antiseptic-impregnated central venous catheters for the prevention of catheter-related bloodstream infection. JAMA 1999;282:554.
36. O'Grady N, Alexander M, Dellinger E, et al. Guidelines for the prevention of intravascular catheter-related infections. Am J Infect Control 2002;30:476.
37. Raad I, Hohn D, Gilbreath B, et al. Prevention of central venous catheter-related infections by using maximal sterile barrier precautions during insertion. Infect Control Hosp Epidemiol 1994;15:231.
38. Maki D, Ringer M, Alvarado C. Prospective randomized trial of povidone-iodine, alcohol, and chlorhexidine for prevention of infection associated with central venous and arterial catheters. Lancet 1991;338:339.

Home Parenteral Nutrition Support for Intestinal Failure

Kristen M. Rhoda, RD[a], Sree Suryadevara, MD[b],
Ezra Steiger, MD[a,c],*

KEYWORDS

- Home parenteral nutrition • Adults • Vascular access device
- Intestinal transplantation

A successful technique of parenteral nutrition (PN) was developed by Dudrick[1] at the University of Pennsylvania in the 1960s. It has been used in a variety of clinical conditions to maintain a patient's nutritional status, allowing for time to heal or for the patient to tolerate surgical or medical therapeutic interventions. It was adapted for use in the home or outpatient settings for patients with various conditions that interfered with absorption of nutrients needed to maintain adequate nutrition and return to a near-normal lifestyle.

Initiation of home parenteral nutrition (HPN) is typically done in the hospital setting by clinicians specializing in nutrition support. In some facilities, comprehensive nutrition support teams (NSTs) have evolved that include dietitians, pharmacists, nurses, and physicians who assess the patient's nutritional status, prescribe the PN solution, and determine the appropriate vascular access device (VAD). It is the goal of the home NST (HNST) to assist in transferring PN management from the hospital to the outpatient setting with the assistance of homecare agencies.

Homecare services have evolved over the past 30 years allowing the provision of parenteral nutrients in the home setting. Ideally, HPN is managed by the HNST in conjunction with the homecare services to keep patients well nourished and hydrated in their homes.

The authors have nothing to disclose.
[a] Intestinal Rehabilitation and Transplant, Digestive Disease Institute, Cleveland Clinic, 9500 Euclid Avenue/A100, Cleveland, OH 44195, USA
[b] Nutrition Support Team, Digestive Disease Institute, Cleveland Clinic, 9500 Euclid Avenue/A100, Cleveland, OH 44195, USA
[c] Cleveland Clinic Lerner College of Medicine of Case Western Reserve University, Cleveland Clinic, 9500 Euclid Avenue/A100, Cleveland, OH 44195, USA
* Corresponding author. Cleveland Clinic Lerner College of Medicine of Case Western Reserve University, Cleveland Clinic, 9500 Euclid Avenue/A100, Cleveland, OH 44195.
E-mail address: steigee@ccf.org

Surg Clin N Am 91 (2011) 913–932
doi:10.1016/j.suc.2011.04.010
0039-6109/11/$ – see front matter © 2011 Elsevier Inc. All rights reserved.

INDICATIONS FOR HOME PN

Medical and surgical teams requesting HPN are referred to the NST staff physician to determine the appropriateness of the therapy. HPN is indicated for patients with intestinal failure (IF) extending beyond the hospital stay. IF is defined as a loss of absorptive capacity secondary to obstruction, dysmotility, surgical resection, congenital defect, or mucosal disease resulting in chronic diarrhea, dehydration, electrolyte abnormalities, micronutrient imbalance, and malnutrition.[2]

Conditions that can lead to long-term IF (>90 days) that are commonly accepted as indications for HPN are listed below.[3]

1. Short bowel syndrome
2. Inflammatory bowel disease
3. Bowel ischemia
4. Radiation enteritis
5. High-output gastrointestinal fistulae
6. Hyperemesis gravidarum
7. Nonterminal cancer
8. Motility disorders
9. Bowel obstruction
10. Severe pancreatitis
11. Protein-losing enteropathy.

These conditions can lead to IF ranging from weeks to years with some patients suffering from permanent IF. It is common to use HPN as a short-term treatment ($\leq$ six weeks) for patients who are severely malnourished with IF before a surgical intervention if the insurance provider will agree to coverage. In all cases, the NST should establish a care plan before hospital discharge to ensure that the patient is knowledgeable in managing the therapy and understands the risks before implementation. This care plan includes identifying the indication for HPN, length of therapy, and the end point or goals of therapy.

Once the care plan has been established, a thorough evaluation process by the multidisciplinary NST should ensue. This process is typically initiated by reviewing insurance coverage, establishing homecare needs, starting the education process, placing the appropriate VAD, stabilizing the PN formula, and evaluating the home environment. Electricity, adequate refrigeration, telephone availability, running water, and a sanitary and safe living environment are necessary to provide proper care for a HPN patient.[4]

EVALUATING INSURANCE COVERAGE AND HOMECARE SERVICES

Evaluating candidates for homecare and insurance coverage is best facilitated by a discharge coordinator (case manager and/or social worker) who is knowledgeable in HPN. In 1992, it was reported that direct costs associated with HPN were as high at $140,000 per year, with Medicare patients being responsible for up to 20% of these costs, if the patient has no secondary insurance coverage.[5] Because of the high cost of the therapy, the discharge coordinator must determine the patient's eligibility for reimbursement and provide the necessary documentation as needed.

Private insurers provide coverage based on the employer's overall company plans. Typically, HPN is a reimbursable therapy, as private insurers tend to follow Center for Medicare Service (CMS) criteria.

CMS requires documentation that the condition causing the need for HPN is of long and indefinite duration, defined as 90 days or a lifetime, as judged to the best of the attending physician's ability.[6] Coverage eligibility often requires IF to be documented as one of the following: a massive small bowel resection (>5 feet), short bowel syndrome with significant enteral losses (>50% intake), the need for bowel rest, significant weight loss ($\geq$10% with an albumin $\leq$3.4) with fat malabsorption and/or dysmotility, and failed enteral nutrition (EN).[6] Documentation of weight and strength, together with the patient's corresponding overall health status, must prove that intravenous nutrition is required because use of all other approaches (ie, enteral trial, pharmacologic means) has failed.[3]

Once insurance coverage is documented, the discharge planner working with the patient identifies a homecare infusion pharmacy and nursing agency for each patient requiring HPN before hospital discharge. The collaboration of homecare services with the HPN clinician promotes effective patient care in the home by coordinating nursing care, supply delivery, and preparation of the PN solution. Although this process is largely insurance-driven, selecting the best agency can provide these patients with a smooth transition from hospital to home.[7]

PSYCHOSOCIAL EVALUATION AND PATIENT EDUCATION

It is known that psychological concerns arise in patients with inflammatory bowel disorders and anatomic loss of small bowel such as grief, depression, drug dependency, and body image issues[8]; and that depression has been deemed the most prominent psychological disturbance in HPN patients.[9] Identification of psychosocial issues in the hospital can virtually eliminate patients being discharged unsafely home from the hospital. The NST nurse and social worker can identify these issues during their assessment by the use of a mini-mental examination[10] that assesses cognitive skills and identifies major mental, psychiatric, or depression disorders.[11] The NST nurse or social worker, or a psychiatrist, can then work with the patient and assess the patient's ability to cope with both the HPN therapy and the underlying disease.

Once the patient is cleared from a psychosocial aspect, the NST nurse begins the education process by discussing the management of HPN and the expectations of the primary caregiver. The nurse provides education and training on the care of the VAD, maintaining intake and output records, and the use of the infusion pump with the goal of achieving patient autonomy. It is recommended that patient education should be initiated in the hospital and continued in the home setting.[12] Home infusion pumps and catheter supplies differ from the equipment used in the hospital; therefore, providing hands-on education together with written and/or video materials is required to reduce complications in HPN patients.[13]

VAD

Selection and maintenance of the VAD is essential to optimal management of the HPN patient to prevent rehospitalizations and potential catheter-associated deaths. VADs used for HPN can be categorized into three groups: tunneled central venous catheters, peripherally inserted central catheters (PICCs), and implanted ports. Each has distinct advantages and disadvantages (**Table 1**). Selection of the VAD depends on patient preference, length of planned therapy, venous anatomy, body habitus, and the skill of the clinician placing the catheter.

Tunneled catheters, such as Hickman or Broviac catheters, are placed under the skin with the external lumen typically located on the chest wall. These catheters are constructed with a subcutaneously positioned Dacron cuff to anchor the catheter in place. This cuff reduces the migration of microorganisms from the exit site, resulting in fewer catheter-related blood stream infections (CRBSIs).[14] Tunneled catheters

Table 1
Characteristics of central catheters used for HPN

Catheter Type	Placement	Comments
Tunneled cuffed catheters Peripherally inserted central catheter (PICC)-nontunneled Implanted ports	Percutaneous placement via subclavian, internal jugular or femoral vein Percutaneous placement via peripheral vein Percutaneous placement via subclavian, internal jugular or femoral vein A subcutaneous pocket required	Cuff inhibits migration of organisms into catheter tract; lower rate of infection than nontunneled CVC. Long term usage, home care, self care easy Lower rate of infection than nontunneled CVCs. Used in acute and home care for therapy ranging from weeks to months Lowest risk for CRBSI; no need for local catheter-site care. For long-term therapy, but required weekly recannulation

Abbreviations: CRBSI, catheter-related blood stream infection; CVC, central venous catheter.
Adapted from Centers for Disease Control and Prevention. Guidelines for the prevention of intravascular catheter-related infections. MMWR Recomm Rep 2002;51(RR-10):1–29.

are advantageous due to ease of self-care and repair, the capacity for multiple usable lumens, and the simplicity for placement and removal. Infection rates with tunneled catheters vary depending on the site of placement, with femoral sites being more prone to infection compared with nonfemoral sites.[15–17]

Implanted ports are silicone rubber VADs within a titanium disk that is placed under the skin. The complexity of placement and removal is a disadvantage compared with other VADs, as it requires surgical creation of a subcutaneous pocket. Younger patients tend to prefer a port as it provides minimal alteration of body image, but the discomfort associated with frequent percutaneous needle cannulation of the port continues to discourage others.

PICCs are most commonly used as short-term catheters (<3 months) that are inserted into the basilic, brachial, or cephalic vein on the forearm and advanced until the tip is in the lower third of the superior vena cava (SVC). The PICC exit site makes it difficult for patients to achieve autonomy, as catheter care is difficult to manage with one unencumbered hand. PICCs are also associated with a higher incidence of catheter dislodgement, thrombotic complications, and CRBSIs, when compared with tunneled catheters and implanted ports.[16,18–20] However, the ease of placement and minimal cost associated with PICC lines has enhanced their use in the hospital and home setting for PN.

VAD CARE

Appropriate care of the VADs includes hand hygiene by the use of antibacterial soap and/or a waterless, alcohol-based solution.[17] Impeccable hand hygiene, as well as a clean surface area treated with 70% alcohol solution to complete the HPN procedures, is needed before handling the VAD. Dressings should be changed at least weekly with the use of either a transparent, semipermeable, or gauze dressing.[17] Chlorhexidine-impregnated sponges that lie under the dressing covering the catheter insertion or exit site have shown promising results in reducing infection in short-term catheters, but comparable data are lacking for long-term catheters.[21]

VAD Lock Solutions

Historically, a VAD is flushed before and after each use with saline and/or heparin in an effort to maintain patency, prevent phlebitis, and extend the use of the VAD. With efforts to reduce the incidence of CRBSIs, the approach of using antibiotic lock therapy (ALT) was introduced in the 1980s. The concern over the use of ALT is the development of more virulent microorganisms as well as antibiotic resistance.[22] The use of ethanol lock therapy (ELT) has generated recent interest in preventing CRBSIs. A retrospective chart review and case report[23,24] supports the use of ELT in HPN patients, but the lack of large, randomized, controlled trials prevents many insurance companies from providing reimbursement for this therapy.

HPN SOLUTIONS

In the hospital setting, as VAD selection and education are underway, the NST determines the appropriate PN solution to meet nutrition, fluid, and electrolyte goals. Macronutrient and fluid requirements are established during the hospital stay to meet patient-specific goals (ie, weight gain or stabilization, fistula closure, and healing). Kilocalorie requirements are based on the patient's weight and body mass index. For obese patients, 10 to 20 kcals/kg/day of actual body weight is used, whereas patients requiring weight stabilization may require 20 to 35 kcals/kg/day.[25] When weight gain is the goal, patients may initially require up to 42 kcals/kg/day.[26] A minimum amount of lipid kilocalories must be provided to prevent essential fatty acid deficiency (EFAD). Fluid requirements are calculated to ensure adequate urine output ($\geq$1000 cc/day) while replacing all gastrointestinal and insensible losses. Of note, most PN bags can hold up to 4.5 L of fluid daily; therefore, with excessive gastrointestinal losses, additional intravenous fluids to supplement the PN solution may be necessary. Calculation of these requirements is discussed in Langley's review of fluid, electrolytes and acid-base disorders.[27]

A multivitamin preparation is added daily to prevent vitamin deficiencies. During the 1997 parenteral vitamin shortage, patients receiving a multivitamin dose fewer than three times per week developed vitamin deficiencies.[28] Other than this occurrence, there are few reports of vitamin deficiencies in HPN patients. The current multivitamin preparation (**Table 2**) is of concern to some expert scientists in the field, as recent findings suggest new metabolic functions for several vitamins (C, D, E, and K) that may constitute a need for increased amounts of these nutrients in the multivitamin preparation.[29] Continued research on vitamin status and dosing is needed in the long-term HPN patient.

Current trace element recommendations are to provide a multiple trace element (MTE) solution daily to PN solutions. Adult MTEs contain varying concentrations of zinc, chromium, manganese, copper, and selenium (**Table 3**) and are provided in an attempt to prevent the development of micronutrient deficiencies in long-term HPN patients. Recommended quantities have changed over time,[29] but the US Food and Drug Administration (FDA) has not updated their recommendations for these nutrients since 1979. Discussion of the need to reduce copper, manganese, and chromium levels in the MTE solutions developed after the 2007 study by Howard and colleagues[30] discovered significant concentrations of these nutrients in autopsy tissues. It is known that conditions, such as cholestasis and renal dysfunction, limit the excretion of copper and manganese, respectively; Therefore, they are not needed in the same quantities as other patients. Trace element levels should be monitored every 6 months (**Table 4**) in long-term HPN patients. Signs and symptoms of trace element deficiency include alopecia and skin rash (zinc), anemia (copper),

Table 2
Adult multivitamin MVI solution

Product	Volume	A (IU)	E (mg)	D (IU)	K (mcg)	B1 (mg)	B2 (mg)	B3 (mg)	B5 (mg)	B6 (mg)	B12 (mcg)	C (mg)	Biotin (mcg)	Folic Acid (mcg)
MVI-12 Injection (Hospira)	5 mL	3300	10	200	0	6	3.6	40	15	6	5	200	60	600
MVI-Adult Injection (Hospira)	5 mL	3300	10	200	150	6	3.6	40	15	6	5	200	60	600
Infuvite Adult (Baxter)	10 mL	3300	10	200	150	6	3.6	40	15	6	5	200	60	600

Abbreviation: MVI, multivitamin.

Table 3
Adult MTE solutions per ml

Product	Chromium	Copper	Manganese	Selenium	Zinc
MTE-5 (American Regent)	4	0.4	0.1	20	1
MTE-5 Concentrated (American Regent)	10	1	0.5	60	5
4 Trace Elements (Hospira)	6	0.42	0.37	0	1.67
MTE-4 (American Regent)	4	0.4	0.1	0	1
MTE-4 Concentrated (American Regent)	10	1	0.5	0	5

Abbreviation: MTE, multiple trace element.

cardiomyopathy (selenium), and glucose intolerance (chromium). Manganese levels are often elevated and may be associated with abnormalities of the central nervous system (ie, ataxia, hyperirritability), and manganese may have to be deleted from trace element additives.

PN solution macronutrients can be formulated in two ways: 3-in-1 or 2-in-1. A 3-in-1 solution contains dextrose, amino acids, and lipid compounded as a total nutrient admixture. These solutions are advantageous for patients requiring reduced dextrose concentrations due to abnormal glucose metabolism as seen in inflammatory conditions and diabetes mellitus. A disadvantage in limiting carbohydrate kilocalories lies in the difficulty meeting estimated kilocalorie needs without providing excess lipid kilocalories. Providing intravenous fat emulsion (IVFE) greater than 3 g/kg has been associated with the development of liver disease in HPN patients.[31] Providing a 2-in-1 solution containing only dextrose and amino acids may be superior to 3-in-1 solutions, in part, for this reason. Patients receiving a 2-in-1 solution must consume and absorb adequate dietary fat to prevent the development of EFAD. Because severe malabsorption is common in HPN patients, it may be necessary to provide as much as 500 mL of 20% IVFE weekly to prevent EFAD (100 g/lipid/wk).

IVFE is sensitive to changes in pH, which results in destabilization or "cracking" of the fat emulsion in some 3-in-1 solutions. Destabilization of 3-in-1 solutions is seen with high concentrations of divalent cations (Mg^{2+} and Ca^{2+}) and the presence of any trivalent cations (Fe^{3+}). Therefore, the sum of divalent cations must be less than 21 mEq/l, and iron should not be added to 3-in-1 solutions.

Reduction of calcium phosphate precipitants is important to prevent microvascular pulmonary emboli. The pH, macronutrient concentration, mixing temperature, and calcium phosphate concentration (<200 mg/dL) have all been shown to influence the compatibility of calcium and phosphorus. The FDA mandated the use of PN filtration systems in 1994, which led to the use of in-line filters to prevent the infusion of unwanted particulates. Currently, 1.2 micron filters are used with 3-in-1 solutions and 0.22 micron filters are used with 2-in-1 solutions. Refer to **Table 5** for stability and compatibility guidelines.

SPECIALIZED PRODUCTS

With continued research on intestinal failure, new components of HPN solutions have been found to have potential in reducing the development of long-term complications of HPN. Glutamine is an amino acid that is the preferred energy source for enterocytes. It is essential in times of metabolic stress for maintaining muscle mass and immune function. The route of administration affects the elicited response.

Table 4
Monitoring schedule for HPN patients

Component	Baseline	Daily	Weekly	Monthly	3–6 Months
Intake/Output, Temperature, and Weight	Yes	Yes	—	—	—
Urinary and Blood Glucose Measurements	Yes	Yes	—	—	—
Check Central Line	Yes	Yes	No	No	No
Electrolytes, Blood Urea Nitrogen, and Creatinine	Yes	Yes, progress to next level if stable	Yes	Yes	—
Calcium, Magnesium, and Phosphorus	Yes	Yes, progress to next level if stable	Yes	Yes	—
Albumin or Prealbumin	Yes	Yes, progress to next level if stable	Yes	Yes	—
Liver enzymes, ALP, Aspartate Aminotransferase, Alanine Aminotransferase, and Bilirubin	Yes	Yes, progress to next level if stable	Yes	Yes	—
Prothrombin Time and International Normalized Ratio	Yes	—	—	—	—
Trace Elements	Yes	No	No	No	Yes
Vitamins	As indicated	—	—	—	—
Anthropometrics and Functional Status	Yes	—	—	Yes	Yes

Abbreviation: ALP, alkaline phosphatase.
Data from Shatnawei A, Parekh N, Rhoda K. Intestinal failure management at the Cleveland Clinic. Arch Surg 2010;145:521–7.

Table 5
Compatibility guidelines for 3-in-1 PN solutions

Macronutrients Per Liter	Micronutrients
Standard Amino Acids[a] 20–60 g	The product of mEq/l of calcium and phosphorus must not exceed 200
Lipid 23–67 g	The product of mEq/l of magnesium and calcium must not exceed 20 mEq/L
Dextrose 35–253 g	IV iron is not compatible at any concentration

For 2-in-1 solutions, the product of mEq/l of calcium and phosphorus must not exceed 200.
[a] Essential amino acid solutions (ie, Nephramine) cannot be mixed with lipid emulsions unless this is done in conjunction with standard amino acids.
Data from Lennon E, Speerhas R. Estimating nutritional requirements. In: Parekh N, DeChicco R, editors. Cleveland clinic nutrition support handbook. Cleveland (OH); 2004. p. 34–60.

Intravenous glutamine increases crypt depth and villous height in the gastrointestinal tract, ultimately improving its absorptive capabilities. These changes were not found when glutamine was given orally.[32] Unfortunately, glutamine is not a component of crystalline amino acid solutions and is not readily available as an additive to PN due to its instability in PN mixtures.

Carnitine is synthesized from lysine and methionine and is an amino acid necessary for oxidation of long-chain fatty acids in the liver. The level of plasma carnitine has been described to drop within weeks of PN initiation and remains low in long-term PN patients.[33–35] Deficiency has been linked to the development of hepatic steatosis,[35] but supplementation has not been found to improve these biochemical markers of carnitine deficiency. Therefore, carnitine is not routinely supplemented in HPN solutions. Carnitine, in the form of Carnitor, is compatible with PN solutions, and can be given intravenously in patients experiencing clinical symptoms (ie, muscular weakness, lethargy) with a low-serum carnitine level, although optimal doses are not yet established.[35]

Lipid emulsions available in the United States are soybean oil-based products containing phytosterols and ω-6 polyunsaturated fatty acids, which have been linked to the development of PN-associated liver disease (PNALD) and cholestasis, immune dysfunction, altered pulmonary gas exchange, and hypertriglyceridemia. The ω-6 fatty acids are considered proinflammatory in nature and, therefore, not only enhance the inflammatory response through their immunosuppressive effect,[36] but may worsen hepatic function.[37–39] Although alternative lipid emulsions are manufactured (ie, fish oil, olive, medium chain triglycerides), soybean oil-based emulsions are the only emulsions available in the United States. Fish oil-based lipid emulsions have been available for compassionate use through Children's Hospital Boston for pediatric patients with PNALD. Several reports suggest the ability to reverse liver damage after substituting a fish oil-based emulsion for a soybean oil-based emulsion.[40–43] More research is needed in this area to determine appropriate use of alternative lipid emulsions for preventing PNALD and EFAD.

INFUSION RATES, CYCLING AND TAPERS

Once the PN solution is infusing continuously and the water volume and dextrose load are tolerated over 24 hours, the solution is cycled to a goal of a 12-hour overnight infusion. Cycling not only improves patient quality of life by providing daytime freedom from the intravenous (IV) infusion, but is beneficial for preventing hepatobiliary compli-cations by increasing the mobilization of hepatic fat stores and fatty acid oxidation during the off-cycle.[44]

Transitioning the PN solution from a continuous infusion to a 12-hour infusion can take 24 hours to several days, depending on the complications that arise during the cycling process. Common cycling complications include glucose intolerance and fluid retention. Improvements in glucose tolerance can be seen when tapering the infusion rates at the start and completion of the cycle. Increasing the number of infusion hours may be necessary if glucose homeostasis and euvolemia cannot be obtained on a 12-hour infusion cycle.

PATIENT MONITORING

Monitoring and management of the HPN patient should be coordinated between the HNST, homecare agencies, and the patient. Diligent follow-up is essential to ensure a successful course of therapy and to minimize complications associated with HPN. The American Society for Parenteral and Enteral Nutrition has developed standards for monitoring HPN that include frequent laboratory testing, clinic follow-up to assess the VAD and potential nutrient deficiencies, and patient self-monitoring.[45,46] Moni-toring parameters (see **Table 4**) are established to reach the patient's nutritional goals safely while avoiding metabolic complications.

Ideally, HPN patients should be sufficiently stable at the time of discharge to require initial laboratory testing on a weekly basis and less frequent laboratory testing over time as the therapy progresses. Patients take an active role in their care by recording their daily intake and output, body temperature, weight, and urinary and/or blood glucose to allow for early recognition and treatment of dehydration, infection, and glucose intolerance.[46] Other studies such as a dual-energy x-ray absorptiometry (DXA) to monitor for metabolic bone disease, and determinations of trace elements and essential fatty acids are required less frequently.

Multiple outpatient clinic visits are usually required within the first month after hospital discharge, and then later at established, less frequent periodic intervals, based on the satisfactory progression of the nutritional goals. A physical examination is completed as well as an assessment of the patients VAD at each visit. For patients on long-term HPN (≥6 months), a review of potential long-term HPN complications are also addressed. Between outpatient clinic visits, the homecare nurse and the patient continue to communicate, 24 hours a day, with the HNST when problems arise, to reduce the development and severity of complications.

CATHETER COMPLICATIONS

Catheter complications can be related to infection, mechanical dysfunction, or occlu-sion. Selecting the appropriate VAD and educating the patient regarding its use and maintenance is essential for reducing the incidence of catheter-related complications.

Infectious Complications

Infectious complications have been linked to the material of the catheter, the insertion site, and the number of catheter lumens, and can be local (the insertion or exit site, or along the tunnel) or systemic (within the catheter hub or lumen).

Infectious complications are more frequent for catheters placed in femoral sites versus a subclavian site, as the density and virulence of the skin flora is higher at the femoral sites. Furthermore, studies have shown femoral catheters to be more susceptible to infections compared with nonfemoral sites.[15–17] When compared with multiple-lumen VADs, single-lumen VADs have shown to have a greater risk of developing a CRBSI and, therefore, the number of catheter lumens should be minimized to absolute needs.[47]

Local infections can occur at the exit or insertion site or along the subcutaneous tunnel or pocket. Diagnosis is based on the presence of erythema or induration within 2 cm of the catheter exit site or along the tunnel without the presence of a CRBSI.[48] Patients' typical complaints include erythema, tenderness, swelling, and purulent drainage. Exit or insertion site infections can usually be managed with oral antibiotics and/or topical antibiotic ointment without having to remove the catheter. If the infection involves the cuff or the tunnel, the catheter should be removed. PICCs should always be removed in the presence of a local or systemic infection.

Systemic infections are diagnosed by quantitative blood cultures drawn through the VAD and a peripheral vein. Positive quantitative blood cultures occur when colony counts via the catheter are at least three times greater than those derived from the peripheral blood. Differential time to positivity compares the time to positive culture from peripheral blood with that from the catheter, and can help to establish the presence of a CRBSI.[49] If the catheter is removed, quantitative cultures should be performed on the distal tip and the tunneled or subcutaneous segment to confirm the diagnosis of a CRBSI. Typical symptoms include fever (especially at the onset of the PN infusion), shaking chills, nausea, and generalized malaise. The most common CRBSIs are caused by gram-positive organisms, including coagulase negative staphylococci and *Staphylococcus aureus*. Treatment obviously varies, depending on the organism identified. **Table 6** shows the management approach for most common CRBSIs.

Mechanical Complications

Mechanical complications are related to catheter malposition and/or fracture. Catheter malpositioning occurs when the tip of the VAD migrates away from the cavoatrial junction. Exposure of the Dacron cuff or external elongation of a PICC line can indicate that the VAD has become malpositioned. Patients may complain of pain or discomfort in the neck or shoulder region, or chest swelling or pain related to the PN infusion.[50] Radiologic confirmation of the catheter tip location is recommended, as a malpositioned catheter can erode and perforate the vein, allowing the PN solution to be infused into the pleural or pericardial space.

A VAD may rupture or split, causing blood and/or PN solution to leak out of the lumen of the catheter, and this increases the risk of an air embolism as well as contamination of the inner lumen. The catheter is clamped between the rupture and the patient's skin surface if possible until the catheter can be repaired or replaced.

Obstructive Complications

Obstructive complications can be thrombotic or nonthrombotic in nature. Thrombotic complications have been described resulting from vessel wall damage, blood flow changes, and a systemic alteration in coagulation, and have been associated at times with catheter tip malposition.[51] Catheters positioned with the tip at the cavoatrial junction have a reduced incidence of venous thrombosis, including the development of SVC syndrome.[19,52] SVC syndrome is a serious thrombotic complication that can result in permanent loss of upper torso vascular access. Clinical signs of a central venous thrombosis, including SVC syndrome, can be manifested by prominent chest wall venous collaterals, shortness of breath, arm or facial edema, and axillary tenderness.

Table 6
Management approach for CRBSIs

Organism	Clinical Presentation	Recommendation
All Organisms	1. Tunnel infection or port pocket infection 2. Septic Thrombosis, endocarditis Osteomyelitis	1. Remove catheter, systemic antimicrobials for 7–10 days 2. Remove catheter, systemic antimicrobials ≥4 weeks
Staphylococcus aureus	1. No active malignancy or immunosuppression 2. Diabetic, immunosuppressed, prosthetic Intravascular device or metastatic infection	1. Remove catheter, systemic antimicrobials for 4–6 weeks 2. Remove catheter, systemic antimicrobials >4–6 weeks
Coagulase-negative *Staphylococcus*	1. Uncomplicated 2. Clinical deterioration or persisting bacteremia	1. Retain catheter, antimicrobials and lock therapy for 10–14 days 2. Remove catheter, antimicrobials ≥4 weeks
Enterococcus	1. Uncomplicated 2. Clinical deterioration or persisting bacteremia	1. Retain catheter, antimicrobials, lock therapy for 7–14 days 2. Remove catheter, antimicrobials ≥4 weeks
Gram-negative *Bacilli*	1. Uncomplicated 2. Clinical deterioration or persisting bacteremia	1. (a). Retain Catheter, antimicrobials for 10–14 days. If bacteremia persists, remove catheter and give antimicrobials for 10–14 days (b). Remove catheter, antimicrobials for 7–14 days 2. Remove catheter, antimicrobials for ≥4 weeks
Candida	1. Uncomplicated and/or complicated	1. Remove catheter, antifungal x 14 days after 1st negative blood culture

Data from Mermel L, Allon M, Bouza E, et al. Clinical practice guidelines for the diagnosis and management of intravascular catheter-related infection: 2009 update by the Infectious Disease Society of America. Clin Infect Dis 2009;(49):1–45.

Other thrombotic complications can result from inadequate catheter flushing leading a build-up of blood, lipid, or medication residue within the catheter. Patency can typically be restored with the use of tissue plasminogen activator for thrombus-related occlusions, 70% ethanol for lipid-related occlusions, and 0.1-N hydrochloric or 0.1-N sodium hydroxide for medication-related occlusions.[53]

Nonthrombotic occlusions can be positional in nature, with a common condition referred to as pinch-off syndrome. Diagnosis of pinch-off syndrome is suggested by diminished flow through the catheter with the patient's arm at the side and improved flow with the arm raised. Confirmation of the diagnosis is obtained with a chest radiograph showing indentation of the catheter as it courses between the clavicle and the first rib. A VAD that leads to pinch-off syndrome requires removal as catheter fracture and catheter embolus can occur.[54]

ALUMINUM CONTAMINATION

Aluminum is a known contaminant of PN solutions that can lead to toxicity at amounts greater than or equal to 5 mcg/kg/d.[55] Aluminum contaminants in protein sources, multivitamins, trace elements, some electrolytes, and some medications can contribute to the aluminum content of a PN solution bag. Excess aluminum can deposit in the bone, liver, spleen, brain, and kidney, leading to anemia, metabolic bone disease (MBD), neurologic complications, and developmental delays in children.[56] Due to the significant side effects of aluminum toxicity, especially in neonates, the FDA has mandated that the aluminum content be noted by the manufacturer on the package insert to assist clinicians in assessing the potential for toxicity and in minimizing aluminum delivery.[55]

COMPLICATIONS OF HPN

Although HPN is a life-saving therapy for patients with IF, it is not without its potential adverse consequences. MBD and hepatobiliary complications are long-term complications of HPN and have been studied extensively in efforts to improve patient outcome.

MBD

MBD is characterized by a reduction of total bone mass and includes osteomalacia and osteoporosis. It is a defect of the bone remodeling pathway in which inadequate vitamin D, phosphorus, calcium, magnesium, and/or excessive protein intake affects the formation and mineralization of the collagen matrix.[57]

The development of MBD is likely multifactorial, as it is associated with several disease states, medications, and immobility. IF is one of many conditions associated with MBD, and has a reported prevalence as high as 67%.[58] MBD presents clinically as bone pain, back pain, muscle weakness, or fractures. Biochemically, the patient may have elevated alkaline phosphatase, hypocalcemia, and/or vitamin D deficiency. Confirmation of MBD is assessed by monitoring bone mineral density via DXA and quantitative computed tomography.

The PN factors associated with the pathogenesis of PN-associated MBD include aluminum toxicity (as discussed above), excessive amino acid infusion, and micronutrient deficiencies. Amino acid intake is correlated with calciuria as shown by Bengoa and colleagues.[59] In this report, patients fed 2 g/kg of protein versus those fed 1 g/kg developed an increase in urinary calcium, which is linked to MBD. Micronutrient formulations should be dosed to provide adequate calcium, magnesium, and phosphorus to maintain normal serum levels while avoiding excess sodium that can potentially worsen the bone health through hypercalciuria.[57] Although diagnostic parameters exist, a basic understanding of nutrients is needed to prevent MBD, as additional nutritional factors may also contribute to its development.

Hepatobiliary Complications

Hepatobiliary complications associated with PN include cholestasis, steatosis, steatonecrosis, and cirrhosis. Diagnosis and treatment are difficult to achieve at times because the pathophysiology of liver disease in patients receiving HPN is multifactorial. PNALD is related to substrate imbalance, fat emulsions, the inability to feed patients enterally, small bowel intestinal overgrowth (SIBO), and the occurrence of sepsis or inflammation.

Currently, HPN programs monitor for liver disease by measuring liver-associated enzymes (LAEs) and bilirubin. A 5-year prospective study by Clarke and colleagues[60] in the early 1990s, evaluated LAEs in patients receiving HPN, including alkaline phosphatase, and aspartate transaminase (AST), as well as bilirubin. They demonstrated a progressive rise in LAEs as the duration of HPN increased. Elevated LAEs are a common finding in HPN patients and may be related to macronutrients or micronutrients in the PN solution.

Excessive glucose infusion (>50 kcal/kg/d) increases the rate of fatty acid synthesis, which can lead to the accumulation of triglycerides in the liver. This situation can lead to the progression of fibrosis and cirrhosis.[61] Excessive lipid infusions (>3 g/kg/d) has been associated with severe liver disease in HPN patients[61] and, therefore, should be limited to less than or equal to 1.0 g/kg/d. Some investigators hypothesize that the lack of sulfur-containing amino acids can alter the production of soluble bile salts, leading to the development of cholestasis.[62] Manganese and copper, delivered in the trace element preparations and/or as individual infusions, are hepatotoxic when their excretion by the liver is reduced as in cholestasis, and, therefore, may merit being withheld from the PN solution.[30,31,61]

Cycling HPN solutions may benefit the liver by promoting mobilization of fat stores during periods of fasting. Stout and Cober[44] published a review of 25 reports studying the effects of cyclic PN and patient outcome. Benefits reported included improvements in macronutrient oxidation, decreases in the respiratory quotient, and stabilization of hyperbilirubunemia.[44]

The adage "if the gut works, use it" continues to hold true in patients with IF receiving HPN. Providing EN, even in trophic amounts, has been shown to prevent or minimize the development of cholestasis. A retrospective study of elevated serum bilirubin levels in 12 infants receiving HPN for a ration of 5 plus or minus 1 months, before and after initiation of full EN, showed a 100% normalization of bilirubin levels after full EN was achieved.[63] The gallbladder is stimulated by the use of EN and, therefore, may obviate cholestasis by preventing the accumulation of gallbladder sludge.[61]

Small intestinal bacterial overgrowth (SIBO) (>10^5 cfu/mL of bacteria in the proximal intestine) is associated with dysmotility and can lead to the development of liver disease.[64] The cause of the development of liver disease in SIBO is not fully understood, but appears to be related to intestinal dysmotility[65,66] and has been associated with hepatic steatosis in some patient populations.[67] Symptoms include gas, bloating, steatorrhea, weight loss, and abdominal discomfort[68] and can be treated with the use of promotility agents, probiotics, and antibiotic regimens. The gold standard for diagnosis is a cultured small bowel aspirate but, due to the invasiveness of this approach, empirical treatment is often considered alternatively.

Finally, the prevalence of infection and/or sepsis contributes to the development of liver disease. During septic events, an increase in proinflammatory cytokines leads to a reduction in bile flow. This often presents as an elevation of LAEs and the development of cholestasis. Determining the source of infection and initiation of treatment will minimize and likely reverse the cholestasis. It should be noted that the development of severe liver dysfunction can be minimized by careful attention to the nature and dosages of macronutrients and micronutrients, and preventing and aggressively treating CRBSIs.[69]

TRANSITIONING OFF HPN

Intestinal rehabilitation programs specialize in transitioning patients with IF from HPN to EN in an effort to reduce and/or prevent the development of HPN-related and complications. Therapies used to improve intestinal absorption include diet modification and medication regimens (ie, antidiarrheals, antisecretories, and digestive enzymes). As absorption improves, the reliance on HPN to meet 100% of the estimated nutritional needs is lessened, and a reduction in the infusion of PN solution can be made. The most common method of weaning PN is to reduce the PN fluid volume and kilocalories as enteral intake increases.[70] In the home setting, a reduction in the number of PN infusion days per week is normally used, as this approach allows for a more gradual transition from PN to EN over a period of weeks to months.[71] Because patients must be able to maintain fluid and electrolyte balance from EN on the days when PN is withheld, this method is not suitable for critically ill patients or patients with large enteral fluid losses. Once the patient is fully transitioned to EN and maintaining adequate fluid and electrolyte balance and nutritional status, arrangements can be made to remove the VAD.

Removal of a PICC line can be done in the home by a homecare nurse provided that the length of the PICC line before placement can be confirmed once removed. This will ensure that none of the VAD was left behind in the patient. Removal of a tunneled VAD can be done in an outpatient setting by the surgeon or in an interventional radiology suite, using local anesthesia. For patients who are unable to transition off PN, alternative options should be considered, especially in the setting of HPN failure.

HPN FAILURE AND SURGICAL OPTIONS

Despite appropriate calculation and infusion of PN solutions and using aseptic catheter care techniques, HPN failure can still occur. HPN failure is defined by the following criteria:

1. Impending or overt liver failure because of PNALD
2. VAD-related thrombosis of two or more central veins
3. Frequent episodes of CRBSI (two episodes per year requiring hospitalization, one episode of a fungemia, one episode of septic shock, or acute respiratory distress syndrome)
4. Frequent episodes of severe dehydration despite infusions of intravenous fluid in addition to HPN.

Gastrointestinal surgical options that could decrease the reliance on long-term HPN should be evaluated for all patients. These options include restoring intestinal continuity, intestinal lengthening (ie, Bianchi or serial transverse enteroplasty [STEP] procedures), and relieving bowel obstructions.[72] Patients who are not candidates for these surgical options and are failing HPN should be referred to intestinal transplant centers for evaluation. A 9-year review of waiting list mortality for intestinal transplantation showed the highest mortality compared with other solid organs, with 8.8% mortality for an isolated intestine transplant and 29.8% mortality for a combined liver and intestine transplant, which indicates the need for early referral following a decision to undergo intestinal transplantation.[73]

Increased experience with intestinal transplantation and immunosuppression has increased the demand for transplant as a treatment option for IF. Patient survival at 1 and 5 years after intestinal transplantation is now 89% and 72%, respectively,[74] with a greater chance of survival when requiring an isolated intestinal transplant versus a combined intestine and liver transplant.[75] Late referral continues to decrease the survival rates. Liver disease, if diagnosed early, can be reversed after an intestinal transplant, but as the disease progresses to cirrhosis, a combined liver and intestinal transplant will be required, which has a lower survival rate.[76] Patients failing HPN who meet the criteria for intestinal transplant, but decide to forego transplantation, also have an increased mortality compared with patients who underwent the intestinal transplant.[75] Furthermore, patients with extreme short bowel syndrome (<50 cm of small bowel remaining) with end-stage liver disease and receiving HPN have a reported mortality rate as high as a 100%.[77,78] With improvements in the timeliness of patient referral and immunosuppressive regimens, survival rates may continue to improve, allowing intestinal transplantation to become a viable option for patients with permanent intestinal failure.

SUMMARY

HPN continues to be a life-saving treatment for many patients with IF as a result of the pioneering work of Dr Stanley J. Dudrick[1] at the University of Pennsylvania. Expert placement and care of the VAD will reduce the incidence of access-related complications. Further studies on ideal locking solutions to replace heparin and saline hold the promise of reducing CRBSIs. Careful monitoring of fluid, electrolyte, and macronutrient and micronutrient status can minimize major organ dysfunction and metabolic complications. A multidisciplined, integrated NST, including physicians, nurses, dietitians, pharmacists, and home infusion providers, can allow patients with IF who need HPN maintain a near-normal life.

REFERENCES

1. Dudrick S. Rhoads lecture: a 45-year obsession and passionate pursuit of optimal nutrition support: puppies, pediatrics, surgery, geriatrics, home TPN, A.S.P.E.N., et cetera. JPEN J Parenter Enteral Nutr 2005;29(4):272–87.
2. O'Keefe S, Buchman A, Fishbein T, et al. Short bowel syndrome and intestinal failure: consensus definitions and overview. Clin Gastroenterol Hepatol 2006; 4(1):6–10.
3. Mirtallo J. Overview of parenteral nutrition. In: Gottschlich M, DeLegge M, Mattox T, et al, editors. The A.S.P.E.N. nutrition support core curriculum: a case-based approach—the adult patient. Silver Spring (MD): American Society of Parenteral and Enteral Nutrition; 2007. p. 264–76.
4. Ireton-Jones C, Hennessy K, Howard D, et al. Multidisciplinary clinical care of the home parenteral nutrition patient. Infusion 1995;1:21–30.
5. Howard L. Home parenteral nutrition: survival, cost, and quality of life. Gastroenterology 2006;130:S52–9.
6. Center for Medicare & Medicaid Sevices; US department of Health and Human services. Available at: http://www.cms.gov/center/peoplewithmedicarecenter. asp. Accessed May 5, 2011.
7. Goff K. Enteral and parenteral nutrition transitioning from hospital to home. Nurs Case Manag 1998;3(2):67–74.
8. Stern J. Home parenteral nutrition and the psyche: psychological challenges for patient and family. Proc Nutr Soc 2006;65(3):222–6.
9. Gulledge A, Srp F, Sharp J, et al. Psychosocial issues of home parenteral and enteral nutrition. Nutr Clin Pract 1987;2:183–94.
10. Sharp J, Roncagli T. Ethical and psychosocial aspects of home parenteral nutrition in advanced cancer. Cancer Pract 1993;1(2):119–24.
11. Folstein M, Folstein S, McHugh P. "Mini-mental state". A practical method for grading the cognitive state of patients for the clinician. J Psychiatr Res 1975; 12(3):189–98.
12. Fuhrman M. Preparing the patient for discharge on home nutrition support. In: Ireton-Jones C, Delegge M, editors. Handbook of home nutrition support. Sudbury (Ontario): Jones and Bartlett; 2007. p. 17–26.
13. Smith C, Curtas S, Kleinbeck S, et al. Clinical trial of interactive and videotaped educational interventions reduce infection, reactive depression, and

rehospitalizations for sepsis in patients on home parenteral nutrition. JPEN J Parenter Enteral Nutr 2003;27(2):137–45.

14. Flowers R 3rd, Schwenzer K, Kopel R, et al. Efficacy of an attachable subcutaneous cuff for the prevention of intravascular catheter-related infection. A randomized, controlled trial. J Am Med Assoc 1989;261(6):878–83.

15. Harden J, Kemp L, Mirtallo J. Femoral catheters increase risk of infection in total parenteral nutrition patients. Nutr Clin Pract 1995;10(2):60–6.

16. Kemp L, Burge J, Choban P. The effect of catheter type and site on infection rates in total parenteral nutrition patients. JPEN J Parenter Enteral Nutr 1994;18(1):71–4.

17. Ryder M. Evidence-based practice in the management of vascular access devices for home parenteral nutrition therapy. JPEN J Parenter Enteral Nutr 2006;30(1):S82–94.

18. DeLegge M, Borak G, Moore N. Central venous access in the home parenteral nutrition population. JPEN J Parenter Enteral Nutr 2005;29(6):425–8.

19. DeChicco R, Seidner D, Brun C, et al. Tip position of long-term central venous access devices used for parenteral nutriton. JPEN J Parenter Enteral Nutr 2007;31(5):382–8.

20. Moureau N, Poole S, Murdock MA, et al. Central venous catheters in home infusion care: outcomes analysis in 50,470 patients. J Vasc Interv Radiol 2002;13:1009–16.

21. Maki D, Mermel L, Klugar D, et al. The efficacy of a chlorhexidine impregnated sponge (Biopatch) for the prevention of intravascular catheter-related infection-a prospective randomized controlled multicenter study [abstract]. 40th Interscience Conference on Antimicrobial Agents and Chemotherapy, Toronto Canada. Washington, DC: American Society for Microbiology. September 17–20, 2000.

22. Messing B, Peitra-Cohen S, Debure A, et al. Antibiotic-lock technique: a new approach to optimal therapy for catheter-related sepsis in home-parenteral nutrition patients. JPEN J Parenter Enteral Nutr 1988;12(2):185–9.

23. Metcalf S, Chambers S, Pithie A. Use of ethanol locks to prevent recurrent central line sepsis. J Infect 2004;49:20–2.

24. Dannenberg C, Bierbach U, Rothe A, et al. Ethanol-lock technique in the treatment of bloodstream infections in pediatric oncology patients with Broviac catheter. J Pediatr Hematol Oncol 2003;25:616–21.

25. Lennon E, Speerhas R. Estimating nutritional requirements. In: Parekh N, DeChicco R, editors. Cleveland clinic nutrition support handbook. Cleveland (OH): The Cleveland Clinic; 2004. p. 34–60.

26. Materese L, Steiger E, Seidner D, et al. Body composition changes in cachectic patients receiving home parenteral nutrition. JPEN J Parenter Enteral Nutr 2002; 26(6):366–71.

27. Langley G. Fluid, electrolytes, and acid-base disorders. In: Gottschlich M, DeLegge M, Mattox T, et al, editors. The A.S.P.E.N. nutrition support core curriculum: a case-based approach–the adult patient. Silver Spring (MD): American Society of Parenteral and Enteral Nutrition; 2007. p. 104–28.

28. Mikalunas V, Fitzgerald K, Rubin H, et al. Abnormal vitamin levels in patients receiving home total parenteral nutrition. J Clin Gastroenterol 2001;33(5):393–6.

29. Buchman A, Howard L, Guenter P, et al. Micronutrients in parenteral nutrition: too little or too much? The past, present, and recommendations for the future. Gastroenterology 2009;137:S1–6.

30. Howard L, Ashley C, Lyon D, et al. Autopsy tissue trace elements in 8 long-term parenteral nutrition patients who received the current U.S. Food and Drug Administration formulation. JPEN J Parenter Enteral Nutr 2007;31:388–96.

31. Allardyce B. Cholestasis caused by lipid emulsions. Surgery 1982;154:641–7.
32. Novak F, Heyland D, Avenell A, et al. Glutamine supplementation in serious illness: a systematic review of the evidence. Crit Care Med 2002;30:2022–9.
33. Dahlstrom K, Ament M, Moukarzel A, et al. Low blood and plasma carnitine levels in children receiving long-term parenteral nutrition. J Pediatr Gastroenterol Nutr 1990;11:375–9.
34. Moukarzel A, Dahlstrom K, Buchman A, et al. Carnitine status of children receiving long-term TPN: a longitudinal prospective study. J Pediatr 1992;120:759–62.
35. Bowyer B, Miles J, Haymond M, et al. L-carnitine therapy in home parenteral nutrition patients with abnormal liver tests and low plasma carnitine concentration. Gastroenterology 1988;94:434–8.
36. Clayton P, Bowron A, Mills K, et al. Phytosterolemia in children with parenteral nutrition-associated cholestatic liver disease. Gastroenterology 1993;105(6): 1806–13.
37. Chen W, Yeh S, Huang P. Effects of fat emulsions with different fatty acid composition on plasma and hepatic lipids in rats receiving total parenteral nutrition. Clin Nutr 1996;15:24–8.
38. Aksnes J, Eide T, Nordstrand K. Lipid entrapment and cellular changes in the rat myocard, lung and liver after long-term parenteral nutrition with lipid emulsion. A light microscopic and ultrastructural study. APMIS 1996;104:515–22.
39. Clayton P, Whitfield P, Iyer K. The role of phytosterols in the pathogenesis of liver complications of pediatric parenteral nutrition. Nutrition 1998;14:158–64.
40. Le H, de Meijer V, Zurakowski D, et al. Parenteral fish oil as monotherapy improves lipid profiles in children with parenteral nutrition-associated liver disease. JPEN J Parenter Enteral Nutr 2010;34(5):477–84.
41. Lee S, Valim C, Johnston P, et al. Impact of fish oil-based lipid emulsion on serum triglyceride, bilirubin, and albumin levels in children with parenteral nutrition-associated liver disease. Pediatr Res 2009;66(6):698–703.
42. de Meijer V, Gura K, Le H, et al. Fish oil-based lipid emulsions prevent and reverse parenteral nutrition-associated liver disease: the Boston experience. JPEN J Parenter Enteral Nutr 2009;33(5):541–7.
43. Gura K, Duggan C, Collier S, et al. Reversal of parenteral nutrition-associated liver disease in two infants with short bowel syndrome using parenteral fish oil: implications for future management. Pediatrics 2006;118(1):197–201.
44. Stout S, Cober M. Metabolic effects of cyclic parenteral nutrition infusion in adults and children. Nutr Clin Pract 2010;25(3):277–81.
45. DeLegge M, Ireton-Jones C. Home care. In: Gottschlich M, DeLegge M, Mattox T, et al, editors. The A.S.P.E.N. nutrition support core curriculum: a case-based approach–the adult patient. Silver Spring (MD): American Society of Parenteral and Enteral Nutrition; 2007. p. 725–39.
46. Hamilton C, Seidner D. Home parenteral nutrition in adults. In: Ireton-Jones C, Delegge M, editors. Handbook of home nutrition support. Sudbury (Ontario): Jones and Bartlett; 2007. p. 115–52.
47. McCarthy M, Shives J, Robinson R, et al. Prospective evaluation of single and triple lumen catheters in total parenteral nutrition. JPEN J Parenter Enteral Nutr 1987;11(3):259–62.
48. Centers for Disease Control and Prevention. Guidelines for the prevention of intravascular catheter-related infections. MMWR Recomm Rep 2002;51(RR-10):1–29.
49. Raad I, Hanna H, Alakech B, et al. Differential time to positivity: a useful method for diagnosing catheter-related blood stream infections. Ann Intern Med 2004; 140(1):18–25.

50. Passaro M, Steiger E, Curtas S. Long-term silastic catheters and chest pain. JPEN J Parenter Enteral Nutr 1994;18(3):240–2.
51. Mammen E. Pathogenesis of venous thrombosis. Chest 1992;102:640S–4S.
52. Petersen J, Delaney J, Brakstad M, et al. Silicone venous access devices positioned with their tips high in the superior vena cava are more likely to malfunction. Am J Surg 1999;178(1):38–41.
53. Krzywda E, Andris D, Edmiston C, et al. Parenteral access devices. In: Gottschlich M, DeLegge M, Mattox T, et al, editors. The A.S.P.E.N. nutrition support core curriculum: a case-based approach—the adult patient. Silver Spring (MD): American Society of Parenteral and Enteral Nutrition; 2007. p. 300–22.
54. Mirza B, Vanek V, Kupensky D. Pinch-off syndrome: case report and collective review of the literature. Am Surg 2004;70:635–44.
55. Food and Drug Administration. Aluminum in large and small volume parenterals used in total parenteral nutrition. Fed Regist 2000;65:4103–11.
56. Gura K. Aluminum contamination in products used in parenteral nutrition: has anything changed? Nutrition 2010;26:585–94.
57. Seidner D. Parenteral nutrition-associated metabolic bone disease. JPEN J Parenter Enteral Nutr 2002;26(5):S37–42.
58. Cohen-Solal M, Baudoin C, Joly F, et al. Osteoporosis in patients on long-term home parenteral nutrition: a longitudinal study. J Bone Miner Res 2003;18(11):1989–94.
59. Bengoa J, Sitrin M, Wood R, et al. Amino acid induces hypercalciuria in patients on TPN. Am J Clin Nutr 1983;83:264–9.
60. Clarke P, Ball M, Kettlewell M. Liver function tests in patients receiving parenteral nutrition. JPEN J Parenter Enteral Nutr 1991;15(1):54–9.
61. Jeejeebhoy K. Management of PN-induced cholestasis. Pract Gastroenterol 2005;24:62–8.
62. Schneider S, Joly F, Gehrardt M, et al. Taurine status and response to intravenous supplementation in adults with short-bowel syndrome undergoing long-term parenteral nutrition: a pilot study. Br J Nutr 2006;96:365–70.
63. Javid P, Collier S, Richardson D, et al. The role of enteral nutrition in the reversal of parenteral nutrition-associated liver dysfunction in infants. J Pediatr Surg 2005;40:1015–8.
64. Corazza G, Menozzi M, Strocchi A, et al. The diagnosis of small bowel bacterial overgrowth. Reliability of jejunal culture and inadequacy of breath hydrogen testing. Gastroenterology 1990;98:302–9.
65. Gunnarsdottir S, Sadik R, Shev S, et al. Small intestinal motility disturbances and bacterial overgrowth in patients with liver cirrhosis and portal hypertension. Am J Gastroenterol 2003;98:1362–70.
66. Soza A, Riquel A, Gonzalez R, et al. Increased orocecal transit time in patients with nonalcoholic fatty acid liver disease. Dig Dis Sci 2005;50:1136–40.
67. Sabate J, Jouet P, Harnois F, et al. High prevalence of small intestinal bacterial overgrowth in patients with morbid obesity: a contributor to severe hepatic steatosis. Obes Surg 2008;18:371–7.
68. Dibase J. Nutritional consequences of small intestinal bacterial overgrowth. Pract Gastroenterol 2008;32(12):15–28.
69. Salvino R, Ghanta R, Seidner D, et al. Liver failure is uncommon in adults receiving long-term parenteral nutrition. JPEN J Parenter Enteral Nutr 2006;30(3):202–8.
70. Marian M, McGinnis L. Overview of enteral nutrition. In: Gottschlich M, DeLegge M, Mattox T, et al, editors. The A.S.P.E.N. nutrition support core

curriculum: a case-based approach—the adult patient. Silver Spring (MD): American Society of Parenteral and Enteral Nutrition; 2007. p. 187–208.

71. Wu G, Wu Z, Wu Z. Effects of bowel rehabilitation and combined trophic therapy on intestinal adaptation in short bowel patients. World J Gastroenterol 2003;9: 2601–4.

72. Yannam G, Sudan D, Grant W, et al. Intestinal lengthening in adult patients with short bowel syndrome. J Gastrointest Surg 2010;14:1931–6.

73. Chungfat N, Dixler I, Cohran V, et al. Impact of Parenteral-nutrition associated liver disease on intestinal transplant waitlist dynamics. J Am Coll Surg 2007; 205:755.

74. Mazariegos G, Steffick D, Horslen S, et al. Intestine Transplantation in the United States, 1999–2008. Am J Transplant 2010;10(2):1020–34.

75. Pironi L, Forbes A, Francisca J, et al. Survival of patients identified as candidates for intestinal transplantation: a 3-year prospective follow-up. Gastroenterology 2008;135:61–71.

76. Fiel M, Sauter B, Wu H, et al. Regression of hepatic fibrosis after intestinal transplantation in total parenteral nutrition liver disease. Clin Gastroenterol Hepatol 2008;6:926–33.

77. Cavicchi M, Beau P, Crenn P, et al. Prevalence of liver disease and contributing factors in patients receiving home parenteral nutrition for permanent intestinal failure. Ann Intern Med 2000;132:525–32.

78. Chan S, McCowne K, Bistrian B, et al. Incidence, prognosis, and etiology of end-stage liver disease in patients receiving home total parenteral nutrition. Surgery 1999;126(1):28–34.

Nutritional Supplements in the Surgical Patient

Sidney J. Stohs, PhD[a,b,]*, Stanley J. Dudrick, MD[c,d]

KEYWORDS

- Nutritional supplements • Dietary supplements
- Surgical patients • Vitamins • Minerals • ω-3 Fatty acids
- Proteins • Amino acids

The nutritional status of a patient is a major determinant in achieving a successful surgical outcome. As a consequence, it is essential that patients be in the best possible nutritional and metabolically balanced state, both before and after surgery. The need for appropriate nutrition applies equally to those undergoing a surgical procedure on an outpatient basis as well as an inpatient basis. Because more surgeries are being conducted on an outpatient or overnight hospital stay basis, greater awareness is needed regarding the nutritional status of these patients. The risks of malnutrition include a compromised immune system with increased incidence and severity of infections, poor wound healing, greater frequency of both minor and major complications, longer recovery times, longer hospitalizations, and higher mortality.

Studies have shown that 40% to 55% of hospitalized patients are either malnourished or at risk for malnutrition, and the risks of malnutrition increase with age. Malnourished surgical patients are believed to be 2 to 3 times more likely to experience complications as well as increased mortality.[1] Despite the provision of sufficient food, most hospitalized patients who receive 3 meals per day without artificial nutritional support may not consume sufficient calories to meet their needs.[2] Furthermore, if patients are not consuming sufficient calories, they are also consuming insufficient amounts of other essential nutrients. Insufficient food intake may often be attributed to causes other than disease. However, achieving the optimal nutritional state for

The authors have nothing to disclose.
a Creighton University Medical Center, Omaha, NE, USA
b 4967 Stillwater Trail, Frisco, TX 75034, USA
c Department of Surgery, Saint Mary's Hospital, 56 Franklin Street, Waterbury, CT 06706, USA
d Department of Surgery, Yale University School of Medicine, 333 Cedar Street, New Haven, CT 06510, USA
* Corresponding author. 4967 Stillwater Trail, Frisco, TX 75034, USA.
E-mail address: sstohs@yahoo.com

Surg Clin N Am 91 (2011) 933–944
doi:10.1016/j.suc.2011.04.011
0039-6109/11/$ – see front matter © 2011 Elsevier Inc. All rights reserved.

patients is not always possible because of pathologic, biochemical, emotional, or physical factors that may or may not be related to the surgical procedure involved. In addition, patient nutrition may not be a high priority, particularly if outpatient surgery is involved.

Patients may be overfed and undernourished, with large percentages of the general population being deficient in vitamin A, vitamin B6, vitamin B12, vitamin C, vitamin D, vitamin E, vitamin K, folic acid, zinc, calcium, magnesium, and selenium.[3–9] These nutritional deficiencies can be extrapolated directly to the surgical patient population, with some indications that the incidence of deficiencies may be higher than in the general population.

Approximately two-thirds of the adult American population is overweight, whereas about one-third is considered to be obese.[10] Various studies indicate that up to 600 more kilocalories are consumed by each adult per day than 30 to 35 years ago.[11] A prime reason for the lack of appropriate nutritional balance relates to the increased consumption of refined foods that are high in calories in the form of sugars, starches, and fats, and low in vitamins, minerals, trace elements, and fiber because of the refining and manufacturing processes used. In addition, agricultural practices and soil depletion have resulted in crops with lower mineral, trace element, micronutrient, and vitamin content.[12] Furthermore, average individuals do not perform the same level of physical work, or get the same amount of exercise, as their forebears, and, as a consequence, do not use the amount of calories consumed daily by them. The net effect is that the average individual consumes an excess of calories together with lower levels of essential nutrients, while concurrently burning fewer calories.

Various techniques are used to enhance nutrient intake in surgical patients, including improved institutional diets, total parenteral nutrition, nasogastric feeding tubes, oral feeding tubes, and oral nutritional supplements. This article focuses on the use of orally administered nutritional dietary supplements, with emphasis on their associated applications, advantages, and potential problems.

More than 50% of the adult population reports consuming dietary supplements daily, with women consuming supplements more regularly then men; similar numbers of patients report taking dietary supplements before surgery.[13–15] Some studies indicate that as many as 70% of adults regularly use oral dietary supplements, and the number of patients using dietary supplements before surgery similarly varies between 50% and 70%.[13,15–17]

A recent study indicated that 72% of cardiologists, 59% of dermatologists, and 91% of orthopedists reported recommending dietary supplements to their patients, while reporting that they themselves at least occasionally use dietary supplements almost 70% of the time.[18] A previous study indicated that 70% of physicians and 89% of nurses used dietary supplements, whereas 79% of physicians and 82% of nurses indicated that they had recommended dietary supplements to their patients.[19] Thus, oral nutrition in the form of dietary supplements is a form of nutritional supplementation that is accepted by a large percentage of the general population as well as physicians and other health care providers, and is a system that should be encouraged both before and after surgery.

Several investigations have examined the clinical outcomes and cost benefits of oral nutritional supplements. In general, oral supplements, when given before and after surgery have been shown to result in less weight loss after surgery,[20,21] fewer major and minor complications,[20–22] less fatigue,[20] less muscle wasting,[20,23] shorter length of hospital stay,[24] and lower overall surgery-related costs.[21,22]

USEFUL DEFINITIONS

The term dietary supplement as used in the United States was defined by an act of Congress with the passage of the Dietary Supplement Health and Education Act (DSHEA) of 1994. A dietary supplement is defined as a product taken by mouth that contains a dietary ingredient intended to supplement the diet. Dietary ingredients may include vitamins, minerals, herbs, or other botanic products, amino acids, and substances as enzymes, glandulars, organ tissues, and metabolites. Dietary supplements can be extracts or concentrates, and can occur in forms such as capsules, tablets, liquids, softgels, gelcaps, powders, or bars. They must be labeled as dietary supplements because by law they are a special category of foods, and not drugs. The American definition of dietary supplements differs from that used in Europe, where the term refers to vitamins and minerals; herbal products are regulated separately as herbal medicines or herbal remedies.[25]

DSHEA allows structure/function claims to be made for dietary supplements that describe the role of a nutrient or dietary ingredient intended to affect normal structure or function in humans. Examples of structure/function claims include claims that fiber maintains bowel integrity, calcium builds strong bones, ω-3 fatty acids support heart health, and chromium helps maintain blood glucose levels in the normal range. If a dietary supplement includes a structure/function claim, it must also state that the US Food and Drug Administration has not evaluated the claim, and must further state that the dietary supplement is not intended to "diagnose, treat, cure or prevent any disease," because, by law, only a drug can make this claim.

Daily values (DVs) are printed on all nutrition facts labels, and represent the recommended daily intake (RDI) of a nutrient that is considered to be sufficient to meet the requirements of 97% to 98% of healthy individuals in every demographic in the United States, based on 2000 kcal per day. The RDIs are based on the older recommended dietary allowance (RDA). Each RDA was calculated based on the estimated average requirement (EAR), which is the amount of a nutrient expected to satisfy the needs of 50% of the people in a demographic. The RDA is usually about 20% higher than the EAR. The dietary reference intake (DRI) is a system of nutrition recommendations from the Institute of Medicine of the US National Academy of Sciences, introduced in 1997 and designed to broaden the RDAs.

However, the multiple systems that recommend essential nutrient intake add confusion and questionable clarity to the basic question, "How much is needed for optimal health?" All of the systems are based largely on the lowest amount of a nutrient needed to prevent a deficiency or disease state, and not on the amount required to provide optimal health. They are based on the minimal needs of healthy individuals, with little or no allowance for disease or stressful situations such as surgery. As a consequence, there is a general misconception among not only the lay public but also health professionals that all that anyone needs for good health is 100% of the DV amount of each essential nutrient, which clearly does not provide an amount needed for optimal health. Supplementing with a multivitamin/mineral product formulated with 100% of the DV can decrease the prevalence of suboptimal levels of some, but not all, of these nutrients, and does not enhance the levels of various markers of immune response, antiinflammatory activity, or antioxidant capacity.[4,26]

HOW MUCH OF WHICH NUTRITIONAL SUPPLEMENTS ARE NEEDED?

Many factors are involved in determining how much of the various essential nutrients are required by an individual to meet optimal daily needs. Determining factors include age, weight, gender, physical condition, daily physical activity, stress levels, gastrointestinal health, general health, metabolic rate, disease states, and recovery from injury or surgery. As a consequence, it is apparent that 1 size (amount) does not fit all, and, as previously noted, supplementing with a product that contains 100% of the DVs does not adequately meet the overall needs. Metabolism can be compared with a chain that is only as strong as the weakest link.

An excellent example of interindividual variability in optimal needs is vitamin D. The DV for vitamin D is currently set at 400 IU, and the Institute of Medicine has recommended that this be increased to 600 IU for most adults based on bone health needs. For optimal health, blood levels of 25-hydroxyvitamin D of at least 40 ng/mL are recommended and, to achieve this level of vitamin D intake, individuals may require from 2000 to 4000 IU daily,[27] depending on the various factors cited earlier.

With these considerations in mind, what should a surgeon or other health care provider recommend with respect to a basic, daily multivitamin/mineral product? The average individual should daily consume a dietary supplement that contains at least 200% to 300% of the DV for vitamins and minerals. Alternatively, consuming a product with 100% of the DVs for vitamins and minerals 2 to 3 times daily with meals is appropriate, and may provide better overall absorption of some vitamins and minerals.

The vitamin A should be in the form of β-carotene or mixed carotenoids, and not retinol or its esters retinyl acetate and retinyl palmitate, to avoid vitamin A toxicity. The β-carotene is converted into vitamin A as vitamin A is needed by the body. In addition, in recent years, more people are consuming vegetarian diets and, if they are not taking a vitamin B12 supplement, they may have abnormally low serum levels of this vitamin. Low vitamin B12 levels have implications for increased homocysteine levels, decreased high-density lipoprotein levels, and possibly platelet aggregation,[28] all of which may contribute to surgical and postsurgical complications.

The typical multivitamin/mineral product does not contain appropriate amounts of calcium, magnesium, and vitamin D. As a consequence, patients should be encouraged to take an additional product containing at least 25% of the DV of these components twice a day with meals. A product that contains only vitamin D and calcium is inadequate. The high calcium intake inhibits the absorption of magnesium, and may be 1 of the reasons for the high incidence of magnesium deficiency in this country, which has been reported to be as high or higher that the incidence of calcium deficiency.[29–31]

Calcium and magnesium products that exist in chelated and absorbable forms as calcium citrate, calcium hydroxyapatite, calcium aspartate or other amino acid chelate, and magnesium citrate, magnesium ascorbate, and magnesium aspartate or other amino acid chelate should be recommended. Products that contain magnesium oxide and calcium carbonate (coral calcium or oyster shell calcium), which are poorly absorbed, should be avoided.[32]

In anticipation of surgery, if patients are not currently taking a daily multivitamin/mineral product, they should be urged to begin immediately to do so at the doses recommended earlier. If they are taking a daily multivitamin/mineral product, ensure that they are taking an appropriate amount. For 2 weeks before surgery, it may be appropriate to recommend that the level of intake be increased to 300% to 400% of the DVs for most vitamins and minerals, with the exception of vitamin D, which should be increased to 4000 to 5000 IU per day (1000%–1200% DV) with the addition of a single-entity product. These vitamin and mineral products should be discontinued 24 to 36 hours before surgery. After surgery, ingestion of multivitamin/mineral products should be resumed as soon as possible, usually within 1 or 2 days, and continued indefinitely.

ω-3 Fatty acids are present in every cell in the body and are required for normal cell and organ function. Most of the population in the United States does not consume an adequate daily amount, and an estimated 84,000 people die prematurely each year because of an ω-3 fatty acid deficiency,[33] with vegetarians exhibiting particularly low intake.[28] The beneficial functions of ω-3 fatty acids are extensive, including cardioprotective, immunoprotective, and neuroprotective functions, and enhanced bone density, gastrointestinal health, and protection against muscle wastage in patients who have cancer and the elderly.[34] ω-3 Fatty acids exhibit other health benefits associated with lungs, liver, skin, eyes, hair, joints, and other organs and tissues.[35]

The ω-3 fatty acids primarily responsible for these desirable effects are docosahexaenoic acid (DHA) and eicosapentaenoic acid (EPA), derived primarily from fish oils, although they can be obtained from krill (zooplankton), whereas DHA can be extracted from algae and EPA from yeast. α-Linolenic acid (ALA) is an ω-3 fatty acid derived from plant sources such as flax seed oil, canola oil, soybean oil, nuts, and some berries. However, very little ALA is converted into DHA and EPA, and, as a consequence, it possesses only a small fraction of the health benefits of fish oil.[36]

How much DHA/EPA should adults take per day as a nutritional supplement? The American Heart Association recommends 2 to 3 g per day for general health and wellness. For individuals with health issues including increased blood pressure, triglycerides, cholesterol or glucose, as well as joint or gastrointestinal issues, 3 to 4 g per day of DHA/EPA in divided doses for best absorption may be appropriate.[37] Doses of 5 to 10 g per day of DHA/EPA have been recommended for neurologic issues such as depression, dementia, Alzheimer disease, or decreased cognitive function.[38]

If patients are already using a DHA/EPA product before surgery, they should be encouraged to continue to do so. For patients who are not currently taking a DHA/EPA product, encourage them to take 3 to 4 g per day for 2 to 3 weeks before the surgery, and discontinue taking the product 24 to 36 hours before surgery. As with multiple vitamin/mineral products, the ω-3 fatty acid product should be resumed within several days after surgery and continued indefinitely. There is no need to require that patients use the prescription version of DHA/EPA. Recommend a high-quality product from a reputable manufacturer. Recent studies have shown that concerns expressed about possible contamination of products with heavy metals and pesticides obtained at pharmacies or health food stores are unfounded and do not present a health threat.[39]

Sarcopenia is defined as age-related loss of skeletal muscle mass, strength, and function.[40] After the age of 35 to 40 years, approximately a 0.5% loss in muscle mass occurs per year, which accelerates after the age of 60 years,[41,42] and is primarily caused by a decrease in type 2 (fast glycolytic) muscle fibers. As a consequence, general activities of daily living decline, and mobility gradually becomes impaired. Current research suggests that sarcopenia involves an inflammatory state driven by oxidative stress, cytokines, and decreases in dietary protein intake, activity of anabolic hormones, and physical activity.[43] Furthermore, surgery-induced inflammation is related to decreased muscle strength and endurance, sensation of fatigue, and increased age.[44]

The DRI for protein recommended by the Institute of Medicine for adults including the elderly is 0.8 g/kg body weight, with up to 40% of adults currently having daily protein intakes less than this amount.[45] However, this amount of protein has been shown to be too low to support and preserve muscle mass in older individuals. The recommended daily protein intake for strength and speed athletes is in the range of

1.2 to 1.5 g/kg body weight, an amount that may be more appropriate for the elderly and for individuals undergoing surgery,[46] assuming normal kidney function.

Various studies have shown that the branched-chain amino acids, L-leucine, L-valine, and L-isoleucine inhibit breakdown of skeletal muscle. Of these 3 amino acids, L-leucine has been shown to stimulate muscle protein synthesis, and seems to play the major role in regulating muscle protein metabolism.[47,48] As a consequence, supplementation with L-leucine may be an important adjunct to the preservation of muscle, the amelioration of surgery-related inflammation, and the rate of recovery.

The average diet of the elderly is clearly inadequate in the amount of protein consumed daily. Ideally, the ratio of carbohydrates/protein/fat should be in the range of 40:30:30, with the carbohydrates being derived from whole grains, fruits, and vegetables, whereas the fats are primarily polyunsaturated from plant sources. In preparation for surgery, the amounts of protein and amino acids should be increased.[48,49] Beginning at least 2 to 3 weeks before surgery, the daily intake of protein should be in the range of 1.2 to 1.5 g/kg body weight.[23] A convenient method for doing so is the use of protein shakes that contain 20 to 25 g of protein per serving, equivalent to approximately 3 ounces of fish, chicken, or beef. The protein in these shakes can be from various sources such as whey, soy, or pea.

An alternative mechanism for preserving and supporting muscle is the use of nutritional supplements that contain either a mixture of the 3 branched-chain amino acids (L-leucine, L-valine, and L-isoleucine) or L-leucine as the primary amino acid.[50,51] Products containing these amino acids are available as capsules, shakes, or tablets. A daily intake of 8 to 10 g per day of L-leucine or 12 to 14 g per day of a mixture of the branched-chain amino acids may be appropriate, particularly in patients with compromised renal function who are, therefore, unable to consume high levels of protein.[52] The continued ingestion of protein in amounts that constitute approximately 30% of the total caloric intake should be encouraged after surgery.

Two additional amino acids that should be considered for nutritional supplementation of surgical patients are L-arginine and L-glutamine. Both are conditionally essential amino acids that are particularly beneficial in stressful situations such as surgery. L-Glutamine plays an important role in protein synthesis and wound healing, helps regulate acid-base balance, serves as an energy source, helps maintain gut barrier function and cellular differentiation, and supports the immune system.[53–55] Daily supplementation can be provided with 8 to 10 g of L-glutamine in divided doses 1 to 2 weeks before surgery, discontinuing 24 to 36 hours before surgery, and resuming 1 or 2 days after surgery.

L-Arginine plays an important role in cell division, wound healing, support of the immune system, and removal of ammonia from the body. It serves as a precursor for synthesis of nitric acid and helps decrease blood pressure.[56–59] L-Arginine supplementation can be provided at 10 to 14 g per day in divided doses for 1 to 2 weeks before surgery, discontinuing 24 to 36 hours before surgery, and resuming 1 or 2 days after surgery.

HERBAL PRODUCTS

Various surveys indicate that herbal products and preparations are used by about 22% to 68% of surgical patients,[15–17,60] with several studies indicating that 70% to 80% of the herbs used by the patients are not reported to the caregivers before surgery.[15,60] More than 20% of physicians indicated in a recent survey that they use herbal products themselves.[18] Herbal products are used to address various health-related issues by a large percentage of the population because they are believed to be beneficial, exhibit fewer adverse effects than drugs, and in most cases have a long history or culture of use.

Numerous reviews and journal articles warn of the theoretic and potential complications associated with use of herbal products together with concurrent drug use, particularly with respect to surgical patients.[17,61,62] The reality is that there are few documented cases of clinically significant herb-drug interactions, and most data on herb-drug interactions are based on case reports, animal studies, in vitro assays, and speculation.[63,64] Considering that millions of patients take herbs and are concomitantly taking drugs, or are administered drugs during surgical procedures, the number of clinically relevant adverse reports is minuscule.[63] A stronger case can be made for the adverse effects of drugs on nutrition, vitamin and mineral metabolism, and herbs.[65–67]

Case reports are frequently cited as unequivocal evidence that a dangerous herb-drug interaction exists. For example, all drug interaction software within the health care system warns of potential bleeding disorders that may be caused by ginkgo and garlic when used in conjunction with anticoagulants.[14,61,68] However, in both cases, the only evidence available relates to a small number of published case reports that were incomplete, and involved multiple risk and confounding factors.[63] Human studies have failed to show measurable anticoagulant effects of either ginkgo or garlic,[64] but these warnings continue to persist.[68] As succinctly noted by Karch,[69] "case reports are incomplete, uncontrolled, retrospective, lack operational criteria for identifying when an adverse event actually occurred, and resemble nothing so much as hearsay evidence, a type of evidence that is prohibited in all courts in all of industrialized societies." However, clinical case studies continue to be used and cited as documented evidence.

The American Association of Anesthesiologists has suggested that all herbal products (medicines) should be discontinued at least 2 weeks before surgery,[17] a recommendation that seems to be widely adopted. However, the half-lives of most natural products, including flavonoids, terpenoids, curcuminoids, withanolides, carotenoids, proanthocyanidins, and other polyphenolics that potentially modulate drug absorption and metabolism, are generally in the range of 2 to 6 hours for most of the widely used phytonutrients,[70–73] and are thus cleared from the body within 24 to 36 hours. Herbal constituents are rapidly cleared from the body, which may explain why so few herb-drug interactions are observed in surgical patients in spite of the theoretically large numbers of possibilities. In one study, more than 26% of patients were using herbal products before surgery. Only approximately one-half of these surgical patients ceased using these products before surgery, with no apparent evidence of adverse effects.[13]

Rather than expecting patients to discontinue taking herbal products at least 2 weeks before surgery, a more realistic recommendation, based on the existing evidence, is that patients discontinue use of their herbal products a minimum of 3 days before surgery, unless there are specific and well-documented reasons for extending this time interval. Similarly, patients may consider resuming the use of their herbal products a minimum of 3 days after surgery, again unless there are specific and well-documented reasons for extending this time interval. Using herbal products and phytonutrients to support health in surgical patients is beyond the scope of this article. Various phytonutrients may offer health benefits in particular circumstances.[74] For example, in a study involving 41,620 adult men and women, total dietary antioxidant capacity was associated with a lower risk of ischemic stroke.[75] Surgery, aging, obesity, and disease states are all inflammatory conditions, and a vast array of potent antiinflammatory and antioxidant constituents are present in herbal preparations.

SAFETY ISSUES

The US Poison Control Centers again reported no deaths caused by vitamins/minerals or herbal ingredients and dietary supplements in general in 2009,[76] nor have there been any deaths caused by these potential causes in recent years. When deaths have been caused by the ingestion of herbal products, it has been because of inappropriate use[77] rather than being used in recommended amounts.[78] The numbers of herb-drug interactions and adverse effects caused by nutritional supplements that are reported annually are exceedingly small[76]; much less than the numbers that are predicted by health agencies.

Concerns expressed regarding safety when vitamin/mineral products are used in amounts greater than 100% of the daily value are clearly unfounded, particularly regarding water soluble vitamins and minerals of which excess amounts are readily excreted. Toxicities have not been shown to occur with consumption of vitamins in amounts up to 10 to 20 times the DVs. The recommendations presented earlier are designed not only to meet minimum requirements but also to provide amounts that will address optimum nutritional needs while ensuring a wide margin of safety.

SUMMARY

More than 50% of the adult population of the United States consumes nutritional supplements daily. However, large percentages of the populace are deficient in multiple vitamins and minerals because of poor dietary habits and consumption of foods with inadequate amounts of essential nutrients. These nutritional deficiencies apply to surgical patients in whom malnutrition is a major contributing factor to poor prognosis, higher incidences of postsurgical complications, poor wound healing, compromised immune systems and increased infections, and longer recovery times in general.

Although a large percentage of the adult population consumes multivitamin/mineral products that contain up to 100% of the DV, studies indicate that, for many individuals, this amount of a variety of vitamins and minerals is inadequate to provide blood and tissue levels needed for good nutrition, let alone optimum nutrition. To address the nutritional needs of surgical patients appropriately, consuming up to 400% of the DV for most common vitamins and minerals for several weeks before surgery is recommended, while continuing to consume 200% to 300% of the DV of these nutrients after surgery.

ω-3 Fatty acid deficiency is common throughout the United States. ω-3 Fatty acids are present in every cell in the body and impact the functions of all organs. Surgical patients should be encouraged to take 3 to 4 g of DHA/EPA daily beginning 2 to 3 weeks before surgery if they are not already doing so, and should discontinue their intake 24 to 36 hours before surgery. They can resume taking DHA/EPA within several days after surgery.

Sarcopenia is a common and significant problem in the elderly, and a major determining factor associated with surgical outcomes. High protein intake and exercise are 2 factors that are known to reverse age-related muscle wasting. A protein intake in the range of at least 1.2 to 1.5 g/d for several weeks before surgery, along with an exercise program, should be recommended. When renal function is an issue, or as an alternative approach to preserving and enhancing muscle, a high intake of L-leucine (8–10 g/d), or a combination of the branched-chain amino acids L-leucine, L-valine, and L-isoleucine (12–14 g/d), may be appropriate. These branched-chain amino acids in general, and L-leucine in particular, have been shown to promote protein synthesis.

Two other conditionally essential amino acids that support the immune system, cell division, and wound healing are L-arginine and L-glutamine. Malnourished and physically stressed patients can benefit from ingesting 8 to 10 g of L-glutamine per day and 10 to 14 g of L-arginine per day for 1 to 2 weeks before surgery as well as after surgery.

Numerous articles warn of the theoretic and potential adverse events associated with herb-drug interactions. However, the number of clinically relevant examples that occur annually is small. Large percentages of the population use herbal products immediately before surgery. Because of the short half-lives of the active constituents in herbal products, most herbal products can be safely discontinued a minimum of 3 days before surgery.

In summary, the nutritional status of patients is a major factor in determining the success of surgical procedures. The recommendations in this article are designed to assist physicians in providing safe, knowledgeable, comprehensive, and optimal nutritional support for patients both before and after surgery.

REFERENCES

1. Allred CR, Voss AC, Finn SC, et al. Malnutrition and clinical outcomes: the case for medical nutrition therapy. J Am Diet Assoc 1996;96:361–9.
2. Dupertuis YM, Kossovsky MP, Kyle UG, et al. Food intake in 1707 hospitalized patients: a prospective comprehensive hospital survey. Clin Nutr 2003;22: 115–23.
3. Ahuja JKC, Goldman JD, Moshfegh AJ. Current status of vitamin E nutriture. Ann N Y Acad Sci 2004;1031:387–90.
4. Sebastian RS, Cleveland LE, Goldman JD, et al. Older adults who use vitamin/mineral supplements differ from nonusers in nutrition intake adequacy and dietary attitudes. J Am Diet Assoc 2007;107:1322–32.
5. Ma J, Johns RA, Stafford RS. Americans are not meeting current calcium recommendations. Am J Clin Nutr 2007;85:1361–6.
6. Park S, Johnson M, Fischer JG. Vitamin and mineral supplements: barriers and challenges for older adults. J Nutr Elder 2008;27:297–317.
7. Schleicher RL, Carroll MD, Ford ES, et al. Serum vitamin C and the prevalence of vitamin C deficiency in the United States: 2003–2004 National Health and Nutrition Examination Survey (NHANES). Am J Clin Nutr 2009;90: 1252–63.
8. Nelson FH. Magnesium, inflammation, and obesity in chronic disease. Nutr Rev 2010;68:333–40.
9. McCann JC, Ames BN. Adaptive dysfunction of selenoproteins from the perspective of the triage theory: why modest selenium deficiency may increase risk of diseases of aging. FASEB J 2011. DOI: 10.1096/fj.11-180885.
10. Flegal KM, Carroll MD, Ogden CL, et al. Prevalence and trends in obesity among US adults, 1999-2008. JAMA 2010;303:235–41.
11. Hyman MA, Ornish D, Roizer M. Lifestyle medicine: treating the causes of disease. Altern Ther 2009;15:12–4.
12. Thomas JA, Burns RA. Important drug-nutrient interactions in the elderly. Drugs Aging 1998;13:199–209.
13. Leung JM, Dzankic S, Manku K, et al. The prevalence and predictors of the use of alternative medicine in presurgery patients in five California hospitals. Anesth Analg 2001;93:1062–8.
14. Collins SC, Dufresne RG. Dietary supplements in the setting of Mohs surgery. Dermatol Surg 2002;28:447–52.
15. Glintborg B, Andersen SE, Spang-Hanssen E, et al. Disregarding use of herbal medical products and dietary supplements among surgical and medical patients

as estimated by home inspection and interview. Pharmacoepidemiol Drug Saf 2005;14:639–45.

16. Tsen LC, Segal S, Pothier M, et al. Alternative medicine use in presurgical patients. Anesthesiology 2000;93:148–51.

17. Norred CL. A follow-up survey of the use of complementary and alternative medicines by surgery patients. AANA J 2002;70:119–25.

18. Dickinson A, Shao A, Boyon N, et al. Use of dietary supplements by cardiologists, dermatologists and orthopedists: report of a survey. Nutr J 2011;10:20.

19. Dickinson A, Boyon N, Shao A. Physicians and nurses use and recommend dietary supplements: report of a survey. Nutr J 2009;8:29.

20. Keele AM, Bray MJ, Duncan PW, et al. Two phase randomized controlled clinical trial of postoperative oral dietary supplements in surgical patients. Gut 1997;40: 393–9.

21. Smedley F, Bowling T, James M, et al. Randomized clinical trial of the effects of preoperative and postoperative oral nutritional supplements on clinical course and cost of care. Br J Surg 2004;91:983–90.

22. Lawson RM, Doshi MK, Barton JR, et al. The effects of unselected post-operative nutritional supplementation on nutritional status and clinical outcome of orthopaedic patients. Clin Nutr 2003;22:39–46.

23. Jensen MB, Hessov I. Dietary supplementation at home improves the regain of lean body mass after surgery. Nutrition 1997;13:422–30.

24. Braga M, Gianotti L, Nespoli L, et al. Nutritional approach in malnourished surgical patients. A prospective randomized study. Arch Surg 2002;137: 174–80.

25. Goldstein LH, Elias M, Ron-Avraham G, et al. Consumption of herbal remedies and dietary supplements amongst patients hospitalized in medical wards. Br J Clin Pharmacol 2007;64:373–80.

26. McKay DL, Perrone G, Rasmussen H, et al. The effects of a multivitamin/mineral supplement on micronutrient status, antioxidant capacity and cytokine production in healthy older adults consuming a fortified diet. J Am Coll Nutr 2000;19:613–20.

27. Holick MF. Vitamin D: evolutionary, physiological and health perspectives. Curr Drug Targets 2011;12:4–18.

28. Li D. Chemistry behind vegetarianism. J Agric Food Chem 2011;3:777–84.

29. Gums JG. Magnesium in cardiovascular and other disorders. Am J Health Syst Pharm 2004;61:1569–76.

30. Tong GM, Rude RK. Magnesium deficiency in critical illness. J Intensive Care Med 2005;20:3–17.

31. Nayor D. Widespread deficiency with deadly consequences. Life Ext 2008;77–83.

32. Hanzlik RP, Fowler SC, Fisher DH. Relative bioavailability of calcium from calcium formate, calcium citrate, and calcium carbonate. J Pharmacol Exp Ther 2005; 313:1217–22.

33. Danaei G, Ding EL, Mozaffarian D, et al. The preventable causes of death in the United States: comparative risk assessment of dietary, lifestyle, and metabolic risk factors. PLoS Med 2009;6:1–23.

34. Murphy RA, Mourtzakis M, Chu QS, et al. Supplementation with fish oil increases first-line chemotherapy efficacy in patients with advanced nonsmall cell lung cancer. Cancer 2011. DOI: 10.1002/cncr.25933.

35. Calder PC, Deckelbaum RJ. Omega-3 fatty acids; time to get the message right! Curr Opin Clin Nutr Metab Care 2008;11:91–3.

36. Wang C, Harris WS, Chung W, et al. n-3 Fatty acids from fish or fish-oil supplements, but not α-linolenic acid, benefit cardiovascular disease outcomes in

primary- and secondary-prevention studies: a systematic review. Am J Clin Nutr 2006;84:5–18.

37. Davis M. Broad spectrum cardiac protection with fish oil. Life Ext 2006;37–48.

38. Mazza M, Pomponi M, Janiri L, et al. Omega-3 fatty acids and antioxidants in neurological and psychiatric diseases: an overview. Prog Neuropsychopharmacol Biol Psychiatry 2007;31:12–26.

39. Anon. Fish oil and omega-3 fatty acid supplements. Available at: http://www.consumerlab.com/reviews/fish_oil_supplements_review/omega3/. Accessed March 14, 2011.

40. Muscaritoli M, Anker SD, Argiles J, et al. Consensus definition of sarcopenia, cachexia and pre-cachexia: joint document elaborated by Special Interest Groups (SIG) "cachexia-anorexia in chronic wasting disease" and "nutrition in geriatrics". Clin Nutr 2010;29:154–9.

41. Marcell TJ. Sarcopenia: causes, consequences, and prevention. J Gerentol Med Sci 2003;58:911–6.

42. Dreyer HC, Volpi E. Role of protein and amino acids in the pathophysiology and treatment of sarcopenia. J Am Coll Nutr 2005;24:140S–5S.

43. Jensen GL. Inflammation: roles in aging and sarcopenia. JPEN J Parenter Enteral Nutr 2008;32:656–9.

44. Bautmans I, Njemini J, DeBacker J, et al. Surgery-induced inflammation in relation to age, muscle endurance, and self-perceived fatigue. J Gerontol 2010; 65A:266–73.

45. Paddon-Jones D, Short KR, Campbell WW, et al. Roll of protein in the sarcopenia of aging. Am J Clin Nutr 2008;87:1562S–6S.

46. Tipton KD, Wolfe RR. Protein and amino acids for athletes. J Sports Sci 2004;21: 65–79.

47. Garlick PJ. The role of leucine in the regulation of protein metabolism. J Nutr 2005;135:15535–65.

48. Koopman R, Verdijk L, Manders RFJ, et al. Co-ingestion of protein and leucine stimulates muscle protein synthesis rates to the same extent in young and elderly lean men. Am J Clin Nutr 2006;84:623–32.

49. Fujita S, Volpi E. Amino acids and muscle loss with aging. J Nutr 2006;136: 277S–80S.

50. Desikan V, Mileva I, Garlick J, et al. The effect of oral leucine on protein metabolism in adolescents with Type 1 diabetes mellitus. Int J Ped Endocrinol 2010; 2010:493258. DOI: 10.1155/2010/493258.

51. Baptista IL, Leal ML, Artioli GG, et al. Leucine attenuates skeletal muscle wasting via inhibition of ubiquitin ligases. Muscle Nerve 2010;41:800–8.

52. Laviano A, Muscaritoli M, Cascino A, et al. Branched-chain amino acids: the best compromise to achieve anabolism? Curr Opin Clin Nutr Metab Care 2005;8: 408–14.

53. Novak F, Heyland DK, Avenell A, et al. Glutamine supplementation in serious illness: a systematic review of the evidence. Crit Care Med 2002;30:2022–9.

54. De-Souza DA, Greene LJ. Intestinal permeability and systemic infections in critically ill patients: effects of glutamine. Crit Care Med 2005;33:1125–35.

55. Burrin DG, Stoll B. Metabolic fate and function of dietary glutamate in the gut. Am J Clin Nutr 2009;90:850S–6S.

56. Daly JM, Reynolds J, Thom A, et al. Immune and metabolic effects of arginine in the surgical patient. Ann Surg 1998;208:512–23.

57. Wilmore D. Enteral and parenteral arginine supplementation to improve medical outcomes in hospitalized patients. J Nutr 2004;134:28635–75.

58. Zhou M, Martindale RG. Arginine in the critical care setting. J Nutr 2007;137: 1687S–92S.
59. Buijs N, van Brokhorst-de van der Schueren MAE, Languis JAE, et al. Perioperative arginine-supplemented nutrition in malnourished patients with head and neck cancer improves long-term survival. Am J Clin Nutr 2010;92:1151–6.
60. Kaye AD, Clarke RC, Sabar R, et al. Herbal medicines: current trends in anesthesiology practice, a hospital survey. J Clin Anesth 2000;12:468–71.
61. Ang-Lee MK, Moss J, Yuan CS. Herbal medicines and perioperative care. JAMA 2001;286:208–16.
62. Kumar NB, Allen K, Bell H. Perioperative herbal supplement use in cancer patients: potential implications and recommendations for presurgical screening. Cancer Control 2005;12:149–57.
63. Izzo AA. Herb-drug interactions: an overview of the clinical evidence. Fundam Clin Pharmacol 2004;19:1–16.
64. Haller CA. Clinical approach to adverse events and interactions related to herbal and dietary supplements. Clin Toxicol 2006;44:605–10.
65. Thomas D. The mineral depletion of foods available to us as a nation (1940–2002). Nutr Health 2007;19:21–55.
66. Yarnell E, Abascal BS. Drugs that interfere with herbs. Altern Complement Ther 2009;15:298–301.
67. Mason P. Important drug-nutrient interactions. Proc Nutr Soc 2010;69:551–7.
68. Tachijan A, Jahangir MV. Use of herbal products and potential interactions in patients with cardiovascular diseases. J Am Coll Cardiol 2010;55:515–25.
69. Karch SB. Peer review and the process of publishing adverse event reports. J Forensic Leg Med 2007;14:79–84.
70. Bradamante S, Barenghi L, Villa A. Cardiovascular protective effects of resveratrol. Cardiovasc Drug Rev 2004;22:169–88.
71. Manach C, Williamson G, Morand C, et al. Bioavailability and bioefficiency of polyphenols in humans. I. Review of 97 bioavailability studies. Am J Clin Nutr 2005;81:2305–425.
72. Bailey DG, Dresser GK, Leake BF, et al. Naringin is a major and selective clinical inhibitor of organic anion transporting polypeptide 1A2 (OATP1A2) in grapefruit juice. Clin Pharmacol Ther 2007;81:495–502.
73. Anand P, Kunnumakkara AB, Newman RA, et al. Bioavailability of curcumin: problems and promises. Mol Pharm 2007;4:807–18.
74. Greenlee H, Hershman DL, Jacobson JS. Use of antioxidant supplements during breast cancer treatment: a comprehensive review. Breast Cancer Res Treat 2009; 115:437–52.
75. Del Rio D, Agnolui C, Pellegrini N, et al. Total antioxidant capacity of the diet is associated with lower risk of ischemic stroke in a large Italian cohort. J Nutr 2011;141:118–23.
76. Bronstein AC, Spyker DA, Cantilena LR, et al. 2009. Annual report of the American Association of Poison Control Centers' National Poison Data System (NPDS): 27th Annual Report. Clin Toxicol (Phila) 2010;48:979–1178.
77. Soni MG, Carabin IG, Griffiths JC, et al. Safety of ephedra: lessons learned. Toxicol Lett 2004;150:97–110.
78. Hackman RM, Havel PJ, Schwartz HJ, et al. Multinutrient supplement containing ephedra and caffeine causes weight loss and improves metabolic risk factors in obese women: a randomized controlled trial. Int J Obes 2006;30:1545–56.

Historical Highlights of the Development of Enteral Nutrition

Stanley J. Dudrick, MD[a,b,*], J. Alexander Palesty, MD[b,c]

KEYWORDS

- Enteral nutrition history • Normoglycemia • Immunonutrition
- Early ICU feeding • Glycemic control • Oral nutrition

The past 5 decades have seen great progress in the multitude of approaches to enteral feeding that are rather unique, creative, and increasingly sophisticated, and indeed, especially in more recent years, have included life-maintaining and life-saving methodologies designed and proved to sustain the provision of adequate nutritional support and therapy for a large number and variety of patients. Historically, the application, advancement, and success of enteral nutrition as a safe and effective feeding method has depended on the development of (1) enteral access devices and techniques and (2) enteral nutrient mixtures and defined formulations (**Box 1**). In the broadest sense, enteral nutritional support has been defined as any method of provision of nutrients by tube into the gastrointestinal tract, which would include a portal of entry into the alimentary tract anywhere from the esophagus to the rectum. However, from a practical modern clinical point of view, enteral nutrition is generally understood to imply a technique or method of delivering nutrients to a patient by a tube having its terminus in the stomach, duodenum, or upper jejunum.

Attempts at enteral nutritional therapy are certainly not new and can be documented for more than 3500 years to 1500 BC, when the ancient Egyptians, according to Herodotus, tied animal bladders to small clay or ceramic pipes to deliver nutrients and medications by rectal enemas.[1] More than a millennium later, in 400 BC, Greek physicians, including Hippocrates, used apparatus similar to that of the Egyptians to administer clysters of wine, milk, whey, wheat, and barley broth by rectum.[2] Relatively more recently, but still more than 500 years ago, in 1500 AD Arculanus, Ryff, and Scultetus

The authors have nothing to disclose.

[a] Department of Surgery, Yale University School of Medicine, 333 Cedar Street, New Haven, CT 06510, USA

[b] Department of Surgery, Saint Mary's Hospital/Yale Affiliate, 56 Franklin Street, Waterbury, CT 06706, USA

[c] Department of Surgery, University of Connecticut School of Medicine, 263 Farmington Avenue, Farmington, CT 06030, USA

* Corresponding author. Department of Surgery, Saint Mary's Hospital/Yale Affiliate, 56 Franklin Street, Waterbury, CT 06706.

E-mail address: sdudrick@stmh.org

Surg Clin N Am 91 (2011) 945–964
doi:10.1016/j.suc.2011.05.002
0039-6109/11/$ – see front matter © 2011 Elsevier Inc. All rights reserved.

surgical.theclinics.com

Box 1
Development phases of enteral feeding

1. Rectal feeding 1500 BC to 1950 AD

2. Upper alimentary tract feeding (pharyngeal, esophageal, gastric)

   a. Description: twelfth century

   b. Use: sixteenth century

3. Oroduodenal and orojejunal feeding: 1910

4. Enteral tube feeding techniques: 1939

5. Chemically defined nutrient formulation: 1949

6. Disease- and disorder-specific nutrient formulations: 1970

---

used silver and lead tubes having several small side-holes to retrieve fish bones and other foreign bodies from the esophagus.[3] In 1598, Capivacceus, of Venice, attached a tube to an animal bladder to deliver nutrients through the mouth into the upper esophagus, and in 1617, Fabricius ab Aquapendente poured nutrient solutions into the buccal pouch, or introduced them into the pharynx or upper esophagus by a small silver tube placed through the nose in tetanus patients, saving some lives as a result.[3,4] Flexible leather catheters that were long enough to be advanced into the esophagus were first constructed and introduced by Van Helmont in 1646, and in 1776, John Hunter described the use of a syringe connected with a hollow bougie or flexible catheter of sufficient length to traverse the esophagus and enter the stomach to convey stimulating matter into the stomach without adversely affecting the lungs in treating a nearly drowned patient.[3,4] Later, in 1790, John Hunter reported the ingenious innovation of using a small eelskin, drawn over a flexible whalebone as an obdurator, and advanced through the esophagus into the stomach.[5] The proximal end was attached to a hollow wooden tube connected to a bladder he dissected from an animal. With this hybrid apparatus, he fed a 50-year-old stroke patient with eggs, sugar, milk, wine, and jellies until his paralyzed pharynx regained swallowing function and he could eat safely and effectively.

In the nineteenth century, stomach tubes and pumps for aspiration of gastric contents and for feeding were described in France by Dupuytren in 1803 and by Renault in 1823 and, during this same time period, in Philadelphia by Philip Syng Physick and in London by Sir Astley Cooper.[6,7] In 1878, Brown-Sequard described feeding patients with "esophageal spasm" by rectum with a finely ground mixture of two-thirds beef and one-third hog pancreas for 5 to 8 days.[8] Rectal feeding gained brief notoriety when United States President James Garfield was fed in this manner for 79 days with peptonized beef, broth, whiskey, and defibrinated blood.[9] In the early twentieth century, in 1910, Max Einhorn used his "duodenal pump," a tube with a metal capsule on the end (which was usually used for sampling duodenal content) to introduce milk, eggs, sugar, and water directly into the duodenum in patients who could not be fed by mouth or stomach.[10] He also vigorously condemned rectal feeding because of the high incidence of rectal irritation and the poor absorption of the nutrients. In 1918, Andresen introduced the concept of early postoperative feeding by starting jejunal administration of peptonized milk, dextrose, and alcohol through a Rehfuss tube, which he inserted and advanced well into the jejunum during a gastrojejunostomy operation for pyloric obstruction.[11] This concept was based on his observations that following operation, small bowel peristalsis is preserved despite the stomach remaining immobile for days. Andresen's seminal work and rationale almost 100 years ago formed the basis for the early postoperative enteral feeding, which is increasingly advocated and encouraged to this day.

In 1939, Stengel and Ravdin[12] fed patients postoperatively through an orogastric, orojejunal method by tying two parallel tubes together, using the shorter one for stomach decompression and the longer one for jejunal delivery of casein hydrolysate, glucose, salt, and water. Later that year, Abbott and Rawson[13] advanced and improved the Stengel/Ravdin technique by introducing a sophisticated, specially molded and constructed double-lumen tube, designed to be passed through the nose and advanced and positioned appropriately for both proximal-lumen postoperative gastric decompression and distal-lumen jejunal feeding following gastroenterostomy. Abbott[14] partially digested skim milk for enteral feeding to enhance absorption, but cautioned against completely digesting the infused milk because the higher resultant osmolality caused counterproductive diarrhea. Subsequently, the following year, in 1940, Miller and Abbott introduced a long double-lumen, balloon-tipped tube, together with the concept of delivering enteral feeding distal to a high obstruction, or proximal to a low obstruction of the small bowel.[15] Insertion of their tube was referred to subsequently as a "medical ileostomy." In 1942, Bisgard[16] reported use of a surgically created gastrostomy for subsequent insertion of a gastric tube for decompression; and a postpyloric jejunal tube for feeding. That same year, the first commercially available enteral feeding formula (Nutramigen) was introduced for treatment of children with intestinal allergies or diseases. In 1943, in addition to his landmark work in parenteral nutrition, Elman[17] fed 10% casein hydrolysate (30% small peptides and 70% amino acids) and 10% dextrose together with vitamins and salts by jejunal tube to depleted patients prior to surgery or during radiotherapy. In Europe during that same year, Panikov[18] introduced a trocar into the proximal small bowel following repair of viscera after penetrating abdominal wounds in Russian soldiers. High-calorie mixtures of milk, butter, eggs, sugar, salt, and water were instilled via rubber tubing attached to the trocar, and when the trocar was removed, a previously placed purse-string suture was tied to close the feeding jejunostomy site. In 1944, Tui and colleagues[19] achieved positive nitrogen balance in patients fed a high-calorie, high–amino acid diet by the previously described Abbott-Rawson tube following subtotal gastrectomy for the treatment of duodenal ulcer or pyloric carcinoma. Tui also first introduced the concept and term "hyperalimentation" in describing his attempts to provide maximal tolerable oral and/or enteral nutrition primarily to debilitated, malnourished cancer patients.

In the middle of the twentieth century the modern era of enteral nutritional therapy began, similarly to the modern era of parenteral nutritional therapy, as scientific methods were applied more frequently and successfully to the solution of clinical nutritional problems. In 1947, Riegel and colleagues[20] defined nutritional requirements for achieving nitrogen balance in postoperative patients nourished by various enteral feeding techniques following subtotal gastric resection or craniotomy. These investigators reported that their patients required 0.3 g nitrogen (1.88 g protein) and 30 to 46 kcal/kg body weight per day to achieve positive nitrogen balance or nitrogen equilibrium. Rose,[21] in 1949, defined the amino acid requirements in human beings while feeding highly purified nutrient mixtures of amino acids, sucrose, corn oil, starch, vitamins, and minerals to 4 of his young graduate students who volunteered for the study. In 1952, Boles and Zollinger[22] reported their results of a relatively large series of 103 patients nourished by feeding jejunostomy (16F rubber catheter/Stamm technique) postoperatively. Two years later, in 1954, Pareira and colleagues[7] reported their extensive experience with tube feeding in 240 patients for a total of nearly 7000 tube-feeding days, including 20 patients fed at home. Of note, 12 patients in this series were fed by tube for 3 to 9 months. That same year, 1954, McDonald described the use of a metal cannula for introducing a small polyethylene feeding catheter into the jejunum 12 inches distal to the duodenum in 75 gastrectomy patients.[15] This technique antedated the use of needle-catheter feeding jejunostomies, initiated in 1975 by Page and colleagues and reported in 1977 by Delaney and colleagues,[23] by more than 2 decades.[24] In 1956, Smith and Lee[25] achieved 100% nonoperative closure of fistulas in 11 of 11 patients with "blown duodenal stumps" following subtotal gastric resection with Billroth II reconstruction by feeding partially hydrolyzed lactalbumin, dextrose, alcohol, electrolytes, vitamins, and trace elements through a small-diameter, plastic nasoenteric feeding tube placed well down the efferent jejunal limb through the gastroenterostomy. Starting in 1957 the groups of Greenstein and Winitz, sponsored by the National Aeronautics and Space Administration (NASA), performed an extensive, orderly, rational, and logical series of nutritional studies, particularly in amino acid biochemistry, culminating in 1970 with the development of defined-formula, low-residue diets for possible use in space travel.[26,27] Known also as "space diets," chemically defined diets, and "elemental diets," these diets were considered elemental primarily because their composition of 18 amino acids, simple sugars, essential fats, minerals, and vitamins was precisely formulated from individual components as a semisynthetic, fiber-free diet containing a full range of basic nutrients for the maintenance of normal physiologic functions. Their work formed the basis for the commercial development of these diets for medical purposes and stimulated a still burgeoning enteral formula and food supplement industry (**Box 2**).

A hallmark of progress was achieved in 1959, when Barron[28] and Fallis and colleagues[29] described 10 years' experience in several hundred patients fed through a small-diameter (2.5 mm) polyethylene tube with a mercury-filled balloon tied to the tip. Natural foods were mechanically processed to a fine emulsion or given as strained baby foods and filtered juices. Any gastrointestinal tract drainage from the stomach, intestine, or fistulas was collected, strained, and inserted into the feeding tube together with the food. A mechanical pump designed by Barron[28] to provide slow, constant delivery of the mixture was essential to the success of the technique, and served as a prototype model conceptually for the development of intravenous infusion pumps for parenteral nutrition and delivery of medications. In 1969, Stephens and Randall[30] first introduced chemically defined diets through small-bore (5F or 8F) polyethylene feeding tubes either nasogastrically or via gastrostomy for partial or complete nutritional support of critically ill surgical patients, achieving positive nitrogen balance

---

Box 2
Classification of solutions for enteral feeding

1. Natural foods
2. Polymeric solutions
3. Monomeric solutions
4. Special metabolic solutions
5. Modular solutions
6. Hydration solutions
7. Medical foods
8. Nutritional supplements

in some cases. Their techniques and investigations occurred and were applied concomitantly with those of Dudrick and Rhoads in the development of total parenteral nutrition, and in conformity with the frequently stated principle that "if the gut works, use it."[15] In 1970, Winitz and colleagues[27] reported that they had maintained normal nutritional and physical status in normal volunteer men fed exclusively with chemically defined liquid diets for 6 months.

A major advance in enteral nutritional therapy was made in 1980 when Ponsky[31] first described the technique and early experience with percutaneous endoscopic gastrostomy (PEG) for feeding. Countless patients have benefited from this feeding technology and technique during the past quarter-century. Another giant step forward was made in 1989 by Shike and colleagues,[32] who reported clinical experience with the more challenging technique of percutaneous endoscopic jejunostomy (PEJ) for patients who were at increased risk for aspiration or who had undergone a gastrectomy. In 1989, *Medical Foods* were defined by the United States Food and Drug Administration (FDA); in 1990, Talbot defined and summarized the guidelines for scientific review of enteral food products for medical purposes for the Federation of American Societies for Experimental Biology (FASEB), and presented them to the FDA.[33,34] In 1994, The Dietary Supplement & Health Education Act (DSHEA) exempted dietary supplements from food additive status and allowed some limited claims for products justified by the use of supportive literature.[35] After many years of study and controversy, the FDA, in 1995, defined any supplement which is deemed to diagnose, cure, mitigate, treat, or prevent disease as a drug and not as a food. However, there are still many who believe that all nutritional supplements should be classified as foods, whereas there are equally large numbers of people who believe that any nutrient substances given to patients should be classified as drugs. The debate is likely to continue for some time in the future.

Today, enteral nutrition is being prescribed for patients both in hospitals and in the home at an unprecedented rate.[34] The recent increase in its use during the past two decades is due in part to results of multiple, controlled clinical trials identifying the types of patients likely to receive the greatest benefit from this feeding technique. Improved dietary formulations, technologic advances in enteral access and nutrient delivery, reduced costs, and fewer complications have added support to the clinical adage that the enteral route is the optimal method for feeding most malnourished patients with functioning gastrointestinal tracts and the inability to ingest sufficient quality and quantity of nutrients by mouth. Significant advances have occurred in enteral nutrition therapy since 1990. For example, nutritional pharmacotherapy has become a promising new component of enteral feeding, and is defined as the use of nutrients that have major pharmacologic effects as well as confirmed nutritional benefits; and/or the use of drugs to enhance nutrient use or to modify the nutritional-metabolic environment of the patient. Some examples of these "nutrient drugs" include arginine, glutamine, and the omega-3 fatty acids.

ENTERAL NUTRITION AT THE TURN OF THE MILLENNIUM

As in most other areas of medical science, there has been an explosion of information regarding the effects of enteral nutrients on the molecular mediation of gastrointestinal tract structure and function. Moreover, in the post-genome era, it is now known that nutrients can selectively influence gene expression, and the science of epigenomics is burgeoning and conceptually limitless. This new component of the science of enteral nutrition has great therapeutic promise for the future. The endoscopic placement of feeding tubes for long-term enteral nutrition has become the gold standard for access to the stomach and, more recently, to the jejunum. This avenue of access and technical expertise is safer and less expensive than the traditional methods of open surgical gastrostomy or jejenostomy in seriously ill, malnourished patients. In addition, feeding tubes are now also being inserted minimally invasively by laparoscopic techniques. These innovative approaches to enteral access have greatly stimulated overall clinical nutritional support efforts. Enteral nutrients are also now being used more frequently in malnourished patients with AIDS. The types of diets, rationale for their delivery, and technical expertise required to feed these challenging patients are abundantly available in clinical nutrition textbooks. Moreover, in contrast to traditional teaching, enteral nutrients are now being given increasingly frequently to selected patients with pancreatitis and/or respiratory disease despite the increased potential risks of enteral feeding in these patients. Finally, there is increasing evidence that the presence of nutrients within the gut provides a pharmacologic stimulus to intestinal growth and function, especially of the enterocytes. These findings have significant obvious implications for feeding patients with intestinal failure secondary to short bowel syndrome.[35]

Although the heightened and accentuated interest in providing optimally safe and effective nutritional support has spawned thousands of basic and clinical investigations and subsequent reports during the past two decades, interest can be focused fairly and primarily on 3 dynamic areas of utmost importance, which have stimulated the customary and predictable debates and controversies related to virtually all innovative and advancing areas of scientific endeavor. These 3 areas include the roles, rationale, and results associated with tight glycemic control; immunonutrition; and the route, timing, and combination of feedings most appropriate for meeting target nutritional requirements for critically ill patients, especially those in the intensive care unit (ICU). As Bistrian and McCowen[36] have emphasized, the treatment of hyperglycemia in the ICU has major implications for the use of nutritional support, and is a topic that has been, and currently is, the focus of a variety of multiple conflicting clinical trials. Immunonutrition, which refers specifically to the use, primarily in enteral feedings, of specific nutrient substances alleged to have immunomodulatory benefits independent of, and beyond the capability of, the provision of the usual standard diet, has been touted to have clear advantages in surgical patients in comparison with standard enteral formulas.[36] However, the use of immunonutrition in the ICU has been reported either to increase or to decrease mortality in conflicting studies. Finally, the questionable adage that enteral nutrition is always preferable and superior to parenteral nutrition is continuing to be examined and modulated as data accumulate from a myriad of studies around the world, indicating that the aggressive use of early enteral feeding might improve outcome for patients; and that the combination of early enteral feeding to its maximum tolerance, combined with sufficient early parenteral nutrition supplementation to meet the patients' nutrition needs precisely and adequately, was the most rational, practical, and effective approach for the optimal feeding of critically ill patients.[36]

GLYCEMIC CONTROL AND ENERGY DELIVERY

Berger and Mechanick[37] have recently focused on the latest American and European guidelines for energy delivery and glycemic control issues. These investigators point out the important transatlantic differences between the two parenteral and enteral nutrition societies.[38,39] The American Society for Parenteral and Enteral Nutrition (ASPEN)/Society of Critical Care Medicine (SCCM) experts hesitate to recommend the administration of parenteral nutrition to non-malnourished ICU patients receiving some, but not adequate, amounts of enteral nutrition during the first 7 to 10 days after admission. By contrast, the European Society for Clinical Nutrition and Metabolism (ESPEN) guidelines focus on preventing an early energy debt, preferentially providing enteral nutrition first, but supplementing it with parenteral nutrition if nutritional target needs cannot be met by the fourth day in the ICU. The ESPEN points out that these recommendations are mainly based on observational studies showing a strong correlation between negative energy balance, and morbidity and mortality, and that ongoing prospective studies should clarify this issue when the results become available. Early enteral nutrition remains the recommended feeding route in ICU patients; however, it is often unable to meet nutritional needs totally. Therefore, parenteral nutrition, whether alone or combined with enteral nutrition, is recommended if enteral nutrition is not feasible or is insufficient to meet requirements.[37] Most intensive care nutritionists aim at providing 25 kcal/kg per day, an energy target commensurate with the recent recommendations of ESPEN, using enteral nutrition by nasogastric tube, gastrostomy, or jejunostomy.[40,41] Unfortunately, this goal is rarely reached in patients receiving enteral nutrition exclusively, which results inevitably in underfeeding and progressive nutritional deficiencies.[42–46] Heidegger and colleagues cite evidence that achieving targeted nutritional goals exclusively with enteral nutrition is difficult, especially during the early phase after admission to the ICU.[39,40,42,45,47–49] These studies emphasize further that the inability to deliver adequate calories early results in energy deficits that cannot be compensated for later during the ICU stay, and these deficits have been associated with increased morbidity and mortality.[50,51] The investigators list difficulties in providing early optimal nutrition as being related to a great number of factors, which include setting insufficiently high caloric targets, gastrointestinal dysfunction such as vomiting and diarrhea, repeated procedures and surgical operations associated with interruption of the enteral nutrition, displacement of the feeding tube, inadequate routine nursing procedures with delayed administration of the enteral feedings, or premature withdrawal of the enteral nutrition.[40,42,43,52]

The Algorithms for Critical Care Enteral and Parenteral Therapy (ACCEPT) study, conducted in 14 collaborating Canadian Hospitals, showed that survival in ICU patients was improved when evidence-based guidelines for nutrition were followed assiduously and larger amounts of nutrition were delivered more consistently.[39,40,53] In an analysis of the effect of implementing a nutritional support protocol, Spain and colleagues,[54] demonstrated that only 58% of ICU patients included in an enteral nutrition protocol achieved their nutritional targets. On the other hand, when good compliance to the enteral nutrition protocol was maintained, more than 80% of the prescribed volume was administered by the third day.[40] Despite several corrective measures proposed during recent years, exclusive enteral nutrition in ICU patients has remained associated with nutritional deficiencies that are correlated ultimately with impaired short-term and long-term clinical outcomes.[40,55,56] Thus, although malnutrition in critically ill patients is known to be associated with a higher ICU morbidity and mortality, and although underfeeding is recognized as a factor in increased morbidity, a significant number of ICU patients receiving enteral nutrition still fail to reach their prescribed caloric goals.[40,57–59] Supplemental parenteral nutrition combined with enteral nutrition should be considered in order to meet the energy and protein targets when enteral nutrition alone fails to achieved the targeted goals. Whether such a combined nutritional support can provide additional benefit to the overall clinical outcome, however, remains to be proved in prospective studies.[40]

In Current Opinion in Clinical Nutrition & Metabolic Care in 2010, Berger and Mechanick[37] eloquently summarized several studies in analyzing the glycemic control controversy issues, which started with a publication of the Leuven trial in 2001, and culminating to date with the Normoglycaemia in Intensive Care Evalution—Survival Using Glucose Algorithm Regulation (NICE-SUGAR) trial.[60,61] The safety of tight glycemic control has been one of the major problems with this concept, and in an analysis of 26 protocols, many differences and similarities were identified, including patient characteristics, target glucose level, time to achieve target glucose level, incidence of hypoglycemia, rationale for adjusting the rates of insulin infusion, and analytical methods.[37] Although several computerized infusion and monitoring protocols seem to promise safer achievement of acceptable glycemic targets, the advocates of nurse-driven protocols maintain that the latter perform best, without any definitive evidence to support either point of view. Subsequent to the initial Leuven trial, 6 subsequent, independent, prospective, randomized controlled studies, involving almost 10,000 patients, were unable to confirm the survival benefit reported in that pioneering trial.[37,61,62] The difficulty in accurately replicating the original "proof of concept" Leuven methodology may be the limiting factor for achieving the benefits the original investigations gained by intensive insulin therapy and tight glycemic control.[61]

EARLY OPTIMAL FEEDING IN INTENSIVE CARE UNITS

This emerging body of data suggests that it is virtually impossible to separate intensive insulin therapy from optimal nutritional management in the ICU. However, this is not discussed candidly, which is most unfortunate and unscientific. Is it because endocrinologists, who can provide expert consultation regarding glycemic control, are not ordinarily formally trained in nutrition support? Or is it because physician nutrition experts, who usually have received formal training in nutrition support, nonetheless are simply not comfortable with aggressive intravenous insulin management, particularly in the difficult, critically ill ICU patients? This most important issue has not attracted sufficient attention in the literature, in training programs, in clinical practice, or in the research endeavors.[37] Again, Berger and Mechanick contend that getting the glycemia right is certainly important in several categories of patients, but getting the patients adequately fed is probably at least as important.[37,63,64] The ASPEN/SCCM guidelines do not address this issue in their 2009 versions, and by not directing sufficient attention to energy delivery, these guidelines actually unintentionally promote and inadvertently condone programmed malnutrition.[38] Indeed, underfeeding remains a major threat to ICU patients, and combined nutritional support of early enteral and parenteral nutrition appears to be a reasonable answer to this problem. The Leuven trial remains the only study in which patients achieved proper feeding, with an average delivery of 19 kcal/kg/d throughout the first 2 weeks, whereas the majority of subsequent trials, including the NICE-SUGAR trial, have been characterized by nutritional failure because of inadequate total energy delivery.[60,62] Therefore, it is extremely difficult to compare these trials, because nutritional deficits, negative energy balance, and attendant catabolic states directly influence gluconeogenesis, intermediary metabolism, the response to tight glycemic control, and ultimately the outcome of critical illness.[37,51] The burden of underfeeding heavily biases the interpretation of the results of tight glycemic control studies.[37] In the NICE-SUGAR trial, only 11 kcal/kg/d was provided on average, corresponding to about 50% of the patients' basal metabolic requirements.[60] The trial by Villet and colleagues[51] provided a mean daily energy delivery of 16 kcal/kg/d, which was lower than the Leuven ration but higher than the NICE-SUGAR ration, and showed that the energy deficit resulting from their low feeding intake was sufficient to cause malnutrition-related complications.[60,62] Committing to tight glycemic control while simultaneously underfeeding the patients does not seem prudent, given the existent data and our understanding of the physiology of ICU patients, and may explain the increased mortality in the tight glycemic control groups studied subsequent to the Leuven trials.[37,61,62]

The following excerpt is taken virtually directly from the thoughtful and expert opinions expressed by Berger and Mechanick.[37]

> *Although knowing that malnutrition is deleterious, we fail to penetrate the minds of our colleagues and nursing teams with the priority constituted by its prevention. Feeding via the enteral route is difficult, indeed, but the absence of daily energy delivery monitoring contributes to the problem; not seeing the problem evolve impeaches the resolution. Computers calculate more accurately than humans, and their outputs can be customized to provide visible progression of energy balances. This has been shown to improve energy delivery significantly, resulting in reduced weight loss.[65] With the pervasive influence of computerized medicine in the ICU, why cannot indirect calorimetry be a routine measurement? Why cannot these devices be built-in to ventilators? In fact, as closed-loop insulin-glucose devices are optimized, commercialized, and popularized, one can easily foresee these relevant metabolic data clearly displayed at the bedside similar to an ECG. Approaches to nutritional assessment, enteral nutrition access, parenteral nutrition access, and tight glycemic control protocols are dependent on idiosyncratic features of the ICU. Perhaps, with more research and a higher quality of data, greater standardization can result for the melding of glycemic control and nutrition support. We should also promote inclusion of training in nutrition early during the education of our young colleagues. The tasks should be better defined; the European Council stated that the absence of clear distribution of responsibilities between the various providers (physicians, nurses, and dieticians) of nutritional support was one of the major causes of underfeeding.[37]*

IMMUNONUTRITION

Ever since the early days of nutritional support, immune function has been shown to be altered following major trauma and/or surgical procedures.[66-68] More recently, impaired acquired immunity has been manifested by T-cell proliferation, cutaneous anergy, decreased production of interleukin-2 and interferon-γ, and abnormalities in the T-cell receptor complex.[69,70] Immunonutrition is a nutritional therapeutic approach in which pathologic alterations in innate and acquired immunity, secondary to acute traumatic, surgical, or medical conditions, are modulated by a feeding formula (usually enteral) supplemented with immune-enhancing or immune-modulating nutrients.[71] Much of the seminal research in immunonutrition was performed in the early 1990s by Alexander and coworkers, who found that an enteral formula supplemented with immune nutrients such as arginine, omega-3 fatty acids, vitamins A and C, and zinc reduced wound infection and length of hospital stay in patients with burn injuries.[71,72] At about the same time, Daly and colleagues studied the potential therapeutic benefit of immunonutrition in patients undergoing major elective surgical procedures for upper gastrointestinal malignancies, and found that postoperative administration of a formula supplemented with arginine, omega-3 fatty acids, and nucleotides was associated with a decrease in wound and other infectious problems, together with an improvement in lymphocyte mitogenesis.[71,73] Multiple clinical studies ensued, confirming the beneficial effects of various "immune formulas" in surgical patients; however, not all populations were shown to benefit equally, and the most favorable responses, for example, decreased infectious wound complications and reduced length of hospitalization, were observed in studies of high-risk patients undergoing upper and lower gastrointestinal surgery for cancer.[71] Few controversies exist with regard to the finding that in patients undergoing major gastrointestinal surgical procedures, in which most patients have a substantial degree of malnutrition, infectious complications can be reduced by use of immunonutrition in comparison with standard enteral feeding formulas.[36] However, most of the uncertainty lies in the use of immunonutrition in the critically ill population in whom a number a trials have been conducted in ICUs with diverse results.[36] In trauma patients, studies involving random assignments of patients to an immune-enhancing formula or to an appropriate isonitrogenous control diet have had limited sample sizes, and the only large study reported used an inappropriately low protein control formula, and thus did not address the question of whether an immune-enhancing formula is superior to an isonitrogenous standard feeding.[36,74] The data were not overwhelmingly in favor of immunonutrition for trauma patients, but they did suggest a benefit. The only two well-controlled trials, by Kudsk and colleagues[75] and Mendez and colleagues,[76] showed radically different outcomes, one positive and the other without effect, on infectious complications.[36,75,76] The major differences were that the negative trial appeared to have more patients with acute respiratory distress syndrome in the treatment group, used an experimental formula that contained substantially less arginine than the control formula (6.6 vs 14 g/L), included α-linolenic acid as the source of omega-3 fatty acids, and did not contain nucleotides, raising the possibility that the exact constituents of the feedings may be of paramount importance.[36]

Bistrian and McCowen[36] have pointed out that heterogeneity of patients is likely to be greater in the general ICU populations than in gastrointestinal cancer or trauma populations and, therefore, varied results should not be surprising. In 4 large studies of ICU patients published, one study used an inappropriate control solution that provided less protein than the immunonutrition formula, and there were actually more deaths in the immunonutrition group, and no benefits to immunonutrition by intention-to-treat analysis. In another study, immunonutrition reduced mortality, whereas the 2 largest studies showed no difference between the immunonutrition group and the control group by intention to treat.[36,77–81] In a subgroup of ICU patients with major burn injuries, 3 studies have examined the utility of immunonutrition, one of which was composed mostly of trauma patients and was actually too small for subgroup analyses.[72,82,83] Of the two other studies, only one had controls randomized to an appropriate formula, and this did not show benefits over the usual enteral feeding.[36,72,82,83]

Attempts at resolution of the immunonutrition controversy through meta-analysis have not been definitive, as somewhat different conclusions from 4 different data sets have been reported together with the overall suggestion that this therapy can lower rates of infection, but not lower the rate of overall mortality.[36,84–87] The usual current recommendation has evolved that immunonutrition should be avoided in seriously ill patients, especially those with sepsis.[88,89] Attempting to modulate the immune system in such patients most likely requires use of stronger agents such as pharmacologic agents or antibodies that block cytokine production or action.[36,90] Accordingly, it is the immunologically vulnerable patients with underlying malnutrition and less life-threatening illnesses in whom the nutritional support, including immunonutrition, is most likely to improve outcome.[36] Finally, exactly what the content of the nutritional support should be has not been satisfactorily resolved, and perhaps many ICU patients are too ill to benefit from immunonutrition as a means of disease manipulation.[36] Additional, prospective, adequately powered, randomized, controlled trials are required to define the composition, timing, and use of immunonutrition feedings. Existing quantitative reviews of immunonutrition have been confounded by grouping different immunoenhancing formulas and different types of patients together, thus introducing undesirable and invalidating heterogeneity, and probably masking potentially beneficial therapeutic effects from specifically well-designed immunoenhancing formulations in appropriately selected individual patients. The evolution of this vital area of endeavor will inevitably continue to advance and to define its utility.

ENTERAL FEEDING SOLUTIONS

At present, more than 100 "solutions" for enteral feeding are commercially available in the United States. In the broadest sense, "solutions" include homogenates, emulsions, suspensions, and powders mixed with water. In addition, regular foods can be blended for use as enteral feedings for infusion into the stomach. The composition of nutrient solutions differs greatly, with some designed for general nutrition and others formulated for specific metabolic or clinical conditions. A classification of solutions for enteral feeding is listed in **Box 2** and described here.

Natural foods consist of blended diets that can be used to provide complete nutrition by the oral route, or through a tube, into the stomach (nasogastric tube, PEG, gastrostomy).

Polymeric solutions are formulations of macronutrients in the form of isolates of intact protein, triglycerides, and carbohydrate polymers designed to provide complete nutrition by oral or tube feeding into the stomach. On the other hand, *monomeric solutions* are mixtures of protein moieties in the form of peptides and/or amino acids; fat as long-chain triglycerides (LCT) or a combination of LCT and medium-chain triglycerides (MCT); and carbohydrates as partially hydrolyzed starch maltodextrins and glucose oligosaccharides, designed primarily for patients with abnormalities of digestion and/or absorption. *Special metabolic solutions* are also available, and are designed for patients who have unique metabolic requirements, such as those related to, or secondary to, renal failure, liver failure, heart failure, pulmonary insufficiency, trauma, inborn errors of metabolism, and so forth. More specifically, some examples of this class of special nutritional therapy include: branched-chain amino acids for patients with liver failure with encephalopathy, as well as for some patients with multiple-systems organ failure, stress, and sepsis; essential amino acid mixtures, useful in some patients with renal failure; high-fat, low-carbohydrate solutions, helpful in nourishing patients with pulmonary insufficiency, especially in assisting weaning patients from ventilators; and most recently, immune-modulating solutions, for example, omega-3 polyunsaturated fat, RNA, and arginine have been shown in some studies to be associated with reduced infections, wound complications, or hospital stays in cancer patients.[35] Other nutrients that have been identified as potentially important components of immune-modulating nutritional solutions include glutamine, taurine, carnitine, N-acetyl cysteine, antioxidant vitamins, and trace elements.

Modular solutions consist of nutritional components, which can be given individually or mixed together to yield solutions to meet the special needs of a patient, such as increased calories, increased nitrogen, various minerals, and so forth. These solutions allow the nutritional support team to tailor or supplement dietary therapy specifically for various patients under a wide variety of conditions. *Hydration solutions* are formulated for providing water, minerals, and small quantities of carbohydrates and/or amino acids as supplementation or as minimal humane support primarily for dehydrated and/or cachectic patients, but also are used by athletes engaged in rigorous fitness or physical activities. *Medical foods* are distinguished from other foods by design for special dietary purposes, or as foods for which health claims (eg, fiber for cancer prevention) have been made and which must be used under medical supervision. Single nutrient products promoted for the treatment of specific disease states (eg, zinc sulfate for acrodermatitis enterohepatica) are regulated as drugs by law, as are all injectable or intravenous nutrients. Basically the following minimal criteria must be met for classification as a medical food: (1) the product is a food for oral and tube feeding; (2) the product is labeled for the dietary management of a medical disorder, disease, or condition; and (3) the product is labeled to be used under medical supervision.

Nutritional supplements, or dietary supplements, are nutrient products that are intended to supplement or fortify the diet with one or more nutrients that otherwise might have been consumed in less than recommended amounts. Such products can be extracts or concentrates, and can be liquids, powders, tablets, capsules, soft gels, and so forth. Supplemental dietary ingredients may include vitamins, minerals, herbs, amino acids, proteins, enzymes, metabolites, and other botanic products, either singly or in various combinations. Multivitamins and minerals, vitamin D and calcium, and the omega-3 fatty acids, eicosapentaenoic acid, and docosahexaenoic acid are among the more frequently recommended nutritional supplements.

FUTURE ENTERAL NUTRITIONAL CHALLENGES AND OPPORTUNITIES

The following are some of the future challenges and investigative opportunities for enteral nutritional support: (1) minimizing or avoiding aspiration, the most severe potential complication of enteral nutritional support; (2) minimizing or avoiding bacterial contamination of enteral feeding formulas; (3) clarifying the optimal use of glutamine in enteral diets in tumor-bearing patients; (4) increasing the efficacy and safety of immune-enhancing enteral formulas in favorably modulating the therapy and outcomes in the management of patients who are critically ill secondary to trauma, sepsis, cancer, AIDS, or complications; (5) increasing the efficacy and safety of immune-inhibiting enteral formulas in favorably modulating the therapy and outcomes in the management of transplant patients; (6) further studies of specific nutrient requirements (amino acids, fats, energy sources, vitamins) in stressed and septic patients to prevent deficiencies and overload; (7) further studies to compare wound healing, complication rates, resistance to infection, length of hospital stay, and convalescent time in fed and unfed surgical patients previously not malnourished to justify costs and risks of enteral nutritional support; (8) further studies to define more precisely the interactions among the various mediators and modulators of the inflammatory response and enteral nutritional support formulations; (9) further studies to determine the risk:benefit and cost:benefit ratios of attempts to enhance enteral nutrient efficacy with supplemental growth factors, anabolic steroids, erythropoietin, and so forth; (10) studies to establish clearly that intensive nutritional support, enteral and/or parenteral, significantly alters the ultimate outcomes of many diseases and injuries for which such data are currently inadequate or not available; (11) studies to define optimal enteral nutrient formulations for the prevention, arrest, and/or reversal of atherosclerosis; (12) studies to determine nutrient regulation of gene expression in the intestine (epigenomics); (13) molecular biological studies to provide new information regarding the regulatory events that determine intestinal and systemic responses to specific nutrients in enteral formulations; (14) studies to determine the genetic basis (genomics) for susceptibility to common nutritional disorders, such as obesity and diet-induced atherogenesis, to develop better enteral formulations; (15) evaluation of the intestine as a major route for the introduction of novel genetic material (prebiotics, probiotics); (16) studies directed at the controlled modulation of transgenes by specific enteral nutrients.

A BRIEF PRIMER OF ORAL NUTRITION

Although the vast majority of nutritional therapy for seriously malnourished and/or ill hospitalized patients is by the parenteral route for those with complete compromise of alimentary tract function and by the enteral route for those with partially or completely functioning gastrointestinal tracts, volitional oral nutrition is the ultimate goal in all of these patients, and is also used for nutritional maintenance in the greater number of generally healthy, non-malnourished patients with less serious or stressful pathophysiologic conditions. Nurses, dieticians, and other nutritionists are ordinarily available to provide expertise and science-based advice to promote health and reduce risk for major chronic diseases or disorders through diet and physical activity. A basic premise of the dietary guidelines generally available in all hospitals in all countries is that nutrient needs should be met primarily through consuming foods that provide an array of nutrients and other compounds that may have beneficial effects on health. In some patients, especially the elderly, fortified foods and dietary supplements may be useful sources of one or more nutrients that otherwise might be consumed in less than recommended amounts. However, dietary supplements, while recommended and useful in some cases, cannot completely replace a healthful oral diet.

Protein is the fundamental component for cellular or organ function.[91] The diet must contain not only enough protein and amino acids but also enough nonprotein energy to permit optimal use of dietary protein.[91] Protein energy malnutrition (PEM) is quite common in the world as a whole and has been reported by the Food and Agricultural Organization (FAO) of the United Nations to have been associated with 6 million deaths in children worldwide in 2000.[92–95] In the industrialized world, PEM is seen predominantly in hospitals and in association with disease.[91,96,97] Protein deficiency has adverse effects on all organs and may have long-term adverse effects on brain function, especially in infants and children.[98,99] Patients with PEM have reduced immune function and are more susceptible to infection.[96] Total starvation will result in death in 70 days in an adult whose weight was initially normal, and because these persons still have some adipose tissue reserves, their deaths can be assumed as primarily secondary to protein deprivation.[100] By contrast, protein and energy reserves are much lower in very low birth weight premature infants, and with total starvation, the survival of 1000-g neonates is usually only 5 days.[101]

The upper limit of protein intake in adults is no more than 30% of total energy intake.[91] In brief, consideration of maximal urea synthesis rates of explorers who lived exclusively on animal-based diets have provided the basis for this recommendation. A prime example is that early American explorers in the winter suffered from "rabbit starvation" when they subsisted necessarily on a diet of rabbit meat, which contains very little fat, resulting in protein intakes greater than 30% of total energy intake.[91,102] The recommended dose of dietary protein in stressed or septic patients without renal dysfunction is 1.5 to 2.0 g/kg per day whether they are fed orally, enterally, or parenterally. Blood urea nitrogen should be monitored during all nutritional therapy and not be allowed to rise much above 40 mg/dL. Diets can be enriched with supplemental arginine and/or glutamine so that more than a total of 2 g/kg of protein per day and amino acids can be delivered while meeting energy requirements. Burn patients usually receive 2.0 to 2.5 g/kg of protein per day because of excessive urinary nitrogen and protein losses from the wound. Administration of protein above this level contributes little to nitrogen retention in critically ill patients, and nutritional support cannot overcome ongoing protein catabolism and wasting of lean tissue mass in the stressed, immobilized patient. The best that can be accomplished, until the patient heals and the hypermetabolic response resolves, is to minimize the nitrogen deficits as much as possible. The nutritional support of such patients provides ample challenges to future basic and clinical investigators if optimal morbidity and mortality results are to be achieved. To paraphrase another old adage, we are not only what we eat but also what we can assimilate, use, and retain. This statement is in itself a challenge for the future.

Regarding energy requirements, the Harris-Benedict formula is used commonly to determine basal energy expenditure (BEE) as follows: in males, BEE = 66.5 + (13.8 × weight in kg) + (5 × height in cm) − (6.8 × age); in females BEE = 655 + (9.6 × weight in kg) + (1.7 × height in cm) − (4.7 × age). These values are traditionally assumed to be increased by various stress and activity factors by 1.25 to 2 times in critically ill patients, but metabolic cart measurements have shown these recommended adjustments to be somewhat excessive. Clinically in hypermetabolic, injured, or septic patients, the BEE is rarely increased more than 15%. From a practical viewpoint, the current clinical recommendation for caloric needs, regardless of the feeding technique, is a total of 25 to 30 kcal/kg per day. Using these general guidelines, 90% of patients will receive their energy requirements, and overfeeding will occur in fewer than 20% of patients.

A brief outline of the key prudent dietary guidelines gleaned from the National and International Dietary Guidelines and Recommendations for 2005, which all physicians, surgeons, and other health care providers should be familiar, follows. (1) Consume a variety of nutrient-dense foods and beverages within and among the basic food groups while choosing foods that limit the intake of saturated and *trans* fats, cholesterol, added sugars, salts, and alcohols. (2) Maintain body weight in a healthy range within energy needs by balancing calories from foods and beverages with the calories expended. (3) Prevent gradual weight gain over time by making small decreases in food and beverage calories while increasing physical activity. (4) Engage in regular physical activity and reduce sedentary activities to promote health, psychological well being, and a healthy body weight. (5) Engage in at least 30 minutes of moderate-intensity physical activity, above usual activity at work or at home, on most days of the week to reduce the risk of chronic disease. (6) Consume a sufficient amount and variety of fruits and vegetables each day while staying within energy needs—select from all 5 vegetable subgroups (dark green, orange, legumes, starchy vegetables, and other vegetables) several times a week. (7) Consume 3 or more ounce-equivalents of whole-grain products per day, with the rest of the recommended grains derived from enriched or whole-grain products. (8) Consume 3 cups per day of fat-free or low-fat milk or equivalent milk products. (9) Consume less than 10% of calories from saturated fats and less than 300 mg per day of cholesterol, and keep *trans* fatty acid consumption as low as possible. (10) Limit total fat intake between 20% and 35% of calories, with most fats derived from sources of polyunsaturated and monounsaturated fats such as fish, nuts, and vegetable oils. (11) Select and prepare meat, poultry, dry beans, and milk or milk products from choices that are lean, low-fat, or fat-free. (12) Choose fiber-rich fruits, vegetables, and whole grains often. (13) Choose and prepare food and beverages with little added sugars and caloric sweeteners. (14) Consume less than 2300 mg (approximately one teaspoon of salt) of sodium per day. (15) Choose and prepare foods with little salt, and at the same time consume potassium-rich foods, such as fruits and vegetables. (16) Choose, if desired, to drink alcoholic beverages sensibly and in moderation—up to 1 drink per day for women, and up to 2 drinks per day for men. (17) Practice pristine hygiene in handling and preparing all foods to avoid microbial food-borne illness.

SUMMARY

It is clear that enteral nutritional support can meet the needs of patients who cannot or will not eat what they require by mouth. Modern technology has enhanced access to the stomach and small intestine and has provided a great variety of formulations that can be tailored to the disabilities of the gastrointestinal tract. Innovative outgrowth and maturation of the enteral nutritional techniques currently available are likely to continue to occur in the future, are most exciting, virtually incredible, and apparently unlimited. If the gastrointestinal tract can function and can be used safely, enteral nutritional support, at least in part, should be used to provide the nutritional and metabolic requirements for patients who cannot ingest the required nutrients normally or adequately. With the resources, technology, and techniques that have developed and advanced throughout the past 50 years, it is no longer justifiable in this twenty-first century that people who cannot eat normally, or at all, should suffer and/or die of starvation.[103]

REFERENCES

1. McCamish M, Bounous G, Geraghty ME. History of enteral feeding: past and present perspectives. In: Rombeau JL, Rolandelli RH, editors. Clinical nutrition, enteral and tube feeding. 3rd edition. Philadelphia: WB Saunders Company; 1993. p. 1–11.
2. Bonsmann M, Hardt W, Lorber CG. The historical development of artificial enteral alimentation. Part I. Anasthesiol Intensivmed 1993;34:207.
3. His W. Zur Geschichte der Magenpumpe. Med Kiln 1925;21:391–3 [in German].
4. Pareira MD. Therapeutic nutrition with tube feeding. Springfield (IL): Charles C. Thomas; 1959.
5. Hunter J. A case of paralysis of the muscles of deglutition cured by an artificial mode of conveying food and medicines into the stomach. Trans Soc Improvement Med Chir Know 1793;1:82–188.
6. Cooper SA. Hospital reports. Lancet 1823;1:277.
7. Pareira MD, Conrad EJ, Hicks W, et al. Therapeutic nutrition with tube feeding. J Am Med Assoc 1954;156(9):810–6.
8. Brown-Sequard CE. Feeding per rectum in nervous affectations. Lancet 1878; 1:144.
9. Bliss DW. Feeding per rectum: as illustrated in the case of the late President Garfield and others. Med Rec 1882;22:64.
10. Einhorn M. Duodenal alimentation. Med Rec 1910;78:92.
11. Andresen AF. Immediate jejunal feeding after gastroenterostomy. Ann Surg 1918;67:565–6.
12. Stengel AJ, Ravdin IS. The maintenance of nutrition in surgical patients with a description of the orojejunal method of feeding. Surgery 1939;6:511–9.
13. Abbott W, Rawson AJ. A tube for use in postoperative care of gastroenterostomy patients. JAMA 1939;112:2414.
14. Abbott WO. Fluid and nutritional maintenance by the use of an intestinal tube. Ann Surg 1940;112:584–93.
15. Randall HT. The history of enteral nutrition. In: Rombeau JL, Caldwell MD, editors. Clinical nutrition, enteral and tube feeding. 2nd edition. Philadelphia: WB Saunders Company; 1990. p. 1–9.
16. Bisgard JD. Gastro-jejunal intubation. Surg Gynecol Obstet 1942;74:239–41.
17. Elman R. Parenteral alimentation in surgery with special reference to proteins and amino acids. New York: Hober Inc; 1947.

18. Panikov PA. Spasokukostki's method of feeding abdominal wounds. Am Rev Sov Med 1943;1:32–6.
19. Tui C, Wright AM, Muholland JH, et al. Studies on surgical convalescence. Ann Surg 1944;120:99–122.
20. Riegel C, Koop CE, Drew J, et al. The nutritional requirements for nitrogen balance in surgical patients during the early postoperative period. J Clin Invest 1947;26(1):18–23.
21. Rose WC. The significance of amino acids in nutrition. Harvey Lect 1934;30:45–65.
22. Boles T Jr, Zollinger RM. Critical evaluation of jejunostomy. AMA Arch Surg 1952;65(3):358–66.
23. Delany HM, Carnevale N, Garvey JW, et al. Postoperative nutritional support using needle catheter feeding jejunostomy. Ann Surg 1977;186(2):165–70.
24. Page CP, Carlton PK, Andrassy RJ, et al. Safe, cost-effective postoperative nutrition. Defined formula diet via needle-catheter jejunostomy. Am J Surg 1979;138(6):939–45.
25. Lee RM, Smith DW. Nutritional management in duodenal fistula. Surg Gynecol Obstet 1956;103(6):666–72.
26. Greenstein JP, Birnbaum SM, Winitz M, et al. Quantitative nutritional studies with water-soluble, chemically defined diets. I. Growth, reproduction and lactation in rats. Arch Biochem Biophys 1957;72(2):396–416.
27. Winitz M, Seedman DA, Graff J. Studies in metabolic nutrition employing chemically defined diets. I. Extended feeding of normal human adult males. Am J Clin Nutr 1970;23(5):525–45.
28. Barron J. Tube feeding of postoperative patients. Surg Clin North Am 1959;39:1481–91.
29. Fallis LS, Barron J. Gastric and jejunal alimentation with fine polyethylene tubes. AMA Arch Surg 1952;65(3):373–81.
30. Stephens RV, Randall HT. Use of concentrated, balanced, liquid elemental diet for nutritional management of catabolic states. Ann Surg 1969;170(4):642–68.
31. Ponsky JL. Techniques of percutaneous gastrostomy. New York: Igaku-Shoin; 1988.
32. Shike M, Berner YN, Gerdes H, et al. Percutaneous endoscopic gastrostomy and jejunostomy for long-term feeding in patients with cancer of the head and neck. Otolaryngol Head Neck Surg 1989;101(5):549–54.
33. Forbes AL. An historical overview of medical foods. Development of medical foods for rare diseases. Proceedings of a Workshop. June 9–11, 1991. Bethesda (MD): Government Printing Office; 1991.
34. Talbot JM. Guidelines for the scientific review of enteral food products for special medical purposes. Prepared for the Center for Food Safety and Applied Nutrition, Food and Drug Administration. JPEN J Parenter Enteral Nutr 1991;15(Suppl 3):99S–174S. p. A171–E172.
35. Rombeau JL, Rolandelli RH. Preface. In: Rombeau JL, Rolandelli RH, editors. Clinical nutrition: enteral and tube feeding. 3rd edition. Philadelphia: W.B. Saunders Company; 1997. p. xix–xxx.
36. Bistrian BR, McCowen KC. Nutritional and metabolic support in the adult ICU: key controversies. Crit Care Med 2006;34(5):1525–31.
37. Berger MM, Mechanick JI. Continuing controversy in the intensive care unit: why tight glycemic control, nutrition support, and nutritional pharmacology are each necessary therapeutic considerations. Curr Opin Clin Nutr Metab Care 2010;13(2):167–9.

38. McClave SA, Martindale RG, Vanek VW, et al. Guidelines for the provision and assessment of nutrition support therapy in the adult critically ill patient: Society of Critical Care Medicine (SCCM) and American Society for Parenteral and Enteral Nutrition (A.S.P.E.N. JPEN J Parenter Enteral Nutr 2009;33(3):277–316.
39. Singer P, Berger MM, Van den Berghe G, et al. ESPEN guidelines on parenteral nutrition: intensive care. Clin Nutr 2009;28(4):387–400.
40. Heidegger CP, Darmon P, Pichard C. Enteral vs. parenteral nutrition for the critically ill patient: a combined support should be preferred. Curr Opin Crit Care 2008;14(4):408–14.
41. Kreymann KG, Berger MM, Deutz NE, et al. ESPEN guidelines on enteral nutrition: intensive care. Clin Nutr 2006;25(2):210–23.
42. Adam S, Batson S. A study of problems associated with the delivery of enteral feed in critically ill patients in five ICUs in the UK. Intensive Care Med 1997; 23(3):261–6.
43. De Jonghe B, Appere-De-Vechi C, Fournier M, et al. A prospective survey of nutritional support practices in intensive care unit patients: what is prescribed? What is delivered? Crit Care Med 2001;29(1):8–12.
44. Reid CL, Campbell IT, Little RA. Muscle wasting and energy balance in critical illness. Clin Nutr 2004;23(2):273–80.
45. Weissman C, Kemper M, Askanazi J, et al. Resting metabolic rate of the critically ill patient: measured versus predicted. Anesthesiology 1986;64(6):673–9.
46. Woodcock NP, Zeigler D, Palmer MD, et al. Enteral versus parenteral nutrition: a pragmatic study. Nutrition 2001;17(1):1–12.
47. Genton L, Dupertuis YM, Romand JA, et al. Higher calorie prescription improves nutrient delivery during the first 5 days of enteral nutrition. Clin Nutr 2004;23(3): 307–15.
48. Heyland D, Cook DJ, Winder B, et al. Enteral nutrition in the critically ill patient: a prospective survey. Crit Care Med 1995;23(6):1055–60.
49. McClave SA, Sexton LK, Spain DA, et al. Enteral tube feeding in the intensive care unit: factors impeding adequate delivery. Crit Care Med 1999;27(7): 1252–6.
50. Dvir D, Cohen J, Singer P. Computerized energy balance and complications in critically ill patients: an observational study. Clin Nutr 2006;25(1):37–44.
51. Villet S, Chiolero RL, Bollmann MD, et al. Negative impact of hypocaloric feeding and energy balance on clinical outcome in ICU patients. Clin Nutr 2005;24(4): 502–9.
52. Roberts SR, Kennerly DA, Keane D, et al. Nutrition support in the intensive care unit. Adequacy, timeliness, and outcomes. Crit Care Nurse 2003;23(6):49–57.
53. Martin CM, Doig GS, Heyland DK, et al. Multicentre, cluster-randomized clinical trial of algorithms for critical-care enteral and parenteral therapy (ACCEPT). CMAJ 2004;170(2):197–204.
54. Spain DA, McClave SA, Sexton LK, et al. Infusion protocol improves delivery of enteral tube feeding in the critical care unit. JPEN J Parenter Enteral Nutr 1999; 23(5):288–92.
55. Koretz RL, Avenell A, Lipman TO, et al. Does enteral nutrition affect clinical outcome? A systematic review of the randomized trials. Am J Gastroenterol 2007;102(2):412–29 [quiz: 468].
56. Stratton RJ, Elia M. Who benefits from nutritional support: what is the evidence? Eur J Gastroenterol Hepatol 2007;19(5):353–8.
57. Berger MM, Chiolero RL. Hypocaloric feeding: pros and cons. Curr Opin Crit Care 2007;13(2):180–6.

58. O'Brien JM Jr, Phillips GS, Ali NA, et al. Body mass index is independently associated with hospital mortality in mechanically ventilated adults with acute lung injury. Crit Care Med 2006;34(3):738–44.

59. Ray DE, Matchett SC, Baker K, et al. The effect of body mass index on patient outcomes in a medical ICU. Chest 2005;127(6):2125–31.

60. Finfer S, Chittock DR, Su SY, et al. Intensive versus conventional glucose control in critically ill patients. N Engl J Med 2009;360(13):1283–97.

61. van den Berghe G, Wouters P, Weekers F, et al. Intensive insulin therapy in the critically ill patients. N Engl J Med 2001;345(19):1359–67.

62. Van den Berghe G, Wilmer A, Hermans G, et al. Intensive insulin therapy in the medical ICU. N Engl J Med 2006;354(5):449–61.

63. Alberda C, Gramlich L, Jones N, et al. The relationship between nutritional intake and clinical outcomes in critically ill patients: results of an international multi-center observational study. Intensive Care Med 2009;35(10):1728–37.

64. Beck AM, Balknas UN, Furst P, et al. Food and nutritional care in hospitals: how to prevent undernutrition—report and guidelines from the Council of Europe. Clin Nutr 2001;20(5):455–60.

65. Berger MM, Revelly JP, Wasserfallen JB, et al. Impact of a computerized information system on quality of nutritional support in the ICU. Nutrition 2006;22(3):221–9.

66. Law DK, Dudrick SJ, Abdou NI. Immunocompetence of patients with protein-calorie malnutrition. The effects of nutritional repletion. Ann Intern Med 1973; 79(4):545–50.

67. Law DK, Dudrick SJ, Abdou NI. The effect of dietary protein depletion on immunocompetence: the importance of nutritional repletion prior to immunologic induction. Ann Surg 1974;179(2):168–73.

68. Law DK, Dudrick SJ, Abdou NI. The effects of protein calorie malnutrition on immune competence of the surgical patient. Surg Gynecol Obstet 1974; 139(2):257–66.

69. Makarenkova VP, Bansal V, Matta BM, et al. CD11b+/Gr-1+ myeloid suppressor cells cause T cell dysfunction after traumatic stress. J Immunol 2006;176(4): 2085–94.

70. Zhu X, Herrera G, Ochoa JB. Immunosuppression and infection after major surgery: a nutritional deficiency. Crit Care Clin 2010;26(3):491–500, ix.

71. Mizock BA, Sriram K. Perioperative immunonutrition. Expert Rev Clin Immunol 2011;7(1):1–3.

72. Gottschlich MM, Jenkins M, Warden GD, et al. Differential effects of three enteral dietary regimens on selected outcome variables in burn patients. JPEN J Parenter Enteral Nutr 1990;14(3):225–36.

73. Daly JM, Lieberman MD, Goldfine J, et al. Enteral nutrition with supplemental arginine, RNA, and omega-3 fatty acids in patients after operation: immunologic, metabolic, and clinical outcome. Surgery 1992;112(1):56–67.

74. Moore FA, Moore EE, Kudsk KA, et al. Clinical benefits of an immune-enhancing diet for early postinjury enteral feeding. J Trauma 1994;37(4):607–15.

75. Kudsk KA, Minard G, Croce MA, et al. A randomized trial of isonitrogenous enteral diets after severe trauma. An immune-enhancing diet reduces septic complications. Ann Surg 1996;224(4):531–40 [discussion: 540–3].

76. Mendez C, Jurkovich GJ, Garcia I, et al. Effects of an immune-enhancing diet in critically injured patients. J Trauma 1997;42(5):933–40 [discussion: 940–1].

77. Atkinson S, Sieffert E, Bihari D. A prospective, randomized, double-blind, controlled clinical trial of enteral immunonutrition in the critically ill. Guy's Hospital Intensive Care Group. Crit Care Med 1998;26(7):1164–72.

78. Bower RH, Cerra FB, Bershadsky B, et al. Early enteral administration of a formula (Impact) supplemented with arginine, nucleotides, and fish oil in intensive care unit patients: results of a multicenter, prospective, randomized, clinical trial. Crit Care Med 1995;23(3):436–49.

79. Galban C, Montejo JC, Mesejo A, et al. An immune-enhancing enteral diet reduces mortality rate and episodes of bacteremia in septic intensive care unit patients. Crit Care Med 2000;28(3):643–8.

80. Kieft H, Roos AN, van Drunen JD, et al. Clinical outcome of immunonutrition in a heterogeneous intensive care population. Intensive Care Med 2005;31(4): 524–32.

81. Braga M, Vignali A, Gianotti L, et al. Immune and nutritional effects of early enteral nutrition after major abdominal operations. Eur J Surg 1996;162(2): 105–12.

82. Chuntrasakul C, Siltham S, Sarasombath S, et al. Comparison of a immunonutrition formula enriched arginine, glutamine and omega-3 fatty acid, with a currently high-enriched enteral nutrition for trauma patients. J Med Assoc Thai 2003;86(6):552–61.

83. Saffle JR, Wiebke G, Jennings K, et al. Randomized trial of immune-enhancing enteral nutrition in burn patients. J Trauma 1997;42(5):793–800 [discussion: 800–2].

84. Beale RJ, Bryg DJ, Bihari DJ. Immunonutrition in the critically ill: a systematic review of clinical outcome. Crit Care Med 1999;27(12):2799–805.

85. Heyland DK, Novak F, Drover JW, et al. Should immunonutrition become routine in critically ill patients? A systematic review of the evidence. JAMA 2001;286(8): 944–53.

86. Heys SD, Walker LG, Smith I, et al. Enteral nutritional supplementation with key nutrients in patients with critical illness and cancer: a meta-analysis of randomized controlled clinical trials. Ann Surg 1999;229(4):467–77.

87. Montejo JC, Zarazaga A, Lopez-Martinez J, et al. Immunonutrition in the intensive care unit. A systematic review and consensus statement. Clin Nutr 2003; 22(3):221–33.

88. Heyland DK, Dhaliwal R, Drover JW, et al. Canadian clinical practice guidelines for nutrition support in mechanically ventilated, critically ill adult patients. JPEN J Parenter Enteral Nutr 2003;27(5):355–73.

89. McCowen KC, Bistrian BR. Immunonutrition: problematic or problem solving? Am J Clin Nutr 2003;77(4):764–70.

90. Bernard GR, Vincent JL, Laterre PF, et al. Efficacy and safety of recombinant human activated protein C for severe sepsis. N Engl J Med 2001;344(10): 699–709.

91. Duffy B, Gunn T, Collinge J, et al. The effect of varying protein quality and energy intake on the nitrogen metabolism of parenterally fed very low birthweight (less than 1600 g) infants. Pediatr Res 1981;15(7):1040–4.

92. Food and Agriculture Organization of the United Nations. The state of food and agriculture 2000. Rome (Italy): FAO; 2000.

93. Carpenter KJ. Protein and energy. A Study of changing ideas of nutrition. Cambridge (United Kingdom): Cambridge University Press; 1994.

94. Korpes JE. Jac. Berzelius: his life and work. Stockhlom (Sweden): Almqvist & Wiksell; 1970.

95. Munro HN. Historical perspective on protein requirements: objectives for the future. In: Blaxter K, Waterlow JC, editors. Nutritional adaptation in man. London: John Libbey; 1985. p. 155–67.

96. Bistrian BR. Recent advances in parenteral and enteral nutrition: a personal perspective. JPEN J Parenter Enteral Nutr 1990;14(4):329–34.

97. Wilson DC, Pencharz PB. Nutritional care of the chronically ill. In: Tsang RC, Zlotkin SH, Nichols BL, et al, editors. Nutrition during infancy: birth to 2 Years. Cincinnati (OH): Digital Education Publishing, Inc; 1997.

98. Corish CA, Kennedy NP. Protein-energy undernutrition in hospital in-patients. Br J Nutr 2000;83(6):575–91.

99. Pollitt E. Developmental sequel from early nutritional deficiencies: conclusive and probability judgements. J Nutr 2000;130(2S Suppl):350S–3S.

100. Allison SP. The uses and limitations of nutritional support The Arvid Wretlind Lecture given at the 14th ESPEN Congress in Vienna, 1992. Clin Nutr 1992; 11(6):319–30.

101. Heird WC, Driscoll JM Jr, Schullinger JN, et al. Intravenous alimentation in pediatric patients. J Pediatr 1972;80(3):351–72.

102. Pencharz PB, Young VR. Protein and amino acids. In: Bowman B, Russell R, editors, Present knowledge in nutrition, vol. 1. Washington, DC: International Life Sciences Institute; 2006. p. 59–77.

103. Dudrick SJ. Presidential address: the common denominator and the bottom line. JPEN J Parenter Enteral Nutr 1978;2(1):13–21.

Index

Note: Page numbers of article titles are in **boldface** type.

Surg Clin N Am 91 (2011) 965–976
doi:10.1016/S0039-6109(11)00085-5
0039-6109/11/$ – see front matter © 2011 Elsevier Inc. All rights reserved.

surgical.theclinics.com

Moving?

Make sure your subscription moves with you!

To notify us of your new address, find your **Clinics Account Number** (located on your mailing label above your name), and contact customer service at:

Email: journalscustomerservice-usa@elsevier.com

800-654-2452 (subscribers in the U.S. & Canada)
314-447-8871 (subscribers outside of the U.S. & Canada)

Fax number: 314-447-8029

Elsevier Health Sciences Division
Subscription Customer Service
3251 Riverport Lane
Maryland Heights, MO 63043

*To ensure uninterrupted delivery of your subscription, please notify us at least 4 weeks in advance of move.

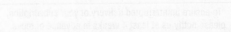

Printed and bound by CPI Group (UK) Ltd, Croydon, CR0 4YY

03/10/2024

01040439-0010